The history of oncology

The history of oncology

Prof. D.J. Th. Wagener

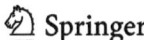 Springer

© 2009 Springer Uitgeverij, Houten, the Netherlands
All rights reserved. No part of this publication may be reproduced, stored in a retrieval system or published in any form or by any means without the prior written permission of the publisher.
Insofar as the copying of parts of this publication is permitted as laid down in article 16b of the Auteurswet 1912 (1912 Dutch Copyright Act), the Order in Council of 20 June 1974 (Statute Book 351) as amended by the Order in Council of 23 August 1985 (Statute Book 471) and article 17 of the Auteurswet 1912, the legally established fees for such copying should be paid to Stichting Reprorecht (P.O. Box 3051, 2130 KB Hoofddorp, the Netherlands). For the reproduction of a part or parts of this publication in anthologies, readers or other compilations (see article 16b of the Auteurswet), please contact the publisher.

The compiler(s) and the publisher are fully aware of their responsibility to ensure the greatest possible reliability in the publications they produce. However, they cannot accept any liability for printing errors and other errors and omissions that may occur in the present publication.

The publisher has made every effort to obtain permission from the legal copyright holders for reproduction of the illustrations included in this publication. Wherever possible, the source of each illustration is given. Those who nevertheless believe that they have any copyright claims in connection with this publication are requested to contact the publisher.

ISBN 978 90 313 6143 4
NUR 870

Cover design: Studio Bassa, Culemborg
Interior design: Bottenheft, Marijenkampen/Arnhem
Drawings: 3D-Elements, Nieuwkoop
Translation: Talencentrum-VU / Ronald Bathgate

Springer Uitgeverij
Het Spoor 2
P.O. Box 246
3990 GA Houten
The Netherlands

www.springeruitgeverij.nl

This book is dedicated to Prof. Pieter H.M. De Mulder
(1949-2007), head of the department of Medical Oncology
at UMC St Radboud, Nijmegen, between 2000 and 2007.
A remarkable man, an excellent colleague, an outstanding
teacher, a great leader and a fine physician and oncologist.

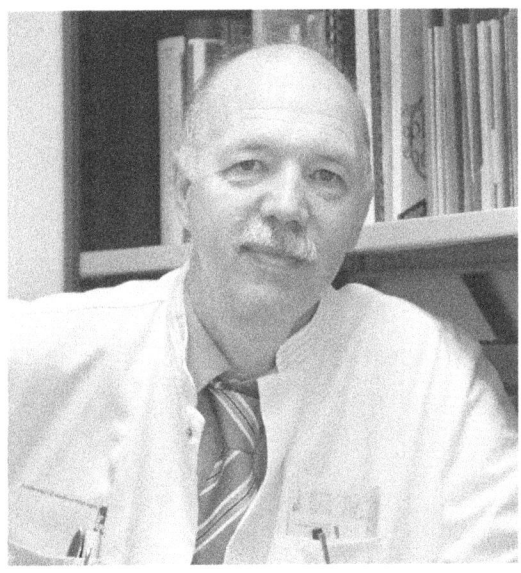

Prof. P.H.M. De Mulder (Photo: F. Franssen)

Contents

Foreword IX

1 Introduction 1

2 The occurrence of cancer in ancient times and the development of ideas about the nature of the complaint 3

3 The treatment of cancer in the past 61

4 The maturing of surgery as a treatment for cancer 69

5 The historical development of radiotherapy 115

6 The development of chemotherapy 145

7 The history of the hormonal treatment of cancer 181

8 The background of targeted therapy and the emergence of a new approach 201

9 Immunotherapy in the past and the present 219

10 The origins of psycho-oncology 239

Glossary 255
Literature 269
Name Index 285
Subject Index 295

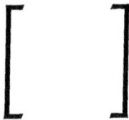

Foreword

When I was invited to give a lecture on the history of oncology and I did some background reading, I discovered that there was no single volume that dealt with the entire history of the subject. Fortunately, however, a great deal of information could be found here and there in the literature.

On reading these sources, I was struck by the fascinating stories that were hidden behind many discoveries. This was the reason that I set about writing this book.

It seemed to me that it would be interesting to the many people involved in the treatment of cancer to see how the current methods of cancer treatment came about. I thought that such information might also be inspiring for the thousands of people working in cancer research, and for all those who are directly or indirectly involved with cancer. The layman who was looking for background information on a particular treatment might also find it useful. A glossary and a few explanatory diagrams have been added for the benefit of this last-mentioned group. It may further be mentioned that each chapter has been written as a separate unit that can be read independently of all the others.

I feel that I should apologize for my temerity in writing a historical account despite the fact that I am no historian, but rather a medical oncologist. Although I have not examined each source in depth, as historians do, considerable effort has gone into checking the accuracy of the facts presented and adding useful background information during the preparation of this book for a wider English-speaking audience.

As I was collecting the literature, it occurred to me that quite a few authors distort the truth they summarize. For example, the humoral theory is sometimes attributed to Galen instead of to Hippocrates, the development of the microscope is often accredited to Antoni van Leeuwenhoek and not to Zacharias Jansen, the introduction of the use of nitrogen mustard as a cytostatic may be ascribed to

FOREWORD

Cornelius Packard Rhoads rather than to James Ewing or Goodman and Gilman of Yale University in the United States, and it is sometimes stated that Sidney Farber rather than Yellapragada SubbaRow first synthesized two substances that blocked the metabolism of folic acid.

I did not restrict my gaze to the past only, but also considered the cancer treatments of the future in order to get as good an insight as possible into cancer as a whole. While this approach would doubtless stop a real historian straight in his tracks, I thought it would be good to include descriptions of recent developments, which are truly spectacular in some fields.

To add some extra color to the history, I have tried to include as many anecdotes as possible. These often come from books rather than peer-reviewed articles.

I have taken a great deal of information from the *Illustrierte Geschichte der Medizin* and from *Medicine, an illustrated history*, from the article 'Cancer: an historical perspective' by G. Diamandopoulos in *Anticancer Research*, from the IPOS Sutherland memorial lecture in *Psycho-Oncology* by J.C. Holland and from assorted chapters of 'Historic milestones in oncology' written by experts in their field and published in a special edition of *Seminars in Oncology* in 1979. The book *A short history of surgery*, written by D. de Moulin, was also a welcome source of information, as was the book *The theory and practice of oncology* by R.W. Raven.

Credits for the illustrations have been given in the accompanying legends. The drawings included provide a simplified representation of theoretical concepts for the layman.

I am most grateful to all those who have read through the manuscript of this book, or parts of it, and given me the benefit of their advice. I would like to mention the following in particular: B. Baks, Dr. L.V.A.M. Beex, Prof. H.P.J. Bloemers, Prof. H. Boonstra, Prof. P. van den Broek, Prof. C.G. Figdor, Prof. A. Geurts van Kessel, Prof. L. Lacquet, Prof. J.W. Leer, J. Smeets, A. Staps and Prof. W. van der Graaf, Dr. F.A.D.T.G. Wagener and Prof. T. Wobbes. Furthermore, my special thanks go to Mrs. E. Peters and the staff of the medical library of the UMC St Radboud at Nijmegen who provided tireless support as I collected the literature, as well as to J.P. Gijselhart from the library of the *Dutch Journal of Medicine* in Amsterdam and S. Bakker from the library of the Dutch Cancer Institute/Antoni van Leeuwenhoek Hospital in Amsterdam and the audiovisual center of that same institution, and to Dr. R.H. Bathgate for valuable suggestions.

Malden nr. Nijmegen, April 2008
Theo Wagener

[1]

Introduction

'Tomorrow was written yesterday.'
(Henriette Roland Holst, Dutch poet and socialist, 1869-1952)

Cancer is a disease that has existed as long as humanity, but is currently increasing in importance. While tuberculosis posed the greatest threat to the health of mankind in the nineteenth century, and cardiovascular disease in the twentieth, it seems likely that cancer will become the leading cause of death in the present century. Nevertheless, great advances have been made in recent times. Today, close to half of cancer patients are cured, whereas a century ago recovery was rare. This may seem splendid from an objective point of view; however, patients see things differently. They want the certainty of cure, not just the hope. It would therefore seem to be a good idea to describe the difficulties that had to be overcome to arrive at the improvements that have already been achieved and the hurdles that remain in the way of further advances, in order to gain some understanding of the very long path that still separates us from full recovery.

Aside from that, a look back to the past allows us to pay due recognition to those who helped to improve the way cancer is treated. We tend to forget them so quickly. It is also valuable for the cancer researchers of today to realize the continued applicability of the statement made by Santayana one hundred years ago: "those who do not remember history are doomed to repeat it" (Char, 1996). Bela Schick's comment says the same thing with a slightly different slant: "People stop citing you in the medical literature after a lapse of twenty years. You see the same ideas republished every couple of decades" (Petrakis, 1979).

Moreover, consideration of past advances can stimulate today's researchers to persevere in their investigations and not to let themselves be discouraged by setbacks. The story of oncology is not only fascinating but also contains many accounts of dead ends, chance discoveries, illusions, mistakes and disappointments alongside the few successes.

CHAPTER 1

One big problem encountered by anyone who wishes to write a historical review is the impossibility of giving everyone the recognition they deserve. Cancer is such a complex complaint that countless people have contributed directly or indirectly to its understanding: not just biologists, virologists, molecular biologists, chemists, physicists, epidemiologists, statisticians and other scientists, but also clinicians like surgeons, radiotherapists, radiologists, pathologists, medical oncologists, and also many other physicians from different specialties. Some have advanced our knowledge by only one small step, but all these small advances were necessary to allow important discoveries to be made later. It would go too far to name every one of these researchers. Churchill said: "history will look kindly on me... for I shall be the one to write it" but the individual researcher makes no personal contribution to an overview like this one (Char, 1996). As a result, many will be forgotten.

The historian also faces another difficulty. He has to rely mainly on written sources. There will be a natural tendency for the author to pay more attention to the publications from his own country, which may make his own account somewhat unbalanced. This approach does however have the advantage of throwing light on background information that might otherwise slip into obscurity, and thus of sometimes creating valuable new insights.

So far, no published book has ever discussed every aspect of the problem of cancer from a historical perspective, which is why I have undertaken this endeavor. The present volume first considers the occurrence of cancer in classical times, and the views that have been held of the nature of this disease in the past. It goes on to discuss the history of treatment, with special reference to the fields of surgery, radiotherapy, chemotherapy, hormone therapy, targeted therapy and immunotherapy, and concludes with a review of advances in the field of psycho-oncology.

'Historians are prophets who stand with their back to the future', said the German philosopher, writer and critic Friedrich von Schlegel in 1798. I adopted the opposite stance when writing some chapters of this book, since I felt it was more instructive to consider the latest developments that offer new opportunities for cures. Targeted therapy is particularly relevant in this context, since it embodies a completely new approach to the problem of cancer.

[2]

The occurrence of cancer in ancient times and the development of ideas about the nature of the disease

Cancer found in animal and human remains

Paleopathology, the study of abnormalities in human and animal remains from the distant past, teaches us that tumors have existed as long as humans and animals have been on this planet. Bones are most resistant to decay. In line with this, the first forms of cancer were found in animal bones. Moodie found part of a dinosaur tail in Wyoming in the United States. One of the tail vertebrae shows a growth that is reminiscent of a vascular tumor. Walker considered this growth to be cancerous, while Calvin Wells believed it to be an exostosis (a benign bone growth). A similar discussion developed in connection with an abnormality found on the shaft of a femur of *Homo erectus* (ape-man), previously called *Pithecanthropus erectus*, discovered on Java in the nineteenth century by the Dutch physician Dubois (Figure 2.1). This is a find from prehistoric times (800,000 years ago). According to Walker, this abnormality was an osteosarcoma, while Wells regarded this too as an exostosis.

A Paleolithic skull with seven holes in it was discovered in the Joan d'Os cave in the Pyrenees. This condition has been ascribed to a multiple myeloma or to lytic metastases of a carcinoma. Prehistoric finds of petrified tumor masses and lytic lesions have also been made elsewhere. For example, a strongly proliferating cancer was discovered on the top part of the upper arm of a human skeleton dating from the last Ice Age in Münsingen in Switzerland. This is doubtless an osteosarcoma. An osteosarcoma has also been found in the femur of a cave bear from the same period.

Nasopharyngeal carcinomas and osteosarcomas have been identified in human mummies from ancient Egypt (Cabanne et al., 1983), and human remains showing traces of cancer have also been found in Peru. It is believed that these are likewise osteosarcomas. Carbon dating indicates that these pre-Colombian patients lived some 2400 years ago.

FIGURE 2.1 Thigh-bone of Homo erectus, with a lesion suspected to be a bone tumor (Naturalis museum of natural history, Leiden, the Netherlands).

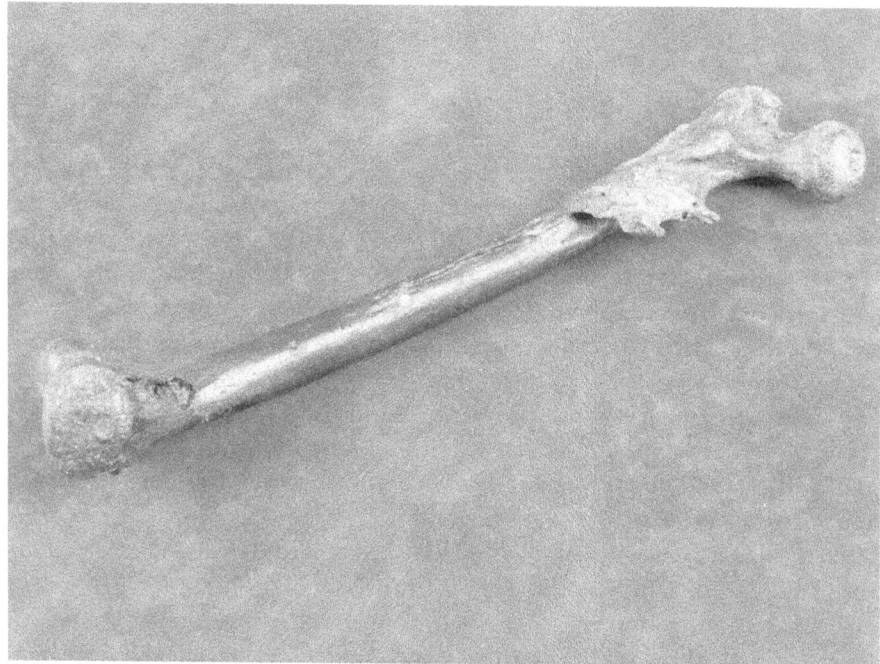

While these paleopathological finds are very interesting and were discovered only with great difficulty, they yield only very limited insights into the problem of cancer. To ascertain what cancer meant to people in the distant past, we have to consult written sources.

Cancer described in ancient documents

The oldest written descriptions of cancer come from ancient Egypt. Descriptions of medical matters have been found on Egyptian papyri dating from about 1950-1550 BC. The best known of these are the Edwin Smith, Ebers and Kahoun papyri.

Edwin Smith was an American who had an antiques business in Cairo. He bought a papyrus from Mustapha Aga in Luxor in 1862. After his death in 1906, his daughter donated the papyrus to the Historical Society of New York, which had it translated in 1930 by James Henry Breasted, director of the Oriental Institute of the University of Chicago. The translation took Breasted ten years. The papyrus consists of seventeen pages and is 377 lines and five meters long; a fragment is shown in Figure 2.2. The text deals mainly with wounds and their treatment, but also describes eight cases of breast tumor (Kardinal and Yarbro, 1979). It is assumed that most of the information in the Edwin Smith papyrus is derived from documents written around 2650 BC. This was the time of Imhotep, the high priest, physician, architect of the first pyramid and vizier to King Djoser.

The Ebers papyrus was also bought by Edwin Smith in Luxor. The identity of the vendor is not known. It is claimed that the papyrus was found between the legs of a mummy in the Assassif district of the Thebes necropolis. Edwin Smith sold the papyrus in 1872 to the Egyptologist George Ebers, after whom it is now named. The Ebers papyrus is 110 pages long and is the longest of all the medical papyri. It was written about fifty years after the Edwin Smith papyrus, but like it describes prescriptions and medicaments going back to 2500-3000 BC. It was translated in 1937 by Bendix Ebbell (Ebbell, 1937). A number of different tumors are mentioned in the papyrus. At that point in time, no distinction was yet made between tumors and inflammations. However, different types requiring different kinds of treatment were distinguished (Cabanne et al., 1983). The Kahoun papyrus from 1950 BC, the oldest known papyrus, discovered by Flinders Petrie in 1889, contains a description of a uterine carcinoma that mentions the peculiar smell of burnt flesh and the specific pains associated with this condition (Wells, 1964).

The ancient Sanskrit epic *Ramayana*, is part of the Hindu scriptures. It describes events that are supposed to have taken place around 1200-1000 BC and was written down around 400-200 BC. It contains 24,000 verses that were originally written on palm leaves. It also contains descriptions of cancers and their treatment.

CHAPTER 2

FIGURE 2.2 *A fragment from the Edwin Smith medical papyrus (Source: Shimkin, 1979, courtesy of the National Institute of Health, Bethesda, MD, USA).*

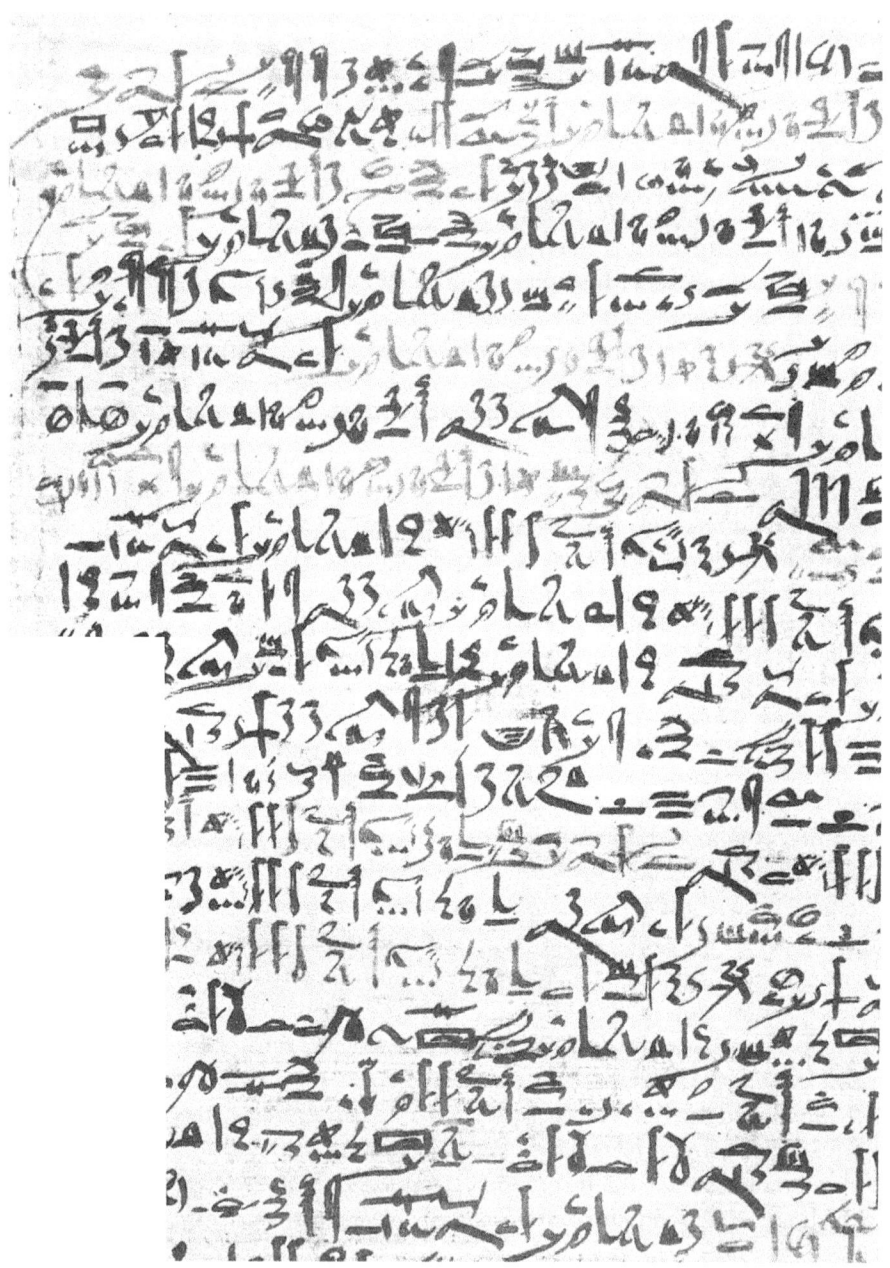

The Hellenistic or Greek period

In order to understand the views held on cancer in the classical Greek period, it is useful to consider them in the context of the ideas and activities that were common in a number of other countries that were important at that time. In ancient China, India, Persia, Babylonia and Egypt, all political power was in the hands of a single man or monarch, generally called an emperor, despot, king or pharaoh. Similarly, all intellectual power – that is, all human knowledge including the knowledge of medicine – was in the hands of a small group of men, the priests, who claimed to have received this knowledge from the gods. This group was far removed from the common people, who were kept ignorant, afraid, poor and deprived. They were told that the 'will of the gods' determined what happened in the world. Natural disasters and the illnesses that plagued people were beyond human understanding and could not be controlled by the common man. The only possible salvation lay in the hands of the priests. In order to control the violence of nature, they offered the cruel, vengeful gods sacrifices – first human, later animal. They treated disease by driving demons out of the persons affected. Religious dogmas overruled rational thinking, hindering advances in all human knowledge including medical science (Diamandopoulos, 1996).

In contrast to the ideas held in the above-mentioned five ancient cultures, the Hellenistic view that 'every free man is master of his own fate' held sway in Greece. This led to the development of democracy – rule by the people themselves – in the political arena and of philosophy ('love of wisdom') in the intellectual domain. This new conviction ultimately meant that all people could think freely and independently, without hindrance in their search for objective scientific truth. The end result of this new attitude was a new intellectual approach based more on knowledge than on belief.

One of the exponents of this new approach was the physician Hippocrates, known as the 'father of medicine'. He was born on the Greek island of Kos around 460 BC (Figure 2.3), and became a famous physician and teacher of medicine. There are many legends about his life, but little is known with any certainty. The only contemporary mention of Hippocrates is in Plato's dialogue *Protagoras*, where he is described as "Hippocrates of Kos, the Asclepiad". It is uncertain who an Asclepiad was. Some theories hold that they were priests of an 'Asclepeion' – a temple of healing, dedicated to Asclepios, the Greek god of medicine. They could also have been a guild of physicians, separate from the healing temples and closely related to the Hippocratic tradition, or a group of people who claimed to be descended from Asclepius. At that time, the teaching of medicine was mainly practical, and the art of medicine was often passed on from father to son. Soranus of Ephesus, a 2nd-century Greek gynecologist, was Hippocrates' first biographer. According to Soranus, Hippocrates was also taught by his father and grandfather. He probably received his initial medical training at the Asclepeion of Kos and later travelled widely, teaching and practicing medicine in Thessaly in northern Greece among other places.

Probably his most important contribution was that he liberated medicine from the shackles of religion, superstition and magic and that he paved the way for a scientific approach based on systematic, accurate observation and logical thinking.

Hippocrates introduced a theory of the cause of disease based on the ideas of the Greek natural philosopher Empedocles (about 490-430 BC), according to whom the universe was built up of four elements: earth, air, fire (energy) and water. Hippocrates thought that the body was built up of the four fluids, known as the humors, that were the biological counterparts of these elements. The blood, formed in the heart, was the counterpart of air; phlegm, originating in the brain, corresponded to water; black bile, originating in the spleen, to earth; and yellow bile from the liver to fire. He regarded health as due to a proper balance in the admixture of these humors, and disease as due to an unbalanced mixture. Too much or too little blood, phlegm or bile was the reason for all diseases. This theory of the constitution of the body and the cause of disease later came to be known as the humoral theory.

Hippocrates postulated that cancer was the result of too much black bile. There are lengthy descriptions of tumors in many of the 70 books of the Hippocratic Corpus. While the authorship of these books is traditionally ascribed to Hippocrates, modern scholarship believes that most or all of them were written by the followers of Hippocrates long after his death. The Greek word for tumor is 'oncos'; the medical term oncology is derived from this. Hippocrates coined the term 'carcinos' for a non-ulcerating tumor and 'carcinoma' for an ulcerating tumor. 'Carcinos' means crab in Greek, while the corresponding Latin word is 'cancer'; in those days, cancer of the female breast was relatively often seen and this is one of the few cancers that are externally visible. It is thought that Hippocrates may have used the term 'crab' because untreated breast cancer is often surrounded by swollen veins resembling the many legs of a crab. It is not entirely certain whether this explanation of the use of the word 'carcinos' actually comes from Hippocrates, or from Paul of Aegina (Kardinal and Yarbro, 1979). We shall be returning to this point later.

Hippocrates also used the term 'scirrhos' ('scirrhus' in Latin) – which means 'hard' – to describe tumors that feel hard on palpation (Cabanne et al., 1983). He was the first to divide tumors into benign and malignant. He probably included swellings due to inflammation as well as less life-threatening tumors under the heading 'benign'.

The Hippocratic oath, written in clear, simple language and based on the principles of absolute respect for human life, helping patients and avoiding doing them any harm, is regarded as the best ethical guide to medical practice of all time.

FIGURE 2.3 Bust of Hippocrates (c. 460-377 BC), found near the Roman port of Ostia. Hippocrates, often called 'the father of medicine', also introduced the humoral theory of the origin of diseases. According to him, cancer was due to an accumulation of black bile. (Source: Shimkin, 1979, courtesy of the National Institutes of Health, Bethesda, MD, USA).

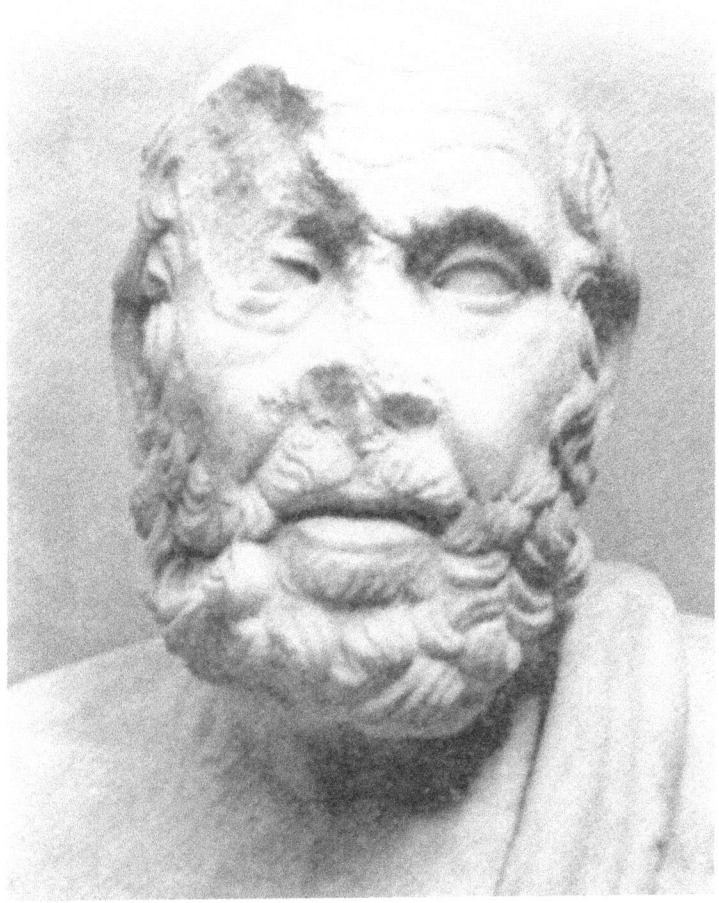

FIGURE 2.4 Galen, another proponent of the humoral theory. His ideas ruled medical science for sixteen centuries. This picture is a sixteenth-century fantasy (probably reproduced from an etching by the Flemish artist Pieter van der Borcht), which was included in the publication: 'Icones veterum aliquot ac, recentium medicorum, philosophorumque elogiolis suis editae, opera I. Sambuci. – Antverpiae, Ex officina Christophori Plantini MDLXXIIII'. ('The Portraits of some physicians and philosophers of past and more recent times, with odes in their praise penned by Johann Sambucus, Antwerp. At the Press of Christopher Plantin, 1574'.) This book was republished by 'De Nederlandsche Boekhandel', Antwerp, in 1901.

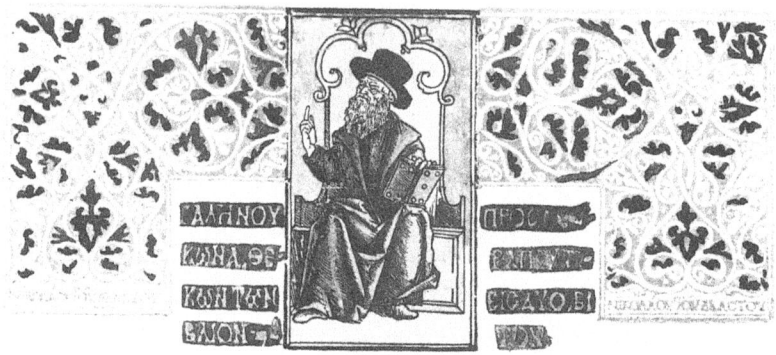

Hippocrates died at an advanced age in Larissa in Thessaly. The exact year of his death is not known; but has been estimated to be about 377 BC (Diamandopoulos, 1996).

It is noteworthy that cancer represented a special threat to women in classical times. While there are no reliable statistical sources to support this view, it was known that the disease often occurred in the breast, womb and other female internal organs. Cancer not only represented a threat to women's lives, but could also be emotionally devastating. Ashamed, oppressed, feeling that they had lost their femininity, women with one of these forms of cancer often kept their terrible secret to themselves, thus reinforcing a virtual conspiracy of silence about the disease that has held sway throughout history (Patterson, 1987).

The Roman period

After the fall of the Greek Empire, Rome took over the task of supporting the development of the scientific knowledge of medicine. Aurelius Cornelius Celsus (c. 30 BC - AD 38) was a member of an aristocratic Roman family, who was probably not a physician but an encyclopedist. He tried to summarize the knowledge of many different fields that was available in his times. He wrote about agriculture, the practice of law, military science, philosophy, rhetoric and medicine. The eight books entitled *De Medicina* (On Medicine) are all that remain of his works. His writings fell into oblivion until Pope Nicholas V (1397-1455) rediscovered them during the Renaissance (Lyons, 1987a). Driven by scientific interest, Celsus drew up a classification of the various forms of cancer. He also described edema due to the pressure of a tumor on the surrounding tissue, and considered the reaction of the lymphatic system as a subsidiary symptom of cancer. He was the first to discover the phenomenon of metastasis (Cabanne et al., 1983).

The most famous physician of this period is Claudius Galenus, normally known as Galen nowadays (see Figure 2.4). His name is derived from the Greek word 'galenios', which means 'calm', and was given him by his father in the vain hope that he would not grow up to be like his mother, who had an irritable, volatile character. Galen was born in AD 130 in Pergamon, the center of parchment production in the district of Ionia on the southwest coast of Asia Minor. His father was an architect, mathematician and landowner. As a boy, Galen was taught by his father. From the age of fourteen, he received instruction in philosophy, mathematics and natural sciences from philosophers. They taught him the importance of anatomy, empirical observation and the doctrines of Hippocrates. Galen relates that he had learned medicine on the advice of his father, who had in his turn got the advice from Asclepius, the god of medicine, in a dream.

Galen began his medical studies in the local temple of Asclepius, an institute of medical education such as were to be found in many cities of ancient Greece.

He continued his studies in a number of other cities after the death of his father and completed his training at the famous university of Alexandria, where he came under the influence of renowned anatomists. He also learned a great deal about the beneficial properties of plants and minerals. He then returned to Pergamon, where he established himself as a physician. He was appointed as the official doctor for the gladiators. Observation of the serious wounds the gladiators often suffered in combat helped to supplement his theoretical knowledge of anatomy with practical examples. Galen was regarded as an excellent physician in Asia Minor. It is not surprising that he felt attracted to the challenge represented by the city of Rome, which was regarded at that time as the capital of the civilized world. However, Rome was not welcoming to foreigners in general, and to people with special skills like Galen in particular. As a result, his first stay was of relatively short duration. But when his renown came to the ears of the Emperor Marcus Aurelius, the latter appointed Galen his personal physician round about AD 157. Galen then settled in Rome, dying there in 200 at the age of 70.

Galen performed no more surgery after he came to Rome, probably as a result of social pressure. He was an erudite man who wrote widely, on mathematics, philosophy, grammar and medicine. He introduced the discipline of experimental physiology. His anatomical descriptions were mainly derived from observations on animals, in particular Barbary Macaques.

Galen further elaborated the medical system originally developed by Hippocrates. He was a proponent of the humoral theory, and believed that the deposition of black bile in certain parts of the body such as the lips, tongue or breast led to the development of tumors that he called 'cancer', the Latin word for crab, He also introduced the term sarcoma (from the Greek *sarcos* = flesh) to describe a tumor that looked meaty when cut through. Galen believed that the human temperament depended on the way the four body fluids or humors were mixed, and divided people up into sanguine, phlegmatic, choleric and melancholic types on this basis. He thought, for example, that depression was the result of an excess of black (*melan* in Greek) bile (*chole* in Greek). This is the origin of the word melancholy. He further stated that many cancer patients were depressed and conversely that many patients who were depressed developed cancer. This idea is still sometimes held, though no scientific proof for it has ever been found.

Galen was less original than Hippocrates, but his ideas continued to dominate medical science for sixteen centuries. To doubt them was a form of heresy. This tenacious adherence to the views of Galen can be explained by stagnation of medical thinking from the time of Galen till the end of the Middle Ages because Christianity, Judaism and Islam had all forbidden post-mortem examination and placed limits on the practice of surgery (Diamandopoulos, 1996). These religions all believed in a life after death. The soul, which remains in the body after death, will be resurrected and the soul of the faithful rewarded with eternal bliss in Paradise. It has often been argued that dissection of the body was forbidden in order not to place this process in jeopardy (Lyons, 1987b). Considerable doubt may be cast on this point of view, however.

For example, James J. Walsh, Professor of the History of Medicine at Fordham University School of Medicine (USA), claimed that Christianity never did forbid autopsies. He believes that many historians have simply copied previous statements to this effect without consulting the original documents, or they cited the Papal bull *De Sepulturis* (On Burials) promulgated by Pope Boniface VIII in 1300 but interpreted the contents incorrectly. It is very difficult to gain access to this bull, but Walsh managed to inspect a copy and stated that there is no mention anywhere in it of a prohibition on autopsies. It does however contain a provision that the bodies of persons who die abroad but wish to be buried at home may not be cut into pieces and boiled so that the bones could more conveniently be transported to the country of origin and buried there. This custom was introduced during the Crusades to make it easier for the remains of kings and noblemen to be brought home for burial. This happened, for example, to the remains of the Holy Roman Emperor Frederick Barbarossa, who drowned in the River Saleph in southeast Anatolia during the Third Crusade in 1190, and to those of the French King Louis IX and his relatives during the unsuccessful crusade of 1270 (Walsh, 1908).

Doubt has also been cast on the claim that Islam prohibited autopsies in the Middle Ages. Emily Savage-Smith has subjected this question to an intensive investigation (Savage-Smith, 1995) and concluded that there was no formal prohibition on the performance of autopsies among Muslims. In her opinion, a whole complex of factors made physicians unwilling to perform post-mortem examinations. She saw the close link between body and soul in Islam, and the wish not to do anything that might disturb the soul of the deceased, as one of the main reasons for this reluctance. The belief in resurrection is one of the fundamental tenets of Islam, and most Muslims believe that this resurrection is not purely spiritual in nature. All discussions of this topic reveal a concern that mutilation before or after death will interfere with this resurrection in some way.

Rabbi Dr. Julius Jakobovits made an in-depth study of the possible prohibition of autopsies in the Judaism of the Middle Ages, and came to the conclusion that there was no decisive evidence for such a prohibition (Jakobovits, 1975).

All in all, it must be concluded that a religious prohibition on post-mortem examinations was not the cause of the slow progress of medical science in the Middle Ages. On the other hand, there can be no doubt that there was a great reluctance to perform autopsies.

The Byzantine Empire

The division of the Roman Empire in AD 395 – initially intended as a mere administrative measure – led in practice to the formation of two independent states: the

Western Roman Empire and the Eastern Roman Empire. The latter came not long after to be called after its capital, Byzantium. After the fall of the Western Roman Empire, the center of medical science moved to the Byzantine Empire (395-1453) and medical science flourished there. This period was characterized by the collection of and writing of commentaries on classical medical texts (medical encyclopedias), in particular those of Hippocrates and Galen. The best known of the many physician/encyclopedists of that time were Oribasius of Pergamon (c. 325-403); Alexander of Tralles(c. 525-605), a Greek physician born in Tralles in Lydia (now Aydin in Turkey); Aetius of Amida in Mesopotamia (502-575); and Paul of Aegina (625-690). While none of these excellent authors added anything original to our knowledge of medicine in general and of cancer in particular, they made a major contribution by ensuring the preservation of many of the ideas and opinions of their predecessors (Diamandopoulos, 1996).

Oribasius, nicknamed 'Galen's ape', stressed the painful nature of cancer. He described the occurrence of cancer on the face, the breast and the genitalia. Aetius pointed out the significance of enlarged lymph nodes in the armpit in cases of breast cancer, and recommended use of poppy extracts to relieve the pain (Cabanne et al., 1983).

The surgeon Paul of Aegina, who was born on the Greek island of Aegina and established himself in Alexandria, shared Hippocrates' views on the origin of the word 'cancer', stating that the swollen blood vessels round an untreated breast tumor often looked like the legs of a crab. As mentioned above, it is uncertain whether Paul of Aegina or Hippocrates actually gave this explanation. Paul of Aegina also considered it possible that the word refers to the fact that a cancer is firmly attached to the body, just as a crab clutches its prey (Diamandopoulos, 1996).

Another suggestion concerning the etymology of the word 'cancer' is that the patient may survive after removal of the tumor, like a crab that has had part of its body cut off.

The Arab World (850-1050)

Physicians in the Arab Empire, which extended from the Indus to the Pyrenees at the peak of its power, were mainly occupied in translating the works of Greek and Roman authors - in particular Galen. He was called the 'Prince of Physicians' because he was regarded by many as the absolute medical authority. Galen was in fact not the only one to hold this title, which has also been accorded to other eminent medical authors such as Avicenna (see below) and the Jewish physician and philosopher Moses Maimonides, who was born in Cordoba, Spain, in 1135 and died in Egypt in 1204.

It is noteworthy that a relatively minor event in the history of the Byzantine Empire had a great impact on medical knowledge. When Nestorius, the Greek-

Orthodox Patriarch of Constantinople, was exiled for heresy in 431, he and his followers – including a large number of physicians – emigrated to Syria. When they continued to be subject to religious persecution there, they moved on further to Persia. Nestorius's heresy lay in his unwillingness to acknowledge that Mary was the mother of God; according to him, she was simply the mother of the human being Jesus (Petrucelli, 1987a). His followers, who came to be known as Nestorian Christians, translated many Greek and Latin medical texts into Syriac for educational purposes, for example at the famous school established at Jundishapur. The Arabs found these old texts when they invaded Persia in the seventh century. They continued this tradition of translating the Greek and Latin scientific classics – this time into Arabic and other languages. Perhaps the most famous center for these activities was the Bait al-Hikma or House of Wisdom, a library and translation institute set up in Baghdad by the Abbassid Caliph Haroun al-Rashid in the ninth century, which continued to exert an important influence throughout the period from the ninth to the thirteenth century.

The most famous Arab physician from this period was Ibn Sina (980-1037) or Avicenna as he was known in the West, who was born in Persia. He wrote the celebrated Canon of Medicine (Canonum medicinae libri V), which – although it was mainly a compendium of old viewpoints (for example that cancer was caused by an excess of black bile) – helped to stimulate renewed interest in the writings of Hippocrates and Galen (Diamandopoulos, 1996). The not very original medical knowledge contained in the Canon helped to lay the foundation of the Golden Age of Arab medicine. The Canon also had an enormous influence on medicine in the West. No fewer than 29 Latin editions of the work appeared between 1473 and 1658 (De Moulin, 1988).

When Arab medicine fell into decline after the Crusades, the original Greek and Latin medical texts and their translations reached Europe by two routes: via North Africa and Spain, and via the Mediterranean Sea and Italy. From there, they spread further to France and then to England, Germany and the rest of Europe, providing a source of inspiration for the revival of a scientific approach to medicine. The medical knowledge of antiquity was thus preserved during Europe's dark Middle Ages by travelling from the West to the East and subsequently returning to the West enriched by the influence of various cultures and traditions (Cabanne et al., 1983).

China

Historical research by Western scholars into the contributions made by Chinese physicians to medicine in general and oncology in particular is still in its infancy. Sun Simiao (581-672) is however worthy of mention here. This prominent physician during the Tang dynasty (618-907) described most diseases, including cancer. He divided tumors into six types: bony, fatty, stony and suppurating, and tumors of the muscles and the blood vessels.

Xue Ji (c. 1488-1558), a physician of the Ming dynasty, published his *Waike Shuyao* (Essentials of external medicine) in 1528. This gives a different classification of cancers than that of Sun Simiao. Xue Ji distinguished tumors of the circulatory system, of the organs of respiration, the muscles, the nerves and the bones. He is cited in the *Illustrierte Geschichte der Medizin* under the distorted name of Sie Kie, and his year of birth is mistakenly given there as the year of publication of the above-mentioned book (Cabanne et al., 1983).

The Middle Ages (10th-14th century)

In the Middle Ages, before the establishment of independent universities, learning in Europe was the exclusive domain of the monastic orders. Driven by their belief in the divine authority of the dogmas of the Catholic Church, the members of these orders suppressed free independent thought. As a result, astrology, alchemy, magic and exorcism replaced a rational approach to the diagnosis and treatment of diseases, including cancer. It is hardly surprising, then, that no advances of any significance were achieved during this whole period. The members of the religious orders who practiced medicine called themselves doctors – a term derived from the Latin verb 'docere', to teach. Their work consisted in praying, the laying on of hands, the expulsion of demons and the use of amulets containing pictures of saints and holy oil, relics of saints and other objects credited by superstition with supernatural powers. Surgery was forbidden. During the Fourth Lateran Council in 1215, it was ordained in decree 18 that the clergy were not permitted to be involved in any form of blood-letting, whether that occurred in connection with a sentence imposed by the court or a duel, or in any form of surgery by cauterization or incision (De Moulin, 1988). Healing was only possible by prayer and divine intervention. The assistance of saints as intermediaries between God and man was invoked in the event of illness. The twin saints Cosmas and Damian, both doctors and both martyrs, were very popular for this purpose, as was the Virgin Mary (Petrucelli, 1987b).

The situation changed with the founding of the medical school of Salerno (tenth century) and of the universities of Bologna (1088) and of Oxford and Cambridge, Paris and Montpellier (all in the thirteenth century). The study of the classical medical texts, in particular those of Galen, resumed. While the practice of medicine flourished in Italy and France, the quality of medical services long remained at a low ebb in Germany – where the power of the Church was still great – and in England – despite the establishment of the universities of Oxford and Cambridge (Diamandopoulos, 1996).

According to the chronicler Salimbene di Adam, the first autopsy since the days of Ptolemy in Alexandria was performed in 1286 in Cremona. The aim of this examination was to trace the cause of a mysterious epidemic (Park, 1995; Jakobovits,

1975). A forensic post-mortem was performed in Bologna in 1302. It was probably no coincidence that this happened in Bologna, since the university there had an important law faculty (De Moulin, 1988). After that time, autopsies were carried out increasingly often, not only to track down diseases or to support court judgments but also for educational purposes. Modino de Liuzzi (1275-1326), attached to the university of Bologna as a physician and anatomist, performed autopsies to support his lectures. He published a textbook on the technique of post-mortem examination, which remained the standard in this field for two centuries (Walsh, 1908).

The Renaissance (14th-17th Century)

As mentioned above, no major advances were made for centuries in the field of cancer after the time of Galen. Things changed during the Renaissance. Countless discoveries were made in this period that had an enormous impact on many branches of science and society. Gutenberg reinvented the art of printing (after it had been in use in China for many centuries) in 1454, and in 1492 Columbus discovered America. Copernicus published his views on astronomy in 1543, including the revolutionary idea that the sun is the center of the solar system and that the planets rotate around it. This was completely at odds with the view that had been held until then, namely that the earth and man formed the center of the universe. The rationalist style of argumentation on a metaphysical basis that had held sway from the time of Galen was now given a more empirical slant, with experiment as the basis.

There were also great advances in the field of medicine. William Harvey (1578-1657) described the circulation of the blood in 1628. Gasparo Aselli (1581-1626) was the first author to publish an account of the lymphatic system. During vivisection on a dog that had been fed shortly before the experiment, he observed white 'cords' secreting a milky fluid on opening the stomach. He reported this observation in his book De lactibus albae et lacteae, which was published posthumously in 1627. Olof (Olaus) Rudbeck (1630-1702), professor of Medicine at Uppsala University in Sweden, studied the lymphatic system in greater detail, and published his findings in 1651.

The Flemish physician and anatomist Andries van Wesel, better known under the name of Vesalius (1514-1564), born in Brussels, was the author of the first complete textbook of anatomy, entitled De humani corporis fabrica libri septem (Seven books on the Workings of the Human Body), with elegant anatomical drawings by his compatriot Johan Stefan van Kalkar. Although it was still officially forbidden to carry out research on corpses at that time, autopsies were allowed for legal reasons (for example to determine the cause of death under suspicious circumstances) or on medical grounds (for example, to establish the cause of a disease, especially if there were fears of the spread of an infection). Two of the illustrations in Vesalius'

CHAPTER 2

FIGURE 2.5 *Woodcut by Johan Stefan van Kalkar showing the muscles of a man, taken from the book* De humani corporis fabrica *by Andreas Vesalius (published in Basle in 1543). The noose round the man's neck indicates that this is the corpse of an executed criminal, on which autopsies were permitted.*

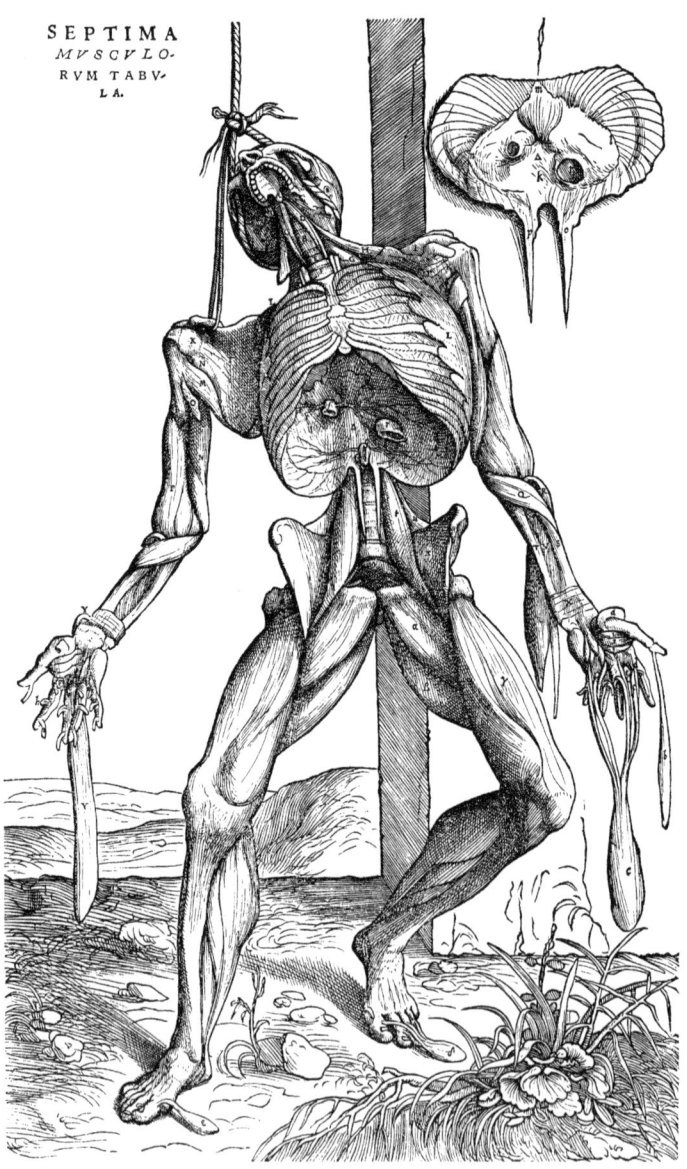

atlas show a body with a noose round its neck, doubtless to underline the fact that the examination had been performed on an executed criminal (Figure 2.5). Autopsies for educational purposes were forbidden. Nevertheless, a guide to the University of Padua related that this did happen. Students were taught anatomy during the winter months, with reference to dissections on corpses that were secretly exhumed in the middle of the night, carried to the anatomy theatre and laid on the demonstration table. A teaching assistant stood on guard. In an emergency, he would give a sign to two helpers who were sitting next to the table. They would turn the tabletop over, dropping the corpse into the river that flowed under the anatomy theatre and revealing a half-dissected rabbit mounted on the underside of the tabletop. This would suggest to any inspectors who made their way into the anatomy theatre that the students were being taught with reference to dissections on animals. Vesalius was unable to discover black bile in the course of his experiments, though there was plenty of blood and lymph. This obviously raised serious questions about the validity of the humoral theory, and consequently his book generated fierce opposition from the followers of Galen.

The discovery of lymph gradually caused this fluid to replace black bile in medical thinking. The new findings led the French philosopher and mathematician René Descartes (1596-1650) to put forward his 'lymph theory' of the etiology of cancer. He postulated that when lymph leaks out of the lymph ducts, the fluid gives rise to a benign tumor. When however the lymph is subject to local fermentation or degeneration, a malignant tumor is produced. This theory held sway for a hundred and fifty years, and was supported by Georg Ernst Stahl, Friedrich Hoffman and John Hunter (1728-1793), a Scottish surgeon who was regarded as one of the most eminent scientists and surgeons of his day. His scientific collection formed the basis of the Hunterian Museum of the Royal College of Surgeons, which is still in existence in Lincoln's Inn Fields, London, today. Hunter also claimed that tumor tissue, like normal tissue, receives its nourishment from the host and develops in accordance with the same fundamental biological laws (Diamandopoulos, 1996). He further stated that 'coagulated lymph', later identified as fibrin, was the omnipotent 'blastema' from which both normal and pathologic organisms grew (Rather, 1978).

The most serious attack on the black bile theory was mounted by the Parisian surgeon Henri François le Dran (1685-1770; Figure 2.6). In a treatise published in 1757, he rejected the humoral doctrine in favor of the theory that cancer is a local complaint – at least in its early stages. Le Dran arrived at his ideas on the basis of his own observations in the autopsy theatre. He further described the dissemination of breast cancer via the lymph ducts to the lymph nodes in the various parts of the body, and stressed the likelihood of relapses in this disease (Bett, 1954). According to le Dran, the passage of a single drop of cancerous lymph through one of the neighboring lymph nodes was enough to contaminate the entire system.

FIGURE 2.6 Henri François le Dran, French surgeon, who definitively disproved the theory that black bile was the cause of cancer (Source: Shimkin, 1979, courtesy of the National Institute of Health, Bethesda, MD, USA).

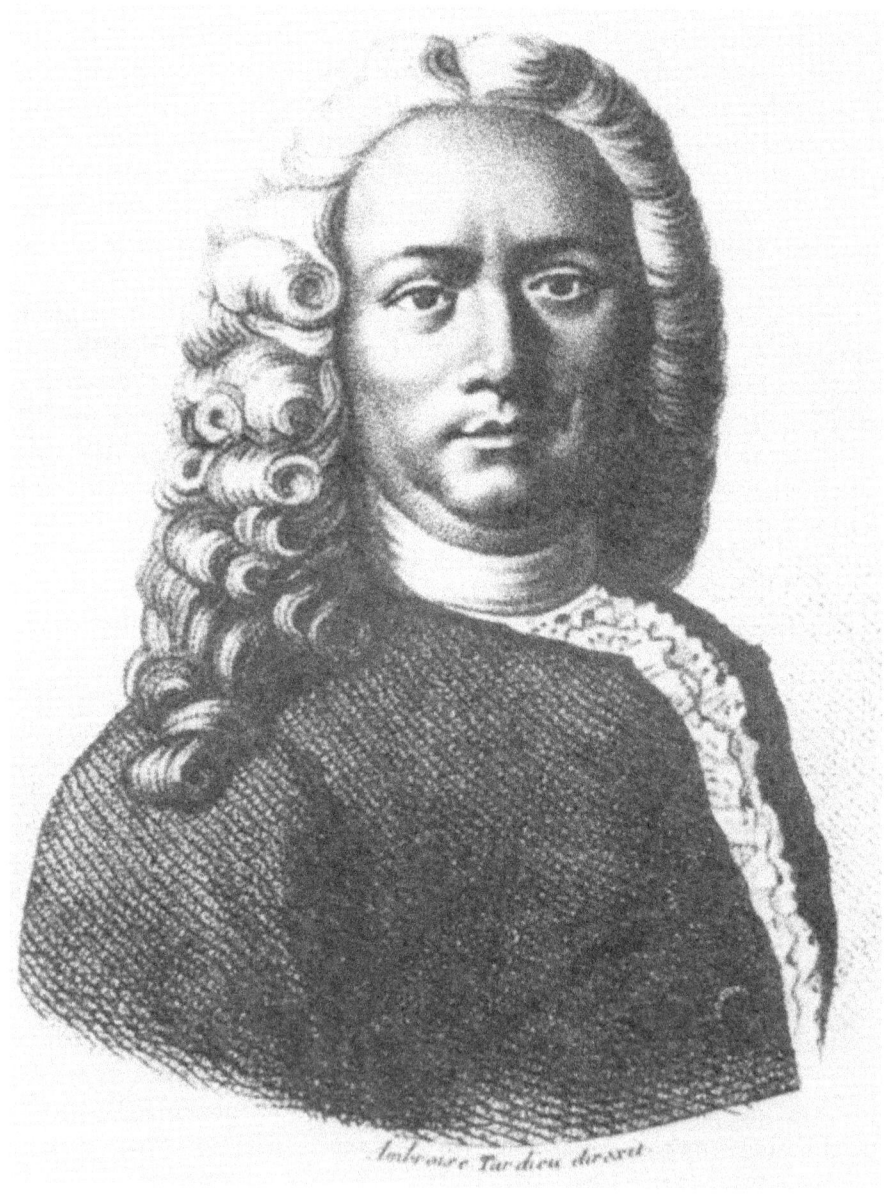

The seventeenth-century medical literature contains a few sparse mentions of the finding of hard, enlarged glands in the ipsilateral armpit in cases of breast cancer. These enlarged glands were ascribed to the same causes as those that had given rise to the cancer in the breast. According to De Moulin, there seem to be no autopsy reports from that time that give an unambiguous description of visceral metastasis. There were also no explicit mentions of cancer as the cause of death, though there was a vague idea that death was due to a toxin secreted by the cancer. The awareness of the possible existence of a specific cancer toxin grew steadily at this time (De Moulin, 1988).

The Dutch surgeon Willem Leurs commented as follows on this point in 1793:

_____ *'The cause of cancer must be sought in a cancer toxin produced by the body itself. The source of this cancer toxin is probably situated in the genitals. Since men in warmer climates have a stronger and quicker discharge of seed than those in colder climates, cancer occurred less often in savages than in civilized persons. Those who were unmarried had more chance of getting cancer, because of the less frequent discharge of seed'* (Van der Sluis, 1990).

The Italian professor of anatomy Hieronymus Fabricius (1537-1619) drew a distinction between swellings due to inflammation and cancers, and warned against incomplete removal of the tumor. The Italian surgeon Marcus Aurelius Severinus (1580-1656) described the myxosarcoma (a sarcoma of the soft tissues). He distinguished between cancers and benign swellings of the breast. If he operated on the breast, he also removed the lymph nodes (Ewing, 1919).

The decline of Galen's authority led to the rise of all kinds of strange theories about diseases, including cancer. Paracelsus (1493-1541), whose real name was Philippus Aurelius Theophrastus Bombast von Hohenheim, was the source of one of these unusual ideas. He was a physician and chemist, and one of the most controversial figures in the history of medicine. Some saw him as an important innovator in the field of medical science because of his introduction of ideas derived from chemistry, while others regarded him as a fantasist or even a charlatan (De Moulin, 1988). He believed that a disease could not be cured until its nature was known, and that this nature could be discovered by incinerating some of the affected tissue and subjecting the residue to chemical analysis. Paracelsus concluded on the basis of his experiments that cancer was due to an excess of mineral salts in the blood. According to him, the disease developed at points where various salts concentrate and try to find a way out of the body (Kardinal and Yarbro, 1979).

The eighteenth and nineteenth centuries

An interesting new social development occurred in France during this period. Jean Godinot, a monk from Rheims, was excluded from the university, and from meetings of the monastic order to which he belonged that were attended by the archbishop, because of his Jansenist beliefs. A secret royal decree ordering him into exile was even issued in 1720. In fact, Godinot went into hiding in his domain near Rheims where he devoted himself to the cultivation of his vineyards and the production of wine and finally became rich, just like Dom Pérignon. At the end of his life he divided up his possessions and in 1740, at the age of 69, he overcame a host of difficulties and opposition from his contemporaries to found a hospital for cancer patients with the aim of relieving their physical and mental suffering. According to the statutes that he had drawn up, the hospital would also provide support in meeting the patients' individual and social problems. This was the first dedicated cancer hospital in the world (Cabanne et al., 1983), and the Jean Godinot Institute that developed out of it is still active in Rheims today.

Herman Boerhaave (1688-1738) of Leiden lived in the same period. He deserves mention here not so much because of his contributions in the field of oncology but because he was the most influential physician and teacher of medicine of his time, whose opinions were followed by many. He believed that cancer was the result of an inflammation.

'An inflammation can disappear, suppurate, lead to gangrene (mortification of the tissues) or turn into a scirrhus. This is a hard, painless swelling that only arises in glands and that can turn into cancer under unfavorable conditions. The swelling is caused by blockage of the ducts providing drainage of the tissue in question. An example is the female breast, where milk can clot in the lacteal ducts during lactation. Any hard swelling that is not painful is considered to be a scirrhus' (Shimkin, 1979).

Some advances in the field of oncology were also made in this period. The French physician and professor of Medicine Jean Astruc (1684-1766) distinguished cysts from real tumors. He demonstrated the essential similarity between hard and soft cancers, and pointed out the important differences in prognosis between the various types of cancer. He compared the growth of cancer from lymph with the heating and swelling of plaster of Paris in water (Ewing, 1919).

Another person who was of importance in the history of oncology is Bernard Peyrilhe (1735-1804). In 1774, at the age of 39, he won the prize offered the previous year by the Academy of Letters and Fine Arts in Lyon for the best essay on the subject 'Investigations into the causes of cancer that can lead to determination of its nature and its effects, and to development of the best methods of treating it'. In his *Dissertatio academica de cancro*, Peyrilhe was the first in the literature to suggest that a liquid living agent of infection – later identified as a virus – could be the cause of cancer (Cabanne et al., 1983). He tried to demonstrate the presence of this infectious agent by injecting a tumor emulsion under the skin of a dog. This experiment failed, however, because an abscess developed at the injection site and his laboratory assistant drowned the dog. He is also known to have treated sores successfully with the newly discovered carbonic acid (Ewing, 1919). He demonstrated that cancer starts as a local process and spreads along the lymph ducts. Peyrilhe also attempted to develop an experimental model of cancer, and to gain insights into the pathogenesis of the disease (Cabanne et al., 1983; Bett, 1954).

Eighteenth-century publications on the nature of cancer were the first to demonstrate an incipient understanding of the problem of metastasis. In 1735, De Gorter wrote about 'cancerous substances' which, having gained access to the blood circulation, can give rise to 'a metastasis from one gland to another' (De Moulin, 1988). Joseph Récamier (1774-1852) described the way in which cancer cells could penetrate blood vessels. He is claimed in the literature to have been the first to introduce the term 'metastasis' for a lesion at a distance from the primary tumor, in this case a brain defect in a patient with breast cancer (Cabanne et al., 1983). According to De Moulin, however, De Gorter made his observation earlier. It may be noted, by the way, that Récamier believed cancer to be an inflammatory process and that nerves caused metastases, giving rise to tumors similar to the original at different places (Récamier, 1829). Récamier is further known for his description in 1829 of the tendency of birthmarks (nevi) to degenerate into cancers.

Pathological anatomy

The scientific basis of medicine was greatly strengthened in the period from 1761 to 1845, the main advances being achieved in the field of pathological anatomy. The start of this 'medical renaissance' can be dated to 1761, when Giovanni Battista Morgagni (1682-1771) from Padua published his monumental work *De sedibus et causis morborum per anatomen indagatis libri quinque* (On the locations and causes of diseases as indicated by anatomy, in five parts), in which he correlated the autopsy findings for seven hundred patients with their clinical data. A systematic description is given of the diseases of the head, the thoracic cavity, the abdomen etc., together with a wealth of what we would call 'case histories'. An example of one of these case histories, taken from the field of oncology, is given below.

———— A 54-year-old man had been suffering from marked emaciation over his whole body for five or six months. He vomited frequently, bringing up a liquid that look like water mixed with soot. An ulcerating cancerous growth consisting of an accumulation of blisters and cysts was found in the stomach near the pylorus (the aperture at the end of the stomach). Pressure on this growth caused it to exude a fluid that resembled male semen. The stomach also contained three glassfuls of a liquid resembling the vomit the man had produced. Two small glandular bodies, each the size of a bean, were found between the stomach and the spleen. They had the same color and substance as the stomach tumor.

Morgagni seems to be describing a signet-ring cell carcinoma of the stomach or a colloid carcinoma here, and it is likely that the two 'beans' were lymph nodes that had been affected by the cancer.

Morgagni, who is sometimes called the father of pathological anatomy, differentiated between malignant tumors and benign swellings due for example to aneurysms and exostoses in the above-mentioned work. He also described cancers of the lungs, esophagus, stomach, rectum and uterus (Kardinal en Yarbro, 1979).

The findings of Marie-François Xavier Bichat (1771-1802) were also interesting. He was a tireless pathologist who had performed six hundred autopsies and who determined the organic structure of the tissues without the aid of a microscope. In cancers, he distinguished between the tumorous parenchyma (or essential element of the growth) and its non-tumorous stroma (framework), thus indicating that one and the same lesion could have two aspects, one malignant and the other benign. His investigations further corroborated previous suggestions that cancers were not built up of black bile or lymph.

René Théophile Hyacinthe Laënnec (1781-1826), a pupil of Bichat and the inventor of the stethoscope, stated that tumors could grow in all types of tissues, and that their structure in general resembled that of the underlying tissue. He regarded cancer as abnormal growth of normal tissue.

The invention of the compound microscope by the Dutch spectacle-maker Hans Janssen from Middelburg and his son Zacharias (c. 1580-1638) made it possible to distinguish between different tissues at a cellular level. The use of the microscope became known largely through the work of Marcello Malpighi (1628-1694), the discoverer of the capillaries, and Antoni van Leeuwenhoek (1632-1723).

Van Leeuwenhoek, a tailor from Delft, made his own primitive microscopes and used them to observe for example blood cells (simply referred to as 'little balls of fat' by Malpighi), spermatozoa and the striations in striated muscle. Nevertheless, the importance of using microscopes in the detection of cancer was insufficiently recognized at that time. It is assumed that this was because of the lack of proper techniques for the examination of tissues (Cabanne et al., 1983).

It was François Raspail (1794-1878) who introduced the freeze-cut technique in 1827, making use of an open tank containing a mixture of ice and salt (Raspail, 1827). This made it possible to cut thin sections of tissue so that they could be studied under a microscope. Raspail observed that tissues were made up of tiny cells. The German physiologist Theodor Schwann (1810-1882) laid the foundation for the cell theory in 1838 together with Mathias Jacob Schleider, by declaring that all plants and animals were made up of cells and cellular products. He also discovered the nucleus and nucleolus of the cell (Ewing, 1919).

Sir Everard Home (1756-1832) was the first to publish a book on cancer containing data obtained with the aid of a microscope. The book, entitled *A short tract on the formation of tumors*, appeared in 1830 and included illustrations showing microscopic sections of cancerous tissue. His studies did not lead to any new insights, however. The next important break-through came in a publication by the German pathologist Johannes Müller (1801-1858). He stated in his monumental work *Über den feinern Bau und die Formen der krankhaften Geschwülste* (On the detailed Structure and Forms of Morbid Cancerous Growths), which appeared in 1838 (Bett, 1954), that there was no essential difference between the structure of cancerous growths and that of normal tissue (Cabanne et al., 1983). This fundamental statement, which supported the macroscopic observations of Laënnec, deserves to be known as 'the first law of oncology'. Müller's remarkable insights were far ahead of his time. He distinguished the different types of tumors on the basis of their microscopic structure and described anaplasia as a widely occurring phenomenon (Bett, 1954). Müller demonstrated definitively that cancers are built up of cells and not of coagulated lymph. He believed, however, that the cancer cells were not derived from normal tissue but grew out of a mass of undifferentiated cells known as blastema that was interspersed between normal tissue. His view that the cell is of importance in the development of cancer made his book very stimulating reading for later researchers in this field. Although his pupil Rudolf Virchow (1821-1902) got most of the credit for suggesting that the cell is the key element in the origin of cancer, Müller must be regarded as the father of microscopic and cellular pathology.

The blastema theory of the origin of cancer was further elaborated by Julius Vogel in 1845 when he posited that each tissue had its own blastema. Vogel assumed that a tumor developed from amorphous blastema, which was converted into cells under the influence of the histological and chemical environment. Friedrich Führer also supported the blastema theory. He distinguished three types of blastema, the albuminous (turbid, proteinoid), the chondromatous (cartilaginous) and the gelatinous, each type being responsible for a particular kind of cancer (Kardinal and Yarbro, 1979).

Adolph Hannover from Copenhagen made a further contribution to the study of the cancer cell with the publication in 1843 of his book *Das Epithelioma*. His observation that cancer cells often resembled epithelial cells led him to coin the term epithelioma for cancer. It may be noted that the word epithelium was introduced as early as 1700 or thereabouts by the Dutch anatomist Frederick Ruys (1658-1731) while he was a professor in Amsterdam, to denote the skin covering the nipple. The term is derived from the Greek epi, meaning on or above, and *thele* meaning nipple. The meaning of this word has gradually expanded to include all tissue covering the skin and internal cavities of the bodies; the endothelium and mesothelium are specialized forms of epithelium. The term epithelioma has been gradually replaced by carcinoma.

It was Virchow who stated 'omnis cellula e cellula' – each cell is formed from another cell – but he did not assume that the initial cell in this line was derived from blastema.

He also laid down another important principle, that 'each tumor originates from the cells of the organ in which it develops'. This may be called 'the second law of oncology'. Virchow was such a prolific worker that several principles that he established in different fields of medicine are known as 'Virchow's law'. They include both the statements mentioned above. According to Virchow, cancers only originated in elements of connective tissue.

Robert Remak (1815-1865) attacked this very popular connective-tissue theory. He reduced the four germ layers proposed by Karl Ernst von Baer (1792-1876) to three: the ectoderm (outermost layer), endoderm (innermost layer) and mesoderm (middle layer), and demonstrated the unchangeable nature of these layers. Remak maintained that epithelial cells can only originate in epithelium. However, Virchow never rejected the mistaken view that cancer grew out of connective-tissue cells, and his authority delayed general acceptance of Remak's ideas by many years.

Remak did on the other hand receive support from Karl Thiersch (1822-1895). Thiersch, a surgeon in Erlangen and Leipzig, studied skin cancers with the aid of serial microscopic sections. He showed in his book *Der epithelial Krebs, namentlich der Haut* (Epithelial Cancer; that is, Cancer of the Skin) that epitheliomas, later known as carcinomas, were of epithelial origin and that metastases were built up out of these cells. Heinrich Wilhelm von Waldeyer-Hastz (1836-1921) came to the same conclusion for gastroenterologic tumors and published his findings in 1874. He also explained how metastases could be formed as the result of the growth of the tumor through the wall of the blood vessels and lymph ducts, and described the formation of cancer-cell embolisms.

Although the lymph theory had largely displaced the black bile theory by the beginning of the eighteenth century, the humoral theory still played a role in determining thinking about cancer. While Virchow did put forward many new ideas, he did not entirely reject the humoral doctrines of his predecessors about the spread of cancer. He regarded metastasis as the result of the circulation of fluids derived from tumors to other tissues, where they formed masses resembling the tissue they were derived from. Virchow formulated a general theory of the origin of cancer. In the first place, the host had to have a constitutional or hereditary predisposition to the disease. Secondly, there must be a chronic source of irritation inducing granulation tissue, which just like embryonic tissue is undifferentiated and can develop into a cancer. The specific nature of the tumor was considered to depend on the nature of the irritation and the susceptibility of the host to the effect in question.

Both Virchow and Müller concluded, just like Bichat but now on the basis of microscopy data, that a cancer was made up of two components, the malignant parenchyma and the benign stroma that consisted of fibrous connective tissue and blood vessels. They classified cancers basically just as we still do today, for example into carcinomas consisting of epithelial cells and sarcomas consisting of mesenchymal tissue (Cabanne et al., 1983). They further distinguished between malignant and benign tumors, on the basis of the way the growths behaved in the patient. In fact, their 'morphologic behavioral classification' closely resembles those of Hippocrates and Galen. The only difference is that they made the diagnosis on the basis of microscopic findings rather than morphologic features visible to the naked eye.

Julius Friedrich Cohnheim (1839-1884), a pupil of Virchow, published another idea on the origin of cancer in 1877. He believed that cancers could be produced by residual cells that had taken the wrong path during embryonic development, or from cells that had retained embryonic features even though they had not necessarily followed a wrong developmental pathway. These cells were, he postulated, distributed between the internal organs and the mucocutaneous zones. According to Cohnheim, the sudden development of cancers from these cells was due to a change in the blood supply, and to the 'bioplastic energy' of the cells (Kardinal and Yarbro, 1979).

A subsequent, more detailed classification of tumors also took this embryologic hypothesis into account. However, it only refers to a small group of tumors that occur mainly in children, and which seem to originate in residual embryonic cells. Examples include retinoblastoma (originating in the retina), neuroblastoma (originating in the sympathetic ganglia), hepatoblastoma (originating in the liver) and nephroblastoma (or Wilms' tumor) originating in the kidney. In adults, on the other hand, practically all tumors originate not in embryonic but in somatic cells (Diamandopoulos, 1996).

In 1886, the French internist Louis Bard (1857-1930) summarized the conclusions of most of his predecessors concerning the genesis of cancer and limited the scope of Virchow's law by rewriting it 'omnis cellula e cellula eiusdem naturae'. This means that as a consequence of cellular specificity, a tissue can only produce a tumor with the same histologic structure as itself. This may be called 'the third law of oncology' or 'Bard's law' (Cabanne et al., 1983).

The availability of vast amounts of new data during the last quarter of the nineteenth and the first quarter of the twentieth century encouraged many researchers to undertake further investigation of the pathologic anatomy and clinical aspects of cancer. Despite all this effort, however, the cause of this disease remained shrouded in mystery.

The description by the German-Swiss pathologist Edwin Klebs (1834-1913) in 1869 of the technique for embedding tissue samples in paraffin wax before cutting sections for microscopic examination represented a major step forward for pathological anatomy. This greatly simplified the procedure for microscopic tissue investigation and led to a considerable reduction in the use of the old freeze-cut technique. However, as clearly demonstrated by William Rutherford FRS (1839-1899), professor of Physiology first at King's College London (from 1869) and later at Edinburgh University from 1874 till his death, the freeze-cut method still retains its practical utility especially in the run-up to surgery, since it facilitates quick diagnosis (Fisher and Hermann, 1979). Freeze-cut sections are therefore still in use for this purpose.

Cytology

Walshe described cytologic techniques for the detection of cancer as long ago as 1844 (Walshe, 1844). These techniques are based on the fact that tumors secrete cells that can be collected by aspiration, smeared out on a glass slide, stained and viewed under the microscope. This makes it possible to determine whether cells are cancerous or not on the basis of their morphology. The initial popularity of these smear tests waned after the introduction of the paraffin wax embedding method, but the tests became important again through the work of the Greek physician George Papanicolaou (1883-1962). After completing his medical studies in Athens, Papanicolaou moved to Germany where he studied philosophy and gained a doctorate in zoology. He then worked for a time as physiologist at a French oceanographic research institute on the Mediterranean, but returned to his native country and worked as a physician during the Balkan War (1912-1913). American volunteers he met there spoke so positively about the career prospects in the United States that he was encouraged to leave for the USA in 1913. After working for a while as a carpet salesman, he found a position at the New York Hospital (Giard, 2007). Papanicolaou refined the smear test and introduced it as a screening method for cervical carcinoma. It is still widely used, and is known variously as the 'Pap test' or the 'cervical smear'. A positive result is an indication that cancer may be present, but a biopsy is almost always required before a definite diagnosis can be made (Diamandopoulos, 1996).

Infection as a cause of cancer

Various theories naming infection as the cause of cancer have appeared in the literature. Amatus Lusitanus (1511-1568) in Lisbon and Daniel Sennert (1572-1637), professor of Medicine at the University of Wittenberg, were the first to claim that cancer was infectious (Ewing, 1919). In the Netherlands, Nicolaes Tulp (1593-1674), physician, mayor of Amsterdam and a friend of Rembrandt (who painted the celebrated *Anatomy Lesson of Dr. Nicolaes Tulp* with him as the central figure), described the case history of an older woman with breast cancer, who was believed to have passed the disease on to her maid (De Moulin, 1988). Since that time, the idea that cancer was infectious became generally accepted (Cabanne et al., 1983). In particular in the seventeenth and eighteenth centuries, cancer was believed to be as infectious as tuberculosis. One result of this belief was that the cancer hospital founded in Rheims by Jean Godinot in 1740 was forced to move in 1779 because it was thought that the patients might infect the inhabitants of the city.

The development of microbiology led to the intensive microbiological study of tumors. Practically every new micro-organism that could be detected was also found in tumorous tissue, and some authors claimed that inoculation with these organisms could lead to the development of cancer. It was subsequently found, however, that all the germs observed came from secondary infections.

Justamond in 1870 ascribed cancer to germs from insect that were taken up by the lymph ducts from the air. He gave full descriptions of these insects, including their length, width and color. Arnaudet, writing in the same year, reported a high incidence of cancer in Normandy, and stated that the disease occurred in several members of the same household. He concluded that cancer was transmitted by infected water. Behla reported in 1892 that families where cancer was found consumed large amounts of home-grown vegetables, and suggested that the cancer was transmitted by infected soil. The London surgeon Alfred Haviland published a number of reports between 1875 and 1892 in which he mapped the distribution of various diseases based on analysis of mortality data for England and Wales. He concluded that the incidence of cancer was particularly high in low-lying regions subject to seasonal flooding, so that the subsoil was always wet. He assumed these conditions to be the cause of the disease. E.N. Nason wrote a letter to the British Medical Journal of 1 January 1898 under the heading 'Cancer Houses', in which he claimed that cancer developed in houses with poor sanitation, while E. Lloyd Jones from Cambridge stated in a longer letter to the same Journal on 1 April 1899 that cancer patients often lived near trees, in particular large ones. This seems to have been a popular topic in the correspondence pages of the British Medical Journal round about this time.

Ernst von Scheurlen (1863-1897) isolated a bacillus from breast cancer in 1887 and claimed that he could induce cancer in dogs with its aid. Thoma and Nils Sjöbring in 1890 described an intranuclear *Coccidia* in cancer tissue, and regarded this as the real cause of cancer. Alexis Korotneff published a description of the protozoa *Rhopalochephalus carcinomatosus* in 1893, while Eisen described *Cancriamoebe macroglossa*. Both these micro-organisms were thought to give rise to cancer. Reginald Harrison observed in 1889 that Egyptians who were infected with bilharzia (more commonly known as schistosomiasis, a disease that is very common in Egypt) were at increased risk of developing bladder cancer. This last-mentioned observation is the only one of those mentioned in this section to have been subsequently confirmed.

The main theory about infection as the cause of cancer was that involving parasites as the carrier of the infection. The parasitic theory reached its heyday with the findings of Johannes Andreas Fibiger (1867-1928), professor of Pathology at the University of Copenhagen. Fibiger found a worm, which he named *Spiroptera neoplastica*, in three wild rats that had developed a spontaneous gastric carcinoma (stomach cancer). After intensive research in the period 1913-1920, he was able to demonstrate that the cockroach was an intermediate host in the life cycle of this worm. After feeding infected cockroaches to laboratory rats, he found that 12 out of the 62 rats that survived for more than sixty days developed a gastric carcinoma. The *Spiroptera* and their eggs were present in the stomach tumor, but not in the metastases. Fibiger was awarded the Nobel Prize for Medicine and Physiology in 1926 for this work, the first publication on which dated from 1913; it may be mentioned, however, that subsequent researchers never managed to replicate Fibiger's results (Kardinal and Yarbro, 1979).

Experimental studies

Many different experimental studies were performed in an attempt to discover the cause of cancer. An important theme in such studies was the transplantation of cancers. In 1851, Joseph Leidy from Philadelphia inserted four fragments of human breast cancer tissue removed from a patient four hours before under the skin of a large frog. He found that three of the grafts took, and that capillaries from the frog penetrated the tumor tissue. This observation received hardly any attention, however. Arthur Nathan Hanau (1858-1900) encountered the same disappointing lack of response in Germany in 1898 after he had succeeded in inducing peritoneal cancer in two rats by implanting tissue fragments taken from a carcinoma in another rat in their vagina. Cabanne et al. (1983) claim that he was so depressed by the lack of interest from other researchers that he committed suicide two years after this experiment. This is not true, however. Hanau underwent two operations for carcinoma of the rectum, and post-mortem examination showed that he had a large stomach tumor (Shimkin, 1979). Moreau was also regarded as a fantasist in France when he reported in 1891 that he had transplanted a mammary carcinoma from one mouse to another and had successfully continued this process over several generations. While these attempts did not get the recognition they deserved at the time, they may be regarded as the start of real experimental oncology.

Many researchers later took up this line of investigation, and countless articles appeared on the transplantation of cancers. It soon became clear that such transplantation is possible between isogenic animals (i.e. animals having the same genes), in particular in mice and rats, and that this method could be used to maintain strains of transplanted cancers with specific characteristics for an indefinite period. Such isogenic mice originated in the 'dancing mice', originally kept at the court of the Chinese emperors for the amusement of the courtiers and later displayed as a curiosity at fairs in Europe, which 'danced' as the result of a neurologic defect maintained for centuries by careful breeding. It was further discovered that heterografting – for example the transplantation of human cancer to one or more different species of animals – was doomed to failure unless special tricks were used to suppress or reduce the immune reaction of the host. The conditions for successful transplantation and the relationship between the graft and the immune response gradually became known. Despite all these advances in our knowledge, the renowned French oncologist Charles Oberling (1895-1960) correctly pointed out that 'the animal to which the tumor is transplanted only provides the nutrient medium for the cells that are foreign to its body and hence will react differently.' He therefore concluded that these transplantation experiments are only of limited utility to man (Cabanne et al., 1983).

In order to achieve progress in the search for the cause of cancer, researchers even tried human-to-human transplantation. For example, Baron Jean-Louis Alibert (1766-1837) injected an extract of human breast cancer into his own arm and the arms of a number of test subjects in 1808. There was no evidence that this procedure gave rise to any cancer. On the other hand, the experiments of Eugène Hahn in Berlin in 1887 and of Victor Cornil (1837-1908) in Paris in 1891 were more successful. They managed to implant fragments of breast-cancer tissue subcutaneously in the arm of patients from whom the tumor was taken. Other researchers performed similar experiments, making it clear that autografting often worked.

Trials of homografting, that is transplanting cancer from one human being to another, were also carried out. After initial experiments on animals and others in which physicians tried out the technique on themselves, the investigations were extended to patients in 1954. Fifteen patients with advanced cancer were found willing to participate in this experiment. Malignant growths were found to develop in thirteen of these patients after transplantation of fragments of the tumor, demonstrating that the body of these patients did not reject the grafts. The next stage of the experiment in 1956 involved fourteen healthy volunteers from Ohio State Prison. Here, none of the grafts was found to have led to malignant tumors. The experiment was repeated five months later, and once again none of the test subjects developed cancer. Southam, the leader of this study, concluded that healthy people possess a defense mechanism against cancer (Cabanne et al., 1983). As a whole, these experiments on the transplantation of cancer in humans unfortunately provided only limited information and brought us no closer to the solution of the problem. It was time to move on to explore other avenues.

The next major step was the attempt to cause cancer in healthy animals by various means. Here again, many researchers have carried out studies of this kind. The advantage compared with the transplantation experiments is that immune reactions in the host organism are largely eliminated. Examination of the cells of the experimental animals in which cancer is induced makes it possible to draw conclusions about how the cancer is induced, how it grows and various pathogenic aspects. This approach has been used to test the carcinogenic effect of many factors, for example chemical substances like tar, physical entities such as ionizing and ultraviolet radiation and biologic agents such as parasites and viruses.

Techniques for growing tissue and cell cultures were developed at the beginning of the twentieth century. Such techniques had their golden age between 1910 and 1926, in the hands of such researchers as M.T. Burrows in America and Alexis Carrel (1873-1944), who worked initially in France and later also in America. Thanks to the use of suitable nutrient media and the availability of antibiotics, it soon became possible to grow cells without limit in an artificial environment, and to maintain the cell lines for practically as long as desired. This gave researchers a powerful tool for the study of the biology of cancer cells (Hill, 1979; Cabanne et al., 1983).

Current views on the cause of cancer

It is assumed at present that many different factors can lead to the development of cancer. Although we are coming increasingly close to the solution of the problem of cancer, we cannot yet state precisely what gives rise to this disease. We are however able to localize the problem and define its limits more exactly. Cancer is essentially a disease of the genes. It was initially held that cancer was a disease of the whole body. Then the focus shifted successively to the tissues and to the cell, while since the final quarter of the previous century we know that the ultimate cause of cancer lies in the DNA of the cell nucleus – to be precise, in the genes that undergo mutation (are damaged).

This damage can be caused by chemicals, radiation or viral infection. Hormones can also play a role. Certain people can also have an inherited predisposition to certain cancers, while random errors in the DNA replication process can also contribute to carcinogenesis. We will be discussing the details of our progress towards the unraveling of the tangled skein of cancer in the remaining sections of this chapter and in Chapter 7, on hormonal treatment.

CHEMICAL CARCINOGENESIS

Our knowledge of chemical carcinogenesis goes back more than two centuries. The London physician John Hill (1716-1775) concluded in 1761 that excessive use of snuff leads to cancer of the nasal cavity, while thirty-four years later Samuel Thomas von Sömmering described the association between carcinoma of the lips and pipe smoking (Miller and Miller, 1979). The London surgeon Sir Percival Pott (1713-1788), is generally credited with being the first to suggest a connection between exogenous risk factors and the development of cancer – though as we have seen, the honor should really go to John Hill. In any case, Pott was the first to describe an occupational cancer, in young chimney-sweeps in England and Wales. As graphically described for example in 'The Water Babies' by Charles Kingsley (1819-1875), it was common at this time and well into the nineteenth century to employ young boys to climb up chimneys to brush out the soot; young boys were well suited for this task, as they were small and agile enough to navigate the often complicated system of interconnected flues involved (Figure 2.7). Many of these chimney-sweeps died of cancer of the scrotum fifteen to twenty years later. Pott established a relationship between the prolonged contact of the skin with soot-impregnated clothing and the subsequent development of skin cancer. He described this in 1775 in his memorandum *Surgical observations relative to the cataract, the polypus of the nose, the cancer*

FIGURE 2.7 English chimney-sweeps, 18th century (Source: Shimkin, 1979, courtesy of the National Institute of Health, Bethesda, MD, USA). The picture shows a master sweep on the right, with his young assistant who would be given the task of actually climbing the chimneys to sweep them.

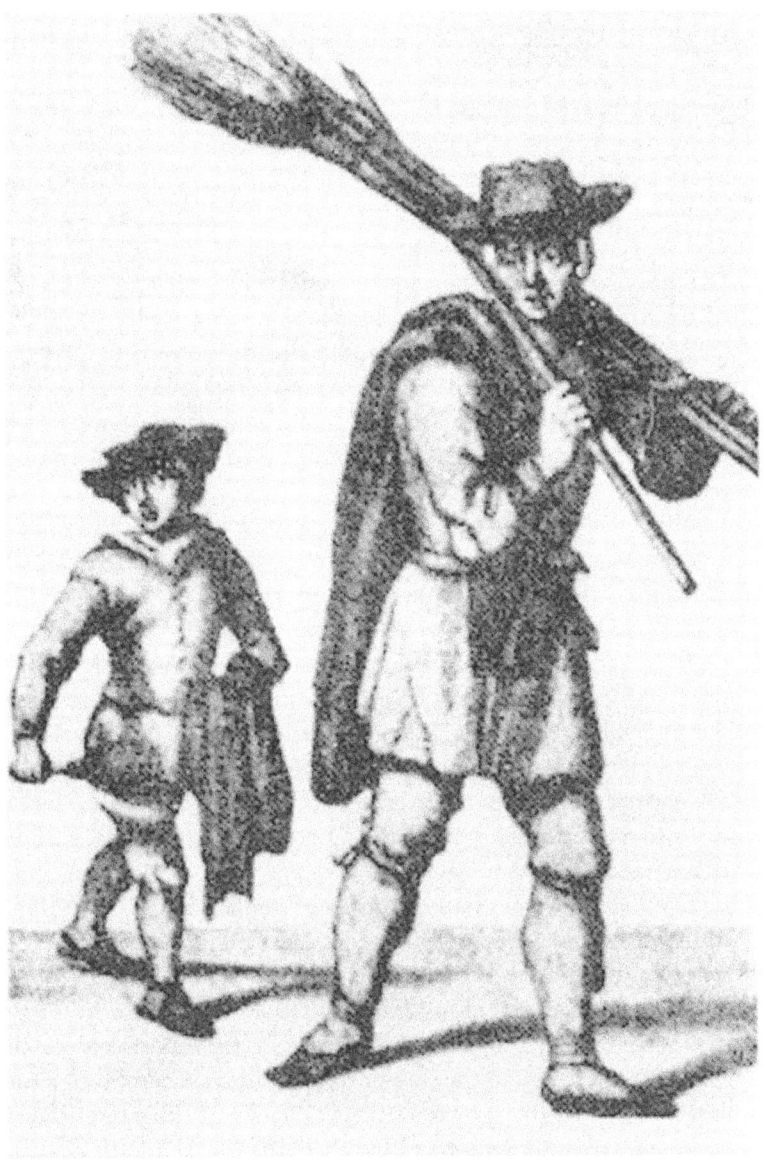

of the scrotum – a publication that was not properly understood, and not given the recognition it deserved, at the time. It was later realized that this cancer found so widely in chimney-sweeps was the first example of a classical occupational disease (Cabanne et al., 1983). When this message was understood, the various European guilds of chimney-sweeps ordered their members to take daily baths. After this regulation came into force, this type of cancer soon became a thing of the past.

The description of cancers caused by soot was followed by accounts of skin cancers due to tar, coal, lignite and lubricating oil. From a histologic point of view, these cancers were all pavement-cell carcinomas, often multiple. They occurred mainly on the hands, arms and scrotum, often being preceded by dermatitis (Petrakis, 1979).

H. Bayon took an experimental approach to the observation that tar was carcinogenic. He induced cancer in rabbits in 1912 by injecting coal-tar into their ears. Two Japanese researchers, Katsusaburo Yamagiwa and Koichi Ichikawa, repeated his experiment in 1915 by repeatedly brushing coal-tar on to the ears of rabbits. They found that cancer developed at the application site after a long latency period. This important observation proved conclusively that coal-tar contained substances that could cause skin cancer (Diamandopoulos, 1996).

Ernest Kennaway (1881-1958), William Mayneord (1902-1988), I. Hieger, J.W. Cook and C. Hewett subjected coal-tar to extensive analysis in the period from the early 1920s to the 1930s, and discovered that it contains the polycyclic hydrocarbons benz' anthracene and benz' pyrene that have a highly carcinogenic effect (Bett, 1954).

The number of substances that were known to be possible causes of occupational cancer grew gradually. Ludwig Rehn (1849-1930) had pointed out the possible relationship between aromatic amines and cancer of the bladder as long ago as 1895, when he found three cases of bladder cancer among workers in a German aniline dye factory. In 1932, ten cases of nasal cancer were described among workers in a nickel refinery. This was the first instance in which a metal derivative was found to have a carcinogenic effect (Miller and Miller, 1979).

It became evident during the 1930s that many more people were dying of lung cancer than in the early years of the twentieth century and during the nineteenth century. This suggested a link with smoking. Moreover, the American surgeons Alton Ochsner (1896-1981) and Michael DeBakey (1908-2008) noticed that there had been a temporary increase in the number of smokers at the beginning of the First World War. This led them to think that there might be a latency period of about twenty years between exposure to tobacco and the development of cancer.

Angel H. Roffo (1882-1947) of Argentina stated in 1937 that most lung cancer patients had smoked . Before that, he had demonstrated experimentally that application of tobacco extracts to the skin or rats and the ears of rabbits gave rise to papillomas (benign wart-like growths). In 1939, Franz H. Müller published the results of a case-control study demonstrating that lung cancer occurred much more often in heavy smokers than in non-smokers (Petrakis, 1979). In the Netherlands, W.F. Wassink (1888-1963), a surgeon at the Antoni van Leeuwenhoek Hospital in Amsterdam, pointed out as early as 1948 that smoking might cause cancer (Wassink, 1948).

A very important case-control study of lung cancer was performed by Ernest L. Wynder (1922-1999) and Evarts A. Graham (1883-1957). Graham was an eminent surgeon who strongly disputed the hypothesis that smoking caused lung cancer until he saw the results of his own investigation. The study was performed by Wynder at the Sloan-Kettering Cancer Center in Manhattan while he was still a student at Washington University School of Medicine in St. Louis, Missouri, in co-operation with his professor and mentor Graham. A total of 605 patients with histologically confirmed lung cancer from St. Louis and the rest of the United States were involved in the study. Detailed data on previous history of smoking and use of alcohol, profession and previous lung diseases were collected for all patients. Analysis of the data showed a very strong association between lung cancer and prolonged heavy smoking, while hardly any lung cancer was found among non-smokers. The results were published in 1950 in the Journal of the American Medical Association (JAMA).

The same issue of the JAMA also contained an article by Morton L. Levin (1904-1995), H. Goldstein and P.R. Gerhardt describing a study with practically identically results, but with the difference that patients were asked about their smoking habits before the diagnosis of lung cancer was made. This was done to exclude interview bias. These two publications inspired many more studies in this field throughout the world. The conclusion was always the same: smoking can cause lung cancer.

One of the most important of these studies was that carried out for the Medical Research Council in England by the epidemiologist Sir Richard Doll (1912-2005) together with the statistician Austin B. Hill (1897-1991). Their two publications in 1950 and 1952 described the results of a case-control study of 1465 lung cancer patients which may be regarded as an extension of the investigation by Wynder and Graham, and which confirmed the conclusions of the latter. Serial studies showed that there was a direct link between the number of cigarettes the patients smoked and the risk of lung cancer (Petrakis, 1979).

The epidemiologic investigations of the carcinogenic effect of asbestos were also important. The mining of asbestos started in 1878, and its industrial use underwent enormous expansion after 1900. The health risks associated with this became evident when it was reported that people working with asbestos were developing pulmonary fibrosis or asbestosis, a condition characterized by sometimes severe shortness of breath due to massive scarring of lung tissue. It is now known that pulmonary fibrosis is not cancer, but it does increase the risk of lung cancer. Kenneth Lynch and William Atmar Smith (1886-1971) in the United States published a paper in 1935 describing the occurrence of lung cancer in a worker in the asbestos industry, while Edward Merewether in 1947 reported that he diagnosed lung cancer in 13.2% of the autopsies he performed on persons who had had a history of long-term work in the asbestos industry. This compares with the finding that autopsies on people who had worked in the silicone industry led to this diagnosis in only 1.3% of the cases.

In 1955, Sir Richard Doll carried out an important retrospective study of 113 men who had been exposed to asbestos dust for more than twenty years. He found that 39 of these subjects died between 1922 and 1953, as compared with an expected mortality of 15.4. This increase could be ascribed in its entirety to lung cancer. In 1953 and 1954, cases of pleural and peritoneal mesothelioma were reported in various countries. On the basis of these findings, Irving J. Selikoff (1915-1992) carried out a prospective study of 632 members of the Asbestos Workers' Union in New York City, which revealed an increase in mortality due to exposure to asbestos. A total of 198 of the workers concerned died in the period from 1943 to 1962, as compared with an expected mortality of 51. Eighty-nine members of the study population died of lung cancer and 35 of mesothelioma, even though the incidence of mesothelioma in the general population is low. An even more striking conclusion was that smoking cigarettes led to a marked increase of the risk of lung cancer in asbestos workers due to a kind of synergy, while exposure to asbestos alone led only to a slight increase in the risk (Selikoff et al., 1968).

Metabolic products of living cells were also found to have carcinogenic properties. This was first reported in 1950 by Cook, Duffy and Schoental. One of the best known substances of this kind is aflatoxin B1, which is produced by *Aspergillus flavus*, a fungus that grows for example on peanut plants. This toxin has been found to be able to cause liver cancer.

Subsequent statistical, clinical and experimental studies showed that a large number of different chemical compounds, including cytostatic agents, had mutagenic properties and were capable of giving rise to cancer in man and in laboratory animals. It could be demonstrated that this chemical carcinogenesis is brought about by the mutagenic effects of the chemicals on the genome DNA of somatic cells (Diamandopoulos, 1996).

In connection with the possible risk of cancer, the United States authorities currently require all new substances to be tested for carcinogenic properties before being used in the foodstuffs industry. The test used in the first instance for this purpose is the Ames test, which is based on the finding that practically all carcinogenic substances are mutagenic. Bruce Ames and co-workers at the University of California, Berkeley, introduced this test in 1973. It makes use of *Salmonella typhimurium*, a bacterial strain that is very sensitive to mutation because its DNA repair capacity is low and the cell wall is readily permeable (Miller and Miller, 1979). Bacteria that have undergone mutation cannot produce histidine. As a result, they can only grow if the culture medium contains histidine. The researcher places the mutated bacteria on a histidine-free culture medium and adds the substance to be tested. If this substance is mutagenic, it can change the DNA of the *Salmonella* back to the form that allows the bacteria to make histidine. These bacteria will then have no problem growing on the histidine-free culture medium, while the bacteria that do not contain back-mutated DNA will be unable to survive. Hence, if the substance being tested is mutagenic, bacteria will grow on the culture medium; while if it is not, the culture medium will be bare. If the Ames test is positive (i.e. if the substance is mutagenic), the substance is not passed for consumption. If the test is negative, the substance can be fed to experimental animals to see whether it is really safe.

A key study for our understanding of the way cancers are caused, which certainly deserves a place in this section on chemical carcinogenesis, is that performed by Isaac Berenblum (1903-1985). He showed in experiments on mice in 1940 that two different types of chemical compounds are needed to induce skin tumors, or in other words that the process of chemical carcinogenesis involves two different steps. He treated the skin of the mice with a carcinogenic substance (3-methylcholanthrene), in a dose that was too low to produce a tumor. He then treated the skin with an extract from the leaves of the croton plant, which has an irritant effect but is not carcinogenic in itself. This gave rise to wart-like growths known as papillomas on the skin of the mice. Further application of croton resin made the growths malignant. Berenblum concluded that the carcinogen caused changes in the skin, which needed a little push before they could grow into cancer cells. He called the first of the two substances involved (the carcinogen) the initiator and the second the promotor (Berenblum, 1940). Further research by Berenblum elucidated the molecular mechanisms involved, and showed the need to assume a third step (latency) to explain the delay involved in the production of a cancer. He found that the cell population had to undergo a number of mutations in key growth-controlling genes before growths can become malignant. The process involved is therefore called multi-step carcinogenesis.

Radiation-induced carcinogenesis

Many articles published throughout the entire twentieth century contained clinical and experimental data demonstrating that radiation energy can cause cancer in both man and animals. For example, it is established that ultraviolet (UV) solar radiation can lead to a form of skin cancer, the malignancy of which depends on the intensity of the radiation and the sensitivity of the skin. Paler skin has been found to be more sensitive than dark skin, because the latter contains larger amounts of the pigment melanin in its melanocytes and thus absorbs the actinic energy (which gives rise to the photochemical effect of solar radiation) better. Some patients, for example those with *xeroderma pigmentosum* (a condition involving excessive dryness of the skin), are more likely to develop skin cancer under the influence of sunlight because their epidermal cells are unable to repair the damage to DNA caused by the sunlight.

Irradiation with particles such as alpha and beta particles, protons and neutrons, and with electromagnetic radiation such as gamma rays and X-rays has been proved to have a carcinogenic effect. Ernst Frieben, a German physician, was the first to describe the carcinogenic effect of X-radiation on humans, as early as 1902. An increased incidence of leukemia and other forms of cancer was subsequently reported after radiotherapy for various conditions such as ankylosing spondylitis (a form of arthritis causing pain and stiffness of the back).

Occupational exposure to radiation was also found to cause cancer. For example, women who were employed to paint watch dials with luminescent radium paint in the early twentieth century developed osteosarcoma many years later. This led to a celebrated legal case in the USA, which eventually had a major impact on health and safety legislation there. It was demonstrated that safety regulations at the plant in question were extremely lax. It has been reported that the young women in question, known as the 'Radium Girls', used to paint their nails, teeth and faces with the deadly paint produced at the factory, sometimes to surprise their boyfriends when the lights went out. They mixed glue, water and radium powder, and then used camel-hair brushes to apply the glowing paint onto dial numbers. The going rate, for painting 250 dials a day, was about one and a half dollar cents per dial. The brushes would lose shape after a few strokes, so supervisors encouraged their workers to point the brushes with their lips, or use their tongues to keep them sharp. Five of the Radium Girls won substantial compensation. Similarly, mineworkers handling ores containing radioactive substances who breathed in small amounts of dust from these ores, were found to develop lung cancer after a latency period of many years. People who survived the atom bombs dropped on Japan at the end of World War II were exposed to gamma radiation and neutrons in Hiroshima and to gamma radiation in Nagasaki. An appreciable number of the survivors developed acute myeloid leukemia in the first few years after the bombardment and various other forms of cancer in the succeeding years. Radiation-induced carcinogenesis, like chemical carcinogenesis, is due to the mutagenic effects on the genome DNA of somatic cells (Diamandopoulos, 1996).

Epidemiology and cancer

Epidemiology has played an important role in establishing the links between carcinogens and cancer. Some epidemiologic studies have already been mentioned in the previous sections, but some key investigations deserve mention here.

Firstly, T.H.C. Stevenson, working at the General Register Office in London, reported in 1922 some clear associations between the incidence of cancer and social class under the conditions prevailing in England.

Herbert L. Lombard and C.R. Doering of the Massachusetts Department of Public Health and the Harvard School of Public Health carried out a series of Massachusetts cancer studies. In 1929, they classified cancers by location and gave a breakdown by country of birth for patients who were born outside the USA. They reported a number of interesting findings. Like Stevenson, they found a link between social class and cancer, but they also reported a high incidence of stomach cancer in those born abroad compared with patients born in the USA. They also found a lower incidence of bowel and breast cancer in women of Italian and Russian origin (Lombard and Doering, 1929).

William M. Haenszel (1911-1998), an epidemiologist at the National Cancer Institute in the USA, published in 1961 an important study of cancer mortality in the United States of people who had been born abroad. He found significant differences between the incidence of cancer among these people and that for the corresponding groups who had remained in the country of origin. These results prompted many studies of the influence of environmental factors on the incidence of cancer.

For example, it was long thought that diet could play a role in influencing the occurrence of cancer. Epidemiologic studies confirmed this idea. As long ago as 1908, W.R. Williams stated in his book *The natural history of cancer* that cancer occurred less often in underdeveloped countries where most people had a vegetarian diet than in countries where a great deal of meat was consumed. To test this idea, studies were carried out in 1959 and in the early 1970s aimed at investigation of the incidence of cancer among Seventh-Day Adventists, East Africans and the Japanese (all of whom have a mainly vegetarian diet) and Western Europeans (who are largely meat-eaters). It was concluded that the vegetarians had a lower incidence of cancer while the meat-eating peoples – particularly those who consume a lot of beef – are at higher risk of bowel cancer and possibly also cancer affecting other parts of the body (Petrakis, 1979).

VIRAL CARCINOGENESIS

Two Danish researchers, Ellerman and Bang, were the first to demonstrate that leukemia in the chicken was caused by a filterable agent – a virus. That was in 1908. Since it was uncertain at that time whether leukemia could actually be regarded as a form of cancer, Francis Peyton Rous (1879-1970) from the Rockefeller Institute in New York subjected the matter to further investigation and demonstrated in 1910 that sarcoma, a solid cancer, is definitely the result of a virus infection in the chicken. He showed that injection of a cell-free extract of a sarcoma in a Plymouth Rock hen into a healthy bird would give rise to a tumor in the latter. However, his superiors rejected the idea that viruses could cause cancer (Wold and Green, 1979). He also got letters from worried people who were afraid that they could catch cancer from their partner who suffered from the disease. The idea was also vehemently criticized by the medical profession. Subsequent investigations carried out in England showed that he was right, however, and he was awarded the Nobel Prize for his work in 1966 – after having been nominated for the prize frequently during the previous twenty years. Despite his advanced age, he flew to Stockholm to accept the prize (Diamandopoulos, 1996). The virus is still known as the Rous sarcoma virus.

More viruses that could cause cancer were gradually discovered. In 1931, Richard Shope, a colleague of Rous at the Rockefeller Institute, showed that benign wart-like tumors (papillomas) in the rabbit could be transmitted by cell-free extracts. Rous and Beard demonstrated that these papillomas often turned into a malignant growth under the influence of the papilloma virus. John J. Bittner of the University of Minnesota Medical School described in 1936 how a virus present in mouse milk could give rise to mammary carcinoma in mice, while Ludwik Gross (1905-1999) of the Veterans Administration Hospital in the Bronx (New York) showed in 1951 that leukemia in mice is caused by a virus. He also described the mouse parotid tumor virus, which serves as a model for the study of cell growth and malignant transformation. Sarah Stewart and Bernice Eddy at the National Cancer Institute, Bethesda, MD, showed that this was a new type of virus, the polyoma virus – often called the SE polyoma virus in honor of its discoverers. It is currently classified as a papovavirus.

The adenoviruses were discovered in 1953 by Wallace Rowe and co-workers at the National Institutes of Health, Bethesda, MD. Two other groups of researchers, Maurice Hilleman and Jacqueline Werner from the Army Medical Service Graduate School in Washington, DC, and Grant Taylor from the University of Texas working with John J. Trentin and Yoshiro Yabe at Baylor University, Waco, Texas, found about a decade later that adenovirus type 12 had a powerful effect in inducing tumors in newborn hamsters. This discovery caused considerable turmoil in the medical world, as it was the first time that a virus widely present in humans was found to have oncogenic properties. So far, however, adenovirus oncogenesis has never been observed in humans.

Herpesviruses were likewise discovered in the previous century. The EBV (Epstein-Barr virus, also known as human herpesvirus 4) attracted particularly great attention. This was discovered in 1964 by Michael Epstein (1921-) and Yvonne Barr (1932-) in London, in tissue from a lymphoma (a malignant tumor) of the jaw in children that had been sent to them by Denis Burkitt (1911-1993) from Kampala (Uganda). A similar condition had been described in 1904 by Albert Ruskin Cook (1870-1951), a missionary doctor also working in Uganda, but the tumor came to be known as Burkitt's lymphoma after its subsequent description by Burkitt. The virus is very strongly associated with the development of this lymphoma. It has subsequently been reported to be present in many patients with nasopharyngeal carcinomas in the Far East (Wold and Green, 1979). EBV occurs very widely in humans, often without any adverse consequences.

There is also good evidence that cervical cancer in women is of viral origin. A brief description of the way our knowledge of this form of cancer developed is perhaps in place here. In 1931, F.R. Smith carried out a case-control study of the incidence of cervical cancer and found a higher incidence in women from lower social classes. His investigation was criticized because it was claimed that the selection procedure for his controls was faulty. However, a report published in 1947 of the Ten Metropolitan Areas Cancer Survey in the USA confirmed his findings, and moreover stated that cervical cancer was the second most frequent form of cancer in women in the country. In his study of the marital status of cervical cancer patients, carried out in 1948 and 1949, the British medical statistician W.P.D. Logan found the lowest incidence of cervical cancer in unmarried women, and the highest in women who had had children and in widows. Other researchers observed that cervical cancer was rare in Jewish women, which suggested that cultural differences played an important role. Herbert L. Lombard (1889-1979) and Evelyn A. Potter of the Massachusetts Department of Public Health published a number of different case-control studies. They found a significantly higher cervical cancer rate among divorced women, and also observed that 54% of the patients were married before the age of twenty, as compared with only 16% in the controls. All this evidence made it increasingly clear that a sex-related factor was involved here. This was confirmed by studies by Ganon and J. Røjel. Ganon found in 1950, after a study covering a large number of nuns in Canadian convents, that no cases of cervical cancer had been observed in this population over a twenty-year period. Røjel surveyed prostitutes in Copenhagen in 1953, and found a higher incidence of cervical cancer in this group than in the controls. Subsequent investigations by Harald zur Hausen, professor of Virology at the university of Freiburg (Germany) and later scientific director and chairman of the board of management of the German Cancer Research Center in Heidelberg, revealed in 1983 and 1984 that this form of cancer is caused by human papillomavirus type 16 and 18 (Petrakis, 1979). Zur Hausen received the Nobel Prize for his work in 2008.

Both statistical and experimental studies have demonstrated that various other viruses can also induce cancer in humans or act as cocarcinogens to promote the disease. These include the hepatitis-B virus, which can cause hepatocellular carcinoma, and the retrovirus HTLV-1 that has been found to give rise to T-cell leukemia in adults in southern Japan.

In order to create some kind of order in the large number of viruses that have been discovered, both oncogenic and non-oncogenic viruses are currently classified on the basis of their nucleic-acid content. A distinction is drawn between viruses that contain DNA, such as papovaviruses, adenoviruses and herpesviruses, and those that contain RNA. A special subset of the RNA viruses is formed by the retroviruses, independently discovered in 1970 by Howard Temin at the University of Wisconsin-Madison and David Baltimore at MIT. After infection, these retroviruses transcribe their RNA into DNA with the aid of the enzyme reverse transcriptase. Temin and Baltimore shared the Nobel Prize for Medicine in 1975 with Renato Delbucco for their discoveries concerning "the interaction between tumor viruses and the genetic material of the cell".

It was Alex van der Eb, professor at the University of Leiden, and the Canadian postdoctoral student Frank Graham who succeeded in 1974 in transforming normal mammalian cells into tumor cells with the aid of purified adenovirus DNA. Working together with Carel Mulder from the Cold Spring Harbor laboratory, they used restriction enzymes to isolate a small fragment from the virus DNA, which could then be used to transform the target cells. This procedure made it possible to obtain the virus genes responsible for the transformation, now known as the E1 genes, in a pure form (Graham et al., 1974). This was the first demonstration that certain sequences from the genome of some adenoviruses are oncogenic.

The process whereby viruses ultimately give rise to cancers is a complicated one, that was elucidated in 1976 for a particular class of viruses by four researchers, Stehelin, Varmus, Bishop and Vogt) (Wold and Green, 1979).

Starting from the above-mentioned finding by Peyton Rous that some viruses can give rise to tumors in poultry, J. Michael Bishop, a virologist at the University of California, San Francisco, and his postdoctoral student Harold Varmus made an important contribution to our understanding of the mysteries of abnormal cell growth almost three-quarters of a century later. The special feature of their study was that they used acute transforming tumor viruses, which have a small genome, for their experiment so that the number of genes that could be considered as possible sources of the carcinogenic properties was limited. Working together with Dominique Stehelin, a visiting researcher from the National Scientific Research Center (CNRS) in France, and Peter Vogt, then at the University of Southern California, Bishop and Varmus investigated which of the candidate DNA fragments in the virus actually disturbed the process of cell growth, thus giving rise to tumors. They focused their attention on retroviruses, which can add the genes of infected cells to their genome thus causing newly infected cells to undergo acute transformation into cancer cells. This approach allowed them to discover the second cancer gene, designated the src gene. They then found that the gene in the virus giving rise to the cancer is practically identical with a gene that occurs not only in normal chicken cells but also in normal cells of other organisms – including man. This gene plays a role in the regulation of the normal process of cell division, by coding for the production of a protein that has a key function in the transmission of growth signals in a cell. As soon as the necessary growth factors have adhered to the outer surface of the cell, this protein starts up the cell division process. The researchers called these genes that are responsible for cell division proto-oncogenes. They are the 'starter motors' for cell division. In (human) cancer cells, the proto-oncogene contains errors (mutations) that bring about changes in the protein produced, which then elicit cell division even in the absence of growth factors. The researchers called this mutated gene, which causes cancer, the oncogene. Bishop and Varmus won the Nobel Prize for this investigation in 1989. Stehelin felt that he had been unfairly treated, claiming that he had proposed the idea on which the prize-winning investigation was based and had actually carried out the key experiments (Kolata, 1989). The Nobel Committee stuck to their decision, however.

A whole series of proto-oncogenes, designated for example as myc, myb, ras and erb, have been identified after the original discovery. When these genes mutate, they can cause cancer. They occur not only in humans but also in animals, and have been in existence for hundreds of millions of years. They have survived because they have evolutionary value: they perform crucial regulatory functions in the cell. However, as described above they can also stimulate the cells to multiply in an uncontrolled manner. Recent studies have shown, on the other hand, that they may also hold the one of the keys to the tantalizing possibility of actually curing cancer (Bazell, 1998).

The Philadelphia chromosome

The first author to demonstrate unequivocally that there was a link between chromosome defects and cancer was Theodor Boveri (1862-1915), professor of Biology at Würzburg in Germany. During a stay in Naples, he studied the development of sea-urchin eggs and observed that an uneven distribution of the chromosomes during cell division led to malformations. On the basis of this finding, he proposed as early as 1914 the modern paradigm that mutations in somatic cells lead to uncontrolled proliferation of cells - that is, to cancer (Boveri, 1914).

Clinical genetics was born in 1956, when Joe Hin Tjio and Albert Levan published an article in which they demonstrated that human cells have 46 chromosomes. Technical advances over the years have made this discipline increasingly important. Within a few years, researchers managed to identify specific cancer-related chromosomal defects. The first important cytogenetic defect to be discovered was described by Peter Nowell, a pathologist from Philadelphia, and David Hungerford in 1960. This 'Philadelphia chromosome' is an abnormally small chromosome found in the blood and bone-marrow cells of 95% of patients with chronic myelogenous (or 'myeloid') leukemia. This discovery was of great importance, because it was the first time a link was established between chromosomal defects and cancer.

Many researchers contributed to an understanding of the mechanism of this relationship, by developing techniques that made it possible to visualize the various bands on the chromosome. With the aid of such techniques, Janet Rowley from Chicago was able to detect a translocation (exchange of different parts of a chromosome) of chromosome 9 and 22 (Rowley, 1973). In 1982, two Dutch students from Groningen, Nora Heisterkamp and John Groffen, discovered while working with John Stephenson in the Viral Carcinogenesis Laboratory of the National Can-

FIGURE 2.8 *The Philadelphia chromosome. This was the first major cytogenetic defect to be discovered. It was described by Peter Nowell, a pathologist from Philadelphia, and David Hungerford in 1960. Translocations between chromosomes 9 and 22 (in other words, exchange of a fragment of chromosome 9 for a fragment of 22) lead to formation of the smaller Philadelphia chromosome bearing the bcr-abl gene.*

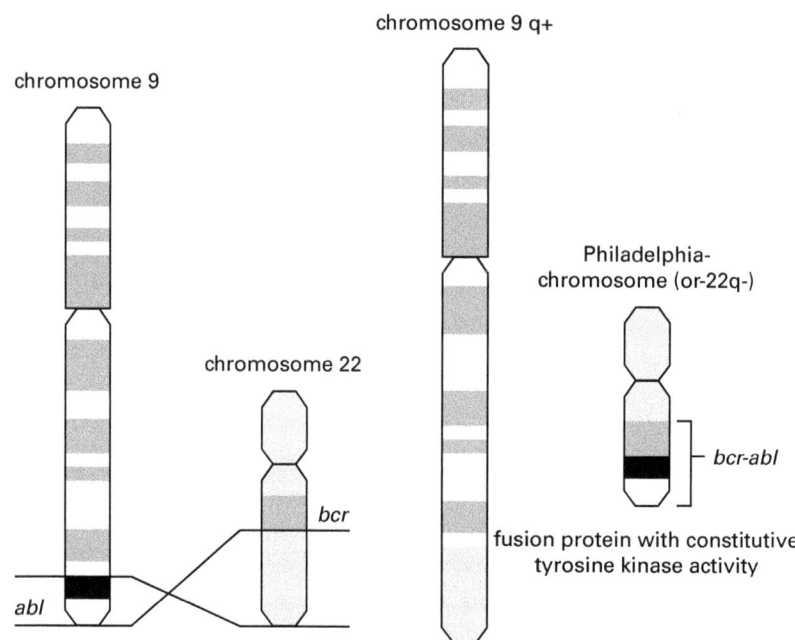

cer Institute in Frederick, Maryland (USA) that the human equivalent van c-abl is located on chromosome 9 (Heisterkamp et al., 1982). Having made this discovery, they contacted Gerard Grosveld and Dick Bootsma from Erasmus University Rotterdam and were able to demonstrate in cooperation with them that the abovementioned translocation involves the move of a small fragment of chromosome 9 bearing the abl proto-oncogene to chromosome 22 (De Klein et al., 1982). Next, Nora Heisterman and co-workers discovered that the c-abl translocation on chromosome 22 is located in the bcr region, and that the exchange of the fragments of chromosome leads to the formation of a new fused gene, bcr-abl (Heisterkamp et al., 1983), which codes for an abnormal protein, the bcr-abl protein. These relationships are illustrated in Figure 2.8.

The definitive proof of the cause of chronic myelogenous leukemia was provided in 1990 by G.Q. Daley, R.A. van Etten and D. Baltimore from MIT, when they reported how they had been able to induce this form of chronic leukemia in mice with the aid of the bcr-abl gene. This finding, in combination with the researches of Owen Witte and co-workers from Los Angeles, established the causal link between the Philadelphia chromosome and chronic myelogenous leukemia (Daley et al., 1990; Lugo et al., 1990).

The circle was finally closed by Brian Druker and co-workers from Oregon Health & Science University, who showed that a specific inhibitor of the activated bcr-abl protein could slow down cell division and bring the patient quickly and simply into remission (we shall be returning to this point in Chapter 8). After this breakthrough, the development of cytogenetic diagnosis for other forms of cancer speeded up considerably (Qumsiyem and Li, 2001).

Heredity and cancer

The cornerstone of the scientific discipline of genetics was laid by the Austrian monk Gregor Mendel (1822-1884). It did not initially look as if Mendel was destined for great things. As the son of a peasant farmer in Silesia, he entered the St. Thomas monastery of the Augustinian Order in Brünn (present-day Brno, in the Czech Republic) as this was the only way he could hope to get a good education. The Augustinians were a teaching order, so they sent Mendel to Vienna for teacher training. However, he failed the examination for his teaching diploma twice. The examiner wrote that he lacked insight and the ability to think clearly and to formulate his ideas coherently. Mendel's worst marks were in biology. Nevertheless, he decided to dedicate his life to practical biological experimentation. With his farming background, this seemed a logical choice. He carried out the experiments in the garden of the Augustinian monastery in Brünn, making use of two different stains of peas (Pisum sativum) with the flower color purple or white. When he crossed the two races, he found that all the plants in the next generation had purple flowers. However, when he crossed these second-generation plants with one another he discovered that some had purple flowers and some had white, in the ratio 3:1. He explained this finding by postulating that the flower color was determined by one factor from each parent plant. He further postulated that the purple factor was dominant, so that all plants in the second generation had purple flowers. Only a quarter of the plants in the third generation would inherit two white factors, thus making their flowers white. He read a paper describing his findings to The Natural History Society of Brünn in 1865 and published the results in the Proceedings of the Society the following year, but no one paid the slightest attention to them until about 1900, when Mendel's work was independently rediscovered by the Dutch botanist Hugo de Vries (1848-1935), the German botanist Carl Correns (1864-1933) and the Austrian agronomist Erich von Tschermach (1871-1962). We now know that the 'factors' mentioned by Mendel are in fact genes, components of the chromosome. The word 'gene' was coined by the Danish botanist Wilhelm Johannsen (1857-1927) to denote the fundamental physical and functional unit of heredity.

The material of which the chromosome is built up, deoxyribonucleic acid or DNA, was discovered in 1869 by the Swiss biochemist Johann Friedrich Miescher (1844-1895). Working in the laboratory of Felix Hoppe-Seyler (1825-1895) at the University of Tübingen, he isolated various phosphate-rich chemical substances from the nuclei of leukocytes, and later also from the nuclei of other types of cells. Since he found this substance only in the cell nucleus, he called it Nuklein (nuclein). The publication of the results was delayed by a couple of years, till 1871, by Hoppe-Seyler who wanted to confirm the findings himself. The importance of the discovery was soon realized, though the precise role of the nuclein was as yet unknown. Miescher's pupil Richard Altmann (1852-1900) changed the name to nucleic acid in 1889, after it had been shown that nuclein had acidic properties.

The Russian-American biochemist Phoebus Levene (1869-1940) played an important – but mainly negative – role in the study of heredity. He postulated, incorrectly, in 1910 that DNA was built up of blocks of the four bases adenine, cytosine, guanine and thymine in a repetitive sequence. This 'tetranucleotide theory' dominated thinking in this field for several decades. He also claimed – again incorrectly – that genes consisted of proteins and that the nucleic acids only had a structural function, serving to hold the chromosome together.

Frederick Griffith (1879-1941) also made an indirect contribution to our knowledge of DNA. He was a British medical officer and geneticist, and was looking for vaccines against pneumonia infections in the 'Spanish flu' pandemic after World War I. He distinguished two strains of pneumococci on the basis of the surface appearance of the colonies they formed on the culture medium he was using: the smooth strain (S strain) and the rough strain (R strain). In the course of his investigations, he injected mice with the different strains. This led to an unexpected observation in 1928. He had injected mice with a mixture of dead S strain and live R strain. A number of mice caught pneumonia and died. Griffith isolated live S bacteria from their lungs. He concluded that a substance from the dead S strain had been transferred to the R strain in the mouse, thus changing the live R bacteria into live S bacteria. The new bacteria retained this phenotype on culture. This means that Griffith's 'transforming principle' was hereditary (Bloemers, 2007). It was not yet clear, however, what caused this effect.

Oswald Avery (1877-1955) and co-workers at the Rockefeller Institute in New York continued this line of investigation. In 1944, they managed to transfer DNA from one strain of bacteria to another, and observed that the recipient bacteria took on the hereditary properties of the donors. This was thus an important indication that DNA played an as yet unspecified role in the storage and transmission of hereditary properties. Erwin Chargaff (1905-2002), a biochemist who had been born in Austria and who worked at nearby Columbia University, established that the four bases – adenine, thymine, guanine and cytosine – in the DNA molecule were present in paired amounts: that is, the molecule contained an equal number of adenine and thymine groups and an equal number of guanine and cytosine. But the precise structure of DNA was still a mystery.

The puzzle was finally solved in 1953 by Maurice Wilkins (1916-2004) and Rosalind Franklin (1920-1958) from King's College London, using X-ray crystallography techniques, and James Dewey Watson (1928-) and Francis Compton Crick (1916-2004) working in Cambridge, who used mainly a molecular modeling approach. It should be noted that while deducing the structure of a complex biological molecule directly from X-ray crystallography data can take years of intricate reasoning, if a plausible structure has been proposed on other grounds it is relatively easy to check whether this would lead to the observed X-ray diffraction images. This is what happened in the present case. Watson's controversial personal account of the events that led up to the discovery, *The Double Helix*, is a classic of popular scientific literature, and has been called one of the 10 best non-fiction books ever written (Watson, 1968).

Lawrence Bragg and his father William laid the foundations for X-ray crystallography or X-ray diffraction, winning the Nobel Prize for this in 1915. They are the only father and son ever to have been awarded the Nobel Prize, while Lawrence at 25 was the youngest person ever to have achieved this distinction. He became director of the Cavendish Laboratory in Cambridge after the Second World War. J. D. Bernal in Cambridge took the first X-ray photos of proteins, in 1934. Wilkins had been working on the structure of DNA for some years in the late 1940s, but without making much progress since his X-ray crystallography skills were not highly developed. In the English scientific community, the structure of DNA was considered to 'belong' to Wilkins and his group, so that it would be improper for researchers from elsewhere to encroach on his terrain. Franklin, who like Wilkins had received her initial training at Cambridge, was added to the team at King's in 1951. She was a highly skilled X-ray crystallographer, and soon started making some very good X-ray photos. It was discovered that there were two forms of DNA, the A and B forms, which differ in the amount of water contained in the crystal. Franklin had initially been working mainly on the A form, which contains relatively little water and did not show clear signs of being helical. It was not until she started working on the B form, with a much higher water content, that she began to get X-ray photos revealing clear signs of the DNA helix. This was later explained as being due to the fact that in the B form, the DNA molecule is as it were floating in water and thus freer to assume its natural helical shape. Unfortunately, relations between Franklin and Wilkins gradually deteriorated to the point that they were barely on speaking terms.

Crick was a problem research student in 1950. He was already 34, and had not yet got his PhD. He had studied physics before the war, and then started to investigate what he himself called the most boring topic imaginable: the viscosity of water at high temperatures. This research was cut off short by the war. During the war, he worked for the navy and was involved in the invention of acoustic and magnetic mines. After the war, he studied biology and in 1950 he joined the group led by Max Perutz (1914-2002) and John Kendrew (1917-1997) at the Cavendish Laboratory in Cambridge. He was a keen, analytical thinker and a skilled mathematician, but was somewhat feared by his colleagues for his booming voice and his critical approach to their investigations.

Watson started to study biology at the University of Chicago at the age of 15. He gained his PhD in 1950 and left for Europe as a postdoctoral student, initially in Copenhagen; but when he heard that interesting work on DNA was going on in England, he applied to move to Cambridge. Perutz related how a young man with a crew cut suddenly came into his room without introducing himself or any form of greeting, and asked, 'Can I come and work here?' He could. He was put in the same room as Crick, in the hope that this would relieve the pressure on the other occupants of the laboratory (Bloemers, 2007). Watson and Crick were both ambitious to make a big discovery, and were fond of taking a discursive approach to a problem, looking at it from various sides and trying to fit widely varying different pieces of information into a meaningful whole. Watson had a wide-ranging knowledge of many aspects of biology, but portrays himself as surprisingly ignorant of many of the scientific techniques he would need to solve the DNA problem. One tool that both Watson and Crick picked on was one that had recently proved its worth in determining the structure of the protein alpha-helix by Linus Pauling, who won the Nobel Prize for Chemistry in 1954 for his work on the chemical bond. This was the building of molecular models, which allowed a wide variety of information to be used to narrow down the possible structures of a complex molecule until hopefully only one correct model was left.

Chemical research had already shown that DNA had a backbone composed of alternating sugar (deoxyribose) and phosphate groups, to which as mentioned above the four bases adenine, thymine, guanine and cytosine were connected in some way or another. It seemed clear for various reasons that the DNA molecule was likely to have a helical structure - though as mentioned above, Franklin doubted this for a long time until she started working on the B form of DNA.

Watson and Crick needed some detailed X-ray data before they could build a proper model. The problem was that, as explained above, they did not feel able just to go to King's and ask Wilkins and Franklin to have a look at their results. The two groups were aware of one another's efforts, especially because Crick and Wilkins had been friends for many years. In fact, in late 1951 Watson and Crick showed Wilkins and Franklin an initial model built on insufficient data, which had three sugar-phosphate chains coiled together, with the phosphate groups in the middle and the bases on the outside. Franklin rightly poured scorn on this abortive model and made it clear that she was convinced that the phosphate groups were on the outside, though she did not show Watson and Crick the X-ray diffraction evidence on which her conclusions were based. The breakthrough came early in 1953, when Watson and Crick were shown X-ray photos of DNA taken by Franklin without her knowledge or permission by their supervisor Perutz, to whom the data had been reported as a member of a committee appointed by the Medical Research Council to look into the research activities of Wilkins' group. Armed with this information, Watson and Crick were soon able to solve the riddle of DNA and come up with the model now known to every schoolchild (Figure 2.9).

The key feature of the model was that the genetic code was stored in a double helix, a sort of twisted ladder with the base pairs adenine-thymine and guanine-cytosine as rungs. Adenine is bigger than thymine and guanine is bigger than cytosine, but together these base pairs are exactly the same length thus permitting a regular structure. The new structure seemed intuitively right: as Watson put it in *The Double Helix*, "a structure this pretty just had to exist". Moreover, it was clear that it had exciting implications for the replication of DNA. Watson and Crick showed their new model to the team at King's, and it took very little time to confirm that its features were in conformity with the X-ray diffraction data. Watson, Crick, Wilkins, Franklin and co-workers quickly prepared brief description of their findings, which were all published in the 25 April 1953 issue of *Nature*. No more than 8 pages in all, these five articles changed the face of biology and medicine. Watson, Crick and Wilkins received the Nobel Prize for this discovery in 1962. Sadly, Rosalind Franklin had died of ovarian cancer before that, in 1958, at the very early age of 37.

Linus Pauling, whose discovery of the alpha-helix had sparked Watson and Crick's interest in helical structures and in molecular modeling, had hoped to add the DNA structure to his trophies, but he was beaten to the post by the Cambridge team. He got no further than publishing a three-chain model very similar to Watson and Crick's earlier abortive model. Due to hasty publication, he did not discover until afterwards that this model contained a number of elementary errors that nullified all chances of validity.

A major step forward in our understanding of how cancer is brought about was made in the 1960s by Henry Harris, born in 1925 in Australia but working at

CHAPTER 2

FIGURE 2.9 Photo of James Watson (left) and Francis Crick in 1953 in the Cavendish Laboratory at Cambridge University, standing in front of the first model of the double helix (Source: Shimkin, 1979, courtesy of the National Institute of Health, Bethesda, MD, USA).

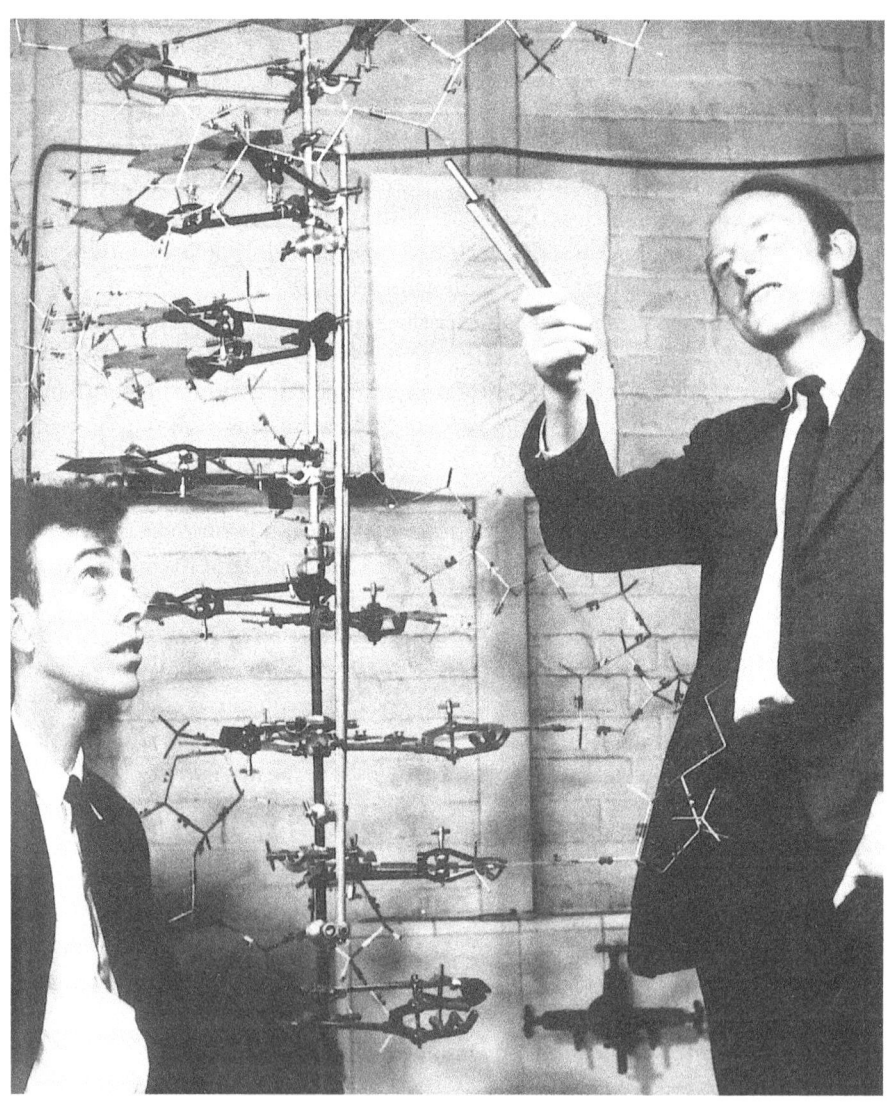

the University of Oxford, and George Klein who had been born in the same year in Budapest and was working at the Karolinska Institute in Stockholm. They fused tumor cells with normal cells and obtained a surprising result. The hybrid cells were no longer malignant; they did however grow well in cell culture, producing offspring that were malignant and losing chromosomes in the process. Harris and Klein concluded that these chromosomes were the carriers of tumor suppressor genes that inhibit cell division. If cell division is initiated, these genes will stop it. If on the other hand the genes are inactivated the cells can keep on dividing and cancer can be produced. These elegant experiments initially failed to get the attention they deserved because their results were at odds with the findings of recent research on retroviruses and oncogenes, which indicated that malignancy and abnormal cell growth properties are dominant (Vogt, 1992). Harris and Klein were eventually proved to be right, however.

The prototype of a cancer caused by a mutation in tumor suppressor gene is the retinoblastoma. This is a malignant tumor of the pigment layer of the eye, which is seen in children. In 40% of the cases, the tumor is family-related. This is the first known human malignant tumor with an autosomal dominant inheritance pattern. Analysis of the results of studies of this patient group led the American geneticist Alfred Knudson to propose the double-hit hypothesis in 1971. One key fact that guided him towards the formulation of this hypothesis was that retinoblastoma was known to occur in two different forms, one family-related and one sporadic.

Children in families with a history of retinoblastoma tend to develop the tumor early and often in both eyes, in contrast to the sporadic form. According to Knudson, children in the former group inherit a germ-cell mutation from one of the parents, with the result that each cell of the retina contains a mutated suppressor gene, thus as it were taking the brake off the carcinogenesis process. A second 'hit' (mutation) will then be sufficient to give rise to a tumor. The likelihood of this happening is so great that it can even occur in several cells independently, thus leading to bilateral tumors and even multiple tumors in the same eye.

In the non-hereditary form of retinoblastoma, both suppressor genes have to be inactivated by mutation before a tumor can be produced. The chance of this happening is much smaller, so that the cancer appears later and only in one eye. This is the essence of Knudson's double-hit model: carcinogenesis requires the inactivation of two separate genes (Schubert et al., 1994). It was later found that in the hereditary form of retinoblastoma, this loss of function is caused by deletion, mutation or inactivation in the long arm of chromosome 13. The gene involved here, known as the retinoblastoma gene, was isolated by Jeremy Squire and co-workers at the University of Toronto in 1986 (Squire et al., 1986). The same loss of function in the retinoblastoma gene is also observed in other forms of cancer, which has led researchers to assume that this gene acts as a universal brake on cell division. Mutations in tumor suppressor genes are also found in frequently occurring forms of cancer such as cancer of the colon.

Physicians in ancient Rome had already documented the fact that breast cancer occurs more often in some families than in others. The first modern record of familial breast cancer dates from 1866, and was penned by the famous French surgeon and anatomist Pierre Paul Broca (1824-1880). He described the occurrence of ten cases of breast cancer in four generations of his wife's family. Four other women in the family died of liver tumors, which were probably metastases of breast cancer. His suggestion that there was a higher risk of breast cancer in certain families was later confirmed by various other researchers. Wick Williams and David Anderson from the University of Texas provided statistical evidence in 1984 of the existence of a gene that caused this higher risk of breast cancer (Couch and Weber, 2002). This point of view was confirmed by Mary-Claire King (1946-), an American human geneticist at the University of Washington.

Mary-Claire King has made a major contribution to the study of chromosomal defects. In 1990 she described the occurrence of the BRCA1 gene on chromosome 17q21 in familial breast cancer (Hall et al., 1990). When she started this investigation, the whole world told her 'Nonsense, you're wasting your time. Breast cancer is multifactorial and cannot be ascribed to a single gene'. She finally managed to find the gene she was looking for, after sixteen years of dedicated research. If this gene is mutated, the risk of getting breast cancer is 60-80%. In 1995, Professor Michael Stratton and Dr Richard Wooster of the Institute of Cancer Research, UK, discovered another gene that plays a role in familial breast cancer, the BRCA2 gene. The Wellcome Trust Sanger Institute just outside Cambridge worked with Stratton and Wooster to isolate the gene. In honor of this discovery, the Wellcome Trust has participated in the construction of a cycle path between Addenbrooke's Hospital site in Cambridge and the nearby village of Great Shelford. It is decorated with over 10,000 lines of 4 colors representing the nucleotide sequence of BRCA2. It makes up part of the English cycle route 11, and can be seen by train passengers travelling from Cambridge to London Liverpool Street (Figure 2.10). The presence of the mutated form of the BRCA2 gene also leads to a risk of 60-80% of getting breast cancer. Mutations in one or both of these genes also lead to a predisposition to ovarian cancer (30-60% for BRCA1 and 5-20% for BRCA2).

Epidemiologic investigation suggests that at least 15% of colorectal carcinomas have a dominant inheritance pattern. The two best defined forms of these complaints are familial adenomatous polyposis (FAP) and hereditary non-polyposis colorectal cancer (HNPCC). The latter is also known as Lynch syndrome.

FAP is an autosomal dominant disease that is found in 1 per 7000 head of population. Patients with FAP typically develop hundreds or even thousands of polyps in their colon before they are 20, and one or more of these polyps are likely to turn malignant in the course of time. This complaint was first observed in the eighteenth century, and its hereditary nature was recognized in the nineteenth.

In 1986, Pedro L. Herrera and co-workers at the University of Geneva described an unusual patient who not only suffered from polyposis but also had severe learn-

FIGURE 2.10 *Cycle path between Cambridge and the village of Great Shelford, decorated over a mile of its length with a series of stripes in four different colors representing the base-pair sequence of the BRCA2 gene. (Courtesy of the Wellcome Trust Sanger Institute, Cambridge).*

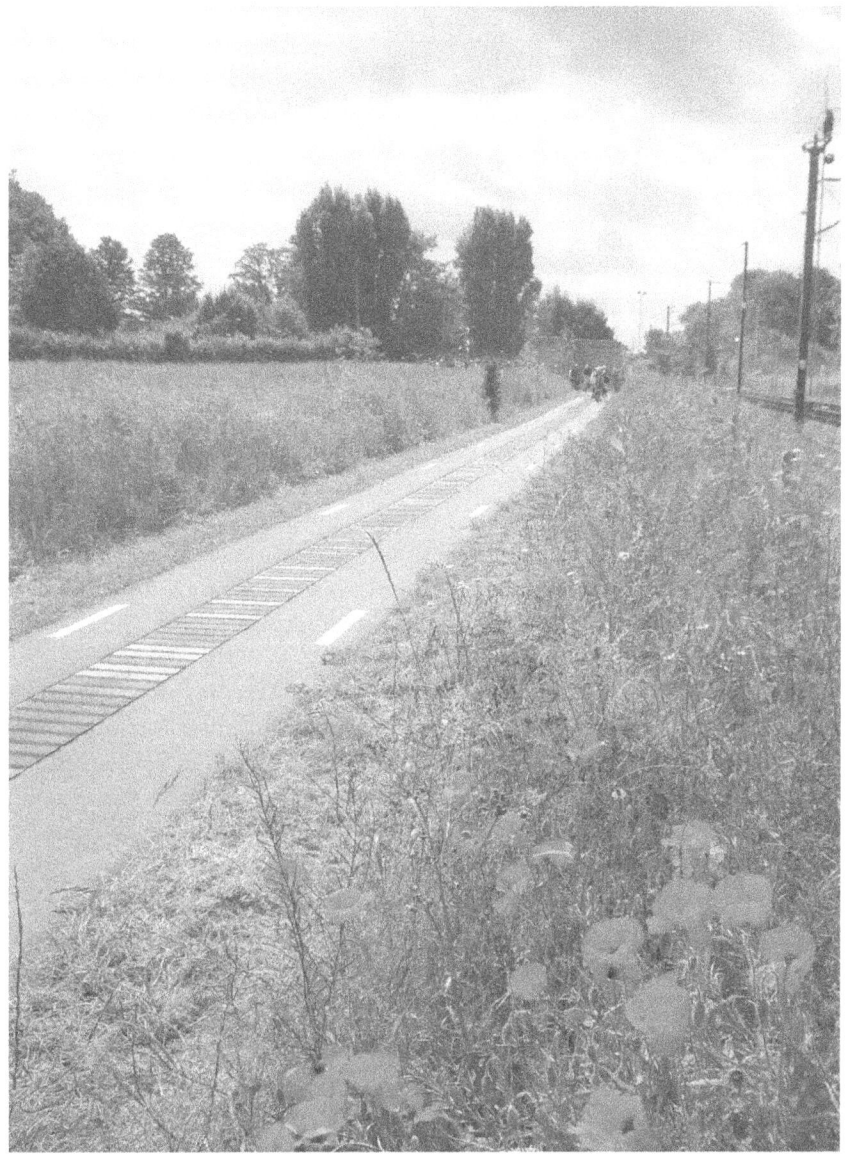

ing difficulties. Investigation of this patient's chromosomes revealed that a small part of chromosome 5 was missing. Further molecular studies by Joanna Groden and co-workers from the University of Utah and Isamu Nishisho and colleagues at Osaka University Medical School showed five years later that the adenomatosis polyposis coli (APC) gene was located at this spot. Mutations in this gene are responsible for causing FAP (Kinzler and Vogelstein, 1996).

Another group of genes, known as the DNA repair genes, that could lead to cancer if mutated was also discovered. The above-mentioned HNPCC is caused by a member of this group. This too is an autosomal dominant complaint, characterized by the occurrence within a single family of several cases of colorectal cancer without polyps. The onset of the cancer is typically found at a relatively young age (round about 45), and the cancer tends to be localized in the proximal part of the colon.

Aldred S. Warthin (1866-1931) was the first to describe this condition. He was professor of Pathology at the University of Michigan at Ann Arbor, and reviewed the reports of the pathology laboratory for the period 1895-1913 after his seamstress had told him that she was sure she was going to die of cancer because so many other members of her family had suffered this fate. Surprisingly, his investigation revealed a number of families with a marked history of cancer. One of these families, that of Warthin's seamstress, was taken as the prototype of families with a strong history of cancer and was subsequently further investigated by Henry T. Lynch (1928-...) under the name of family 'G'. It appeared from Warthin's initial observations that family 'G' also showed a higher than expected incidence of cancers of the uterus and the stomach. More than half a century later, Lynch and co-workers produced a detailed description of these cancer-prone families. Since no other concomitant features such as a high frequency of polyps were found, this syndrome was named hereditary non-polyposis colorectal cancer. The alternative name of Lynch syndrome was proposed in 1984.

The biologic basis of this syndrome was elucidated in the spring of 1993. The research groups headed by Yurij Ionov at Roswell Park Cancer Institute, Buffalo NY, Lauri A. Aaltonen from the University of Helsinki and S.N. Thibodeau at the Mayo Clinic in Rochester (MN) demonstrated replication errors in microsatellites located at various sites along the genome. Microsatellites are relatively short DNA fragments containing a repetitive series of nucleotides. This finding suggested that 'DNA repair genes' are involved in the repair of errors occurring during the replication of DNA, and that NHPCC can occur if something goes wrong with this repair process. In line with this, it was reported that carriers of mutations in these genes run a 30-85% risk of developing colorectal cancer (Marra and Boland, 1995).

The determination of the structure of the human genome was a major step forwards for clinical genetics. This was achieved by a group of academics from various countries, working together in the Human Genome Project at a direct cost of some

800,000,000 US dollars. The group was initially headed by James Watson at the US National Institutes of Health. A private biotechnology company, Celera Genomics, carried out a similar project in parallel. Both groups published their results in 2001. It was established that human DNA contains about 23,000 genes, made up of about three billion nucleotides arranged in a precisely defined sequence. The elucidation of this sequence marked the start of a new era in the study of the genetic background of disease. The function of about half of the genes is known. This will help us to gain much deeper insights into the mechanism of many complaints.

A recent spectacular technological development has made it much easier to determine gene functions. Stephen Fodor from the company Affymetrix in Santa Clara, California, and Patrick Brown from Stanford University introduced the concept of 'massively parallel genomics' in 1996 and 1999 respectively. This approach, which is based on the discovery of the DNA microarray or 'DNA chip', makes it possible to analyze the activity of tens of thousands of genes simultaneously in a very short time. Study of gene expression profiles and DNA copy profiles will yield important new insights into the underlying biology of disease, including cancer (Van der Pouw Kraan et al., 2005). Laura van 't Veer and co-workers at the Dutch Cancer Institute in Amsterdam introduced an important clinical application of this technique in 2002 when they used it to determine a gene expression profile for breast cancer patients that is closely related to the prognosis (Van 't Veer et al., 2002). This seems to make it possible to get a better indication of which patients need adjuvant therapy (see Chapter 6). Further research is still required in this field, however, in order to get a clearer picture.

Apoptosis

The discovery of the oncogene was greeted with great enthusiasm, since it was generally believed that this meant that a cure to cancer was within reach. In fact, however, the situation was not so simple. Five to seven mutations proved to be necessary to produce a cancer cell. Risk analysis clearly showed that it is very unlikely that a whole series of harmful mutations would occur in a single cell without some growth benefit being produced by a beneficial mutation somewhere in the sequence. Apoptosis (defined in the next paragraph) completes the picture. Before a cell divides, a check is carried out to determine whether the DNA is intact. If it is, the cell divides. If it is not, the DNA is repaired. If that turns out to be impossible because the DNA is too badly damaged, apoptosis ensues. Dozens of genes are involved in this entire process. If one of these genes is inactivated by mutation then apoptosis is no longer effective, the cell becomes genetically instable and the mutations accumulate: some cells may be found with five or six mutated genes. The idea of apoptosis explains a lot of hitherto puzzling facts, such as the heterogeneity of tumor material where the function of some cells is found to depend on hormones while others are hormone-independent (see Chapter 7). It therefore seemed to make sense in the context of this book to pay some attention to the history of apoptosis.

The term apoptosis is derived from the ancient Greek prefix apo-, which has the sense of separation, and ptosis which means falling. It seems to have been used originally to denote the falling of leaves from a tree in winter or the sloughing of scabs, but in current medical publications always means programmed cell death. This concept was introduced in 1964 by cell biologist Richard Lockshin (1937-) and physiologist and biologist Carroll Williams (1916-1991) from Harvard to describe the physiological process used to get rid of superfluous cells during insect metamorphosis (Duque-Parra, 2005).

Cell death was long defined on a morphologic basis. The first name given to this concept, necrosis, dates back to Areteus of Cappadocia in the first century AD and Galen a century later (Formigli et al., 2004).

Robert Hooke (1635-1703) studied thin slices of the bark of the cork oak under the microscope in the seventeenth century. The honeycomb-like structures he saw were divided up into small compartments that reminded him of the cells in a monastery. He therefore named these compartments cells, thus introducing the term 'cell' into the scientific literature for the first time. Hooke concluded that these cells had died a natural death (Figure 2.11).

In 1842, the German biologist Carl Vogt (1817-1895) described the natural death of cells in the nervous system of toad embryos (Duque-Parra, 2005). This observation was noteworthy in view of the fact that it was made only three years after Schleiden and Schwann had put forward the cell theory, according to which all living organisms were built up of individual units that they also called cells (Curtin and Cotter, 2003).

Rudolf Virchow took a closer look at the concept of cell death half a century later. He distinguished two types of cell death on the basis of macroscopic examination: necrosis (cell degeneration where the original form of the tissue was preserved) and necrobiosis (a term that he borrowed from K.H. Schultz), which was cell degeneration where the original form of the tissue could no longer be recognized (Formigli et al., 2004).

The above-mentioned Julius Cohnheim reformulated the concept of cell death on the basis of microscopic observations of large masses of fibrin in the tracheobronchial epithelium of diphtheria patients by Carl Weigert (1845-1904), who had been Cohnheim's assistant for a time. Cohnheim introduced the term coagulation necrosis to account for this finding. When it was subsequently demonstrated that the fibrin had nothing to do with the coagulation of tissue, this term was discontinued. However, Weigert's work in the period between 1890 and 1900 led to an enormous increase in studies of cell death and the use of many different names for this phenomenon (Formigli et al., 2004).

FIGURE 2.11 Microscope used by Robert Hooke, with the light source on the left (a). Hooke coined the term 'cell' after microscopic examination of samples of cork (b). (Source: M. Espinasse, Robert Hooke. William Heineman, London, 1956).

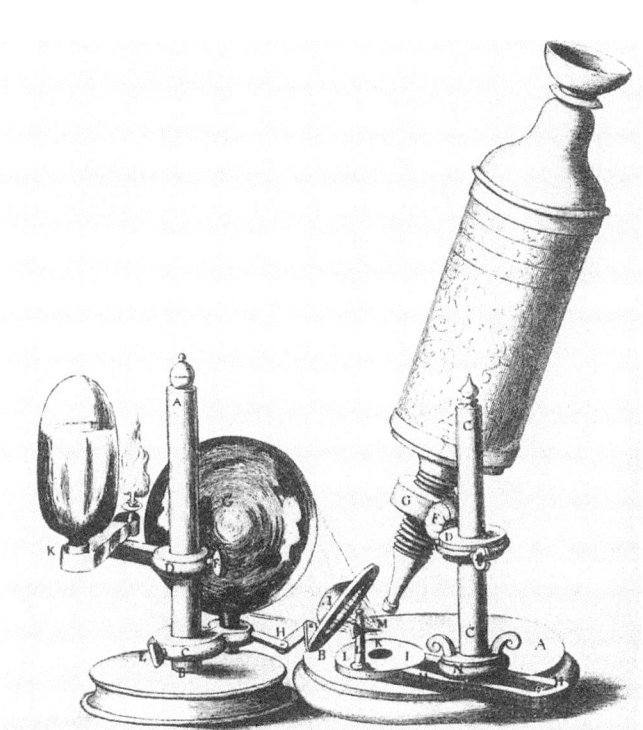

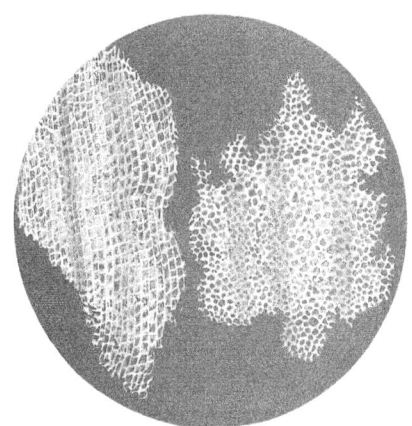

It is noteworthy that the German biologist Walther Flemming (1843-1905), the founder of cytogenetics, identified an unusual form of natural cell death in 1895, while observing the degradation of ovarian follicles with the aid of the *camera lucida*. He called this chromatolysis, a term signifying a reduction in the size of the cells combined with chromatin condensation – the disintegration of the nuclei and the formation of apoptotic bodies. This may be regarded as the first observation of the typical nuclear and cytoplasmic changes now associated with apoptosis.

Interest in apoptosis fluctuated during the first half of the twentieth century. Then, in 1951, A. Glücksmann from the Strangeways Research Laboratory in Cambridge (UK) published an important review article on cell death in which he described karyorrhexis (disintegration of the nucleus) and karyopyknosis (shrinkage of the nucleus) as special forms of cell death. We now know that they are different aspects of apoptosis. Glücksmann's article led to a revival of interest in the mechanism of cell death among some pathologists.

These included the Australian John F. Kerr from Brisbane, who observed an unusual form of cell death in 1965 after artificial ischemic damage to the liver, in which cell components appeared to remain intact within small vesicles. He used the term 'shrinkage necrosis' to describe this phenomenon. Further investigation with the electron microscope identified the earliest morphologic events in this sequence as condensation of the cytoplasm and of the chromatin in the nucleus. Kerr was invited by Professor Alister Currie to spend his sabbatical year in Aberdeen, where he worked with Andrew Wyllie and Currie. During this period, they coined the term apoptosis to replace the initial name shrinkage necrosis. They defined this special form of cell death in 1972, in an important article in the *British Journal of Cancer* (Curtin and Cotter, 2003), where they described cell death as a mechanism that is complementary but opposed to mitosis in the regulation of cell population. They wrote that this form of cell death develops in two distinct phases, the degradation of nuclear and cytoplasmic material to give membrane-bound apoptotic bodies and the subsequent sequestration of these bodies by other cells. Kerr and co-workers stressed the role of what they called the 'intrinsic clock' here, suggesting that a genetic component is involved in the process (Kerr et al., 1972; Kerr, 2002).

The idea that apoptosis could be regulated by genes in the same way as cell proliferation and differentiation was confirmed at the end of the 1990s by studies on the nematode worm *Caenorhabditis elegans*, a tiny transparent creature only 1 mm long. These studies identified at least three genes, designated ced (cell death defective), that were involved in some way in the process of cell death. Ced-3 and ced-4 were found to play a role in the execution of apoptosis, and ced-9 in its inhibition. From that moment, apoptosis was regarded as a highly orchestrated series of events responsible for cell destruction. In view of the greater complexity of higher organisms compared with this tiny worm, it is hardly surprising that a large family of genes involved in apoptosis in man have been discovered. This family includes the p53 tumor suppressor gene and the oncogene c-myc, which permit more sophisticated control of the apoptotic pathway. P53 acts as a cell-cycle checkpoint, allowing the cell to repair DNA damage before proliferation. If the damage is too bad to be repaired, p53 triggers a cell suicide program to prevent the formation of more cells with mutated DNA and hence changed properties.

Sydney Brenner (1927-) and John Sulston (1942-) from the UK and the American Robert Horvitz (1947-) won the Nobel Prize in 2002 for their elucidation of the genetic mechanism of apoptosis. Brenner introduced *C. elegans* as the organism of choice for this study; Sulston laid the foundations for the investigation of the worm and programmed cell death, while Horvitz discovered genetic details of apoptosis that are vital for our current understanding of cancer and other diseases (Curtin and Cotter, 2003). An accurate balance between cell proliferation and programmed cell death proves to be of essential importance for the maintenance of tissue and organ homeostasis (Formigli et al., 2004).

Models of cancer pathogenesis showed that the pathological cell accumulation found in tumors is the result of excessive cell proliferation combined with diminished cell death. The insights gained into the role of apoptosis and the defective control of cell growth in cancer offer hopes of better understanding of the disease and advances in its treatment.

Research into apoptosis is snowballing at the moment. A total of 147,600 articles on this topic had been published by the end of 2006, and a further 17,600 publications were expected in the course of 2006. That comes down to one article every half an hour (Ameisen et al., 2005).

Afterword

If we look at the views about medicine as products of their time, we understand why classical Greek physicians tried to explain health and disease in terms of philosophical concepts. The theory of the four humors, leading to the idea that cancer is the result of an excess of black bile, is then no longer an anomaly but simply a consequence of the philosophical thinking of those days.

It also becomes clear that medieval physicians thought more along theological lines, with the consequence that they believed that cure was only possible through divine intervention, and that the Renaissance ushered in an era characterized by a scientific approach to health and disease. From this perspective, it is equally understandable that disease was ascribed to infection at the end of the nineteenth century and the beginning of the twentieth century, and that during the past couple of decades everything has been viewed in the light of changes in genetic constitution.

[3]

The treatment of cancer in the past

Cancer has always been an aggressive disease. Many different forms of treatment have been devised for it, but until recently the success rate was low. Fortunately, since the start of the new century the tide seems to be turning, with the introduction of targeted therapy, and the prospects for cancer patients are starting to look significantly better.

The present chapter briefly reviews the different forms of cancer treatment that were used before the modern era. The rest of the book is devoted to more detailed discussions of the various types of therapy in separate chapters. Chapter 4 describes the development of surgery as a treatment for cancer, with special reference to the advances made during the past two centuries. The next three chapters deal with the introduction and development of radiotherapy and the history of chemotherapy and hormonal treatment, respectively. These are followed by a chapter on targeted therapy and one on immunotherapy, to illustrate the current scope of therapeutic advances. The final chapter is devoted to a discussion of psychosocial oncology, a discipline that is coming to play an increasingly important role in the treatment of cancer.

The oldest written record of the treatment of cancer is found in the Edwin Smith papyrus, which was mentioned in Chapter 2. It describes eight cases of breast cancer, and states that the tumors were burned out with an instrument called a "fire drill" (Kardinal and Yarbro, 1979). While no precise details of the treatment are given, it is not difficult to imagine what went on. The Ebers papyrus also deals with the treatment of cancer. A distinction is drawn here between different types of tumors, each of which requires a different therapy. An inflamed swelling calls for incision and the drainage of the pus it contains, while a solid mass has to be cut out. This papyrus also contains the following statement:

_____ In the case of breast cancer accompanied by involvement of the lymph nodes, there is nothing more the surgeon can do. It might be fitting to tell the patient that her death is at hand, and to prescribe a laxative prepared from herbs (Forgue and Bouchet, 1980).

The Hindu epic Ramayana likewise devotes some space to the treatment of cancer. The therapies mentioned in it are excision of the tumor or treatment with ointments containing arsenic, which was known to have a caustic effect.

The 70-odd books of the Hippocratic Corpus, believed by modern scholars to have been largely or entirely written by the followers of Hippocrates rather than by Hippocrates himself, contain many references to treatment as well as to medical theory and diagnosis. One of the most famous books attributed to Hippocrates is the *Aphorisms*, which contains short, pithy sayings about medical practice. It was probably intended as teaching material for students who could not afford to buy the expensive handwritten medical textbooks of that time. One of these aphorisms ran as follows:

_____ It is better not to treat patients with invisible cancers, for if they are treated they die quickly and if they are left untreated they live longer.

The Corpus also contained the advice that some tumors could best be removed surgically, while others should be treated with ointments containing copper, lead, sulfur or arsenic. It was further stated that the prognosis was better if the patient was treated early, and that involvement of the lymph nodes was a bad sign (Cabanne et al., 1983). The first description of a rectoscope has also been ascribed to Hippocrates (Riskin et al., 2006).

The encyclopedist Aurelius Cornelius Celsus (c. 30 BC - AD 38) was very pessimistic about the result of all forms of cancer treatment – a view shared by most Roman physicians at that time (Cabanne et al., 1983).

Galen's idea that cancer was due to an accumulation of black bile had the consequence that cancer was regarded as a systemic or metabolic disease rather than a localized complaint. It followed that if cancer was diagnosed, the whole patient needed to be treated. Galen recommended, for example, that the patient should be given a purgative (laxative) and then prescribed a special diet consisting mainly of vegetables, and not containing any walnuts. He also made wide use of drugs, mainly compounded from herbs and often prescribed in the form of a mixture of a number of different remedies (Cabanne et al., 1983).

Leonides of Alexandria (c. AD 180) had a different opinion. He removed the cancer using an ample incision, cutting through plenty of healthy tissue to ensure removal of all the tumor, and then cauterized the wound (Ewing, 1919). The physician Oribasius of Pergamon (c. 325-403) wrote that cancer was incurable. Indeed, he was so pessimistic about the outcome that he advised against any form of operation on cancer patients. Paul of Aegina (625-690) disagreed. He was the author of the seven-book *Epitome of Medicine*, of which the sixth book on surgery is the most noteworthy. He stated there, among other things, that patients should follow a special diet in preparation for a breast cancer operation, and should pray to St. Agatha to strengthen themselves mentally. St. Agatha was a Christian martyr from Sicily, who probably died about AD 250. Legend has it that her persecutor had her breasts cut off as part of the torture she was made to suffer. She is therefore the patron saint of breast cancer patients (Figure 3.1). Paul of Aegina considered the prognosis for breast cancer, if it was operated on, to be better than that for cancer of the uterus. According to him, surgery was always indicated in cases of breast cancer. He recommended ligating the blood vessels to stop bleeding, rather than cauterization which had usually been used up to that time (Cabanne et al., 1983). He also gave a detailed description of the procedure for tracheotomy (making a surgical incision in the windpipe to provide an airway if the patient is suffocating) (Hill, 1979).

The famous Arab physician Avicenna (980-1037) had his own treatment for cancer. He recommended the use of arsenic-based ointments combined with bloodletting, laxatives and a plant extract. Albucassis (1013-1106), a surgeon from Cordoba in Moorish Spain, believed that cauterization with a red-hot iron was better than cutting the tumor out with a knife. It is noteworthy that Avenzoar or Ibn Zuhr (1091-1161), known as the father of experimental surgery, described cancer of the esophagus and stomach together with one of his pupils. The patients did not undergo surgery, but it is interesting that a stomach catheter was already used to feed patients at that time (Cabanne et al., 1983).

The founding of universities in the Middle Ages had a number of important consequences. Apart from rediscovery of the medical works of Galen, a valuable store of new practical knowledge was built up that provided a basis for the clinical evaluation of patients suffering from all kinds of diseases, including cancer (Diamandopoulos, 1996). It may be mentioned for example that Pietro Clerico – also known as Petroncello – at the medical school of Salerno (10th-11th century) recommended the use of a digital rectal examination to detect a carcinoma of the rectum, while Guido Lanfranchi of Milan (c. 1250-1306) who became a popular professor of surgery in Paris taught his students how to distinguish breast cancer from mammary hypertrophy (Cabanne et al., 1983). His teacher, William of Saliceto (or Guglielmo da Saliceto, 1210-1277), wrote a critical commentary on the treatment of breast cancer at that time. He stated, "the affected part must be radically excised with a sharp knife, for this complaint cannot heal well without amputation" (Hill, 1979).

John of Ardenne (1307-1380) was the first English surgeon who is known to have published anything in the field of oncology. He wrote in Latin, the language of learning at that time. He described the symptoms of cancer of the rectum, such as bleeding and obstruction. He was convinced of the serious nature of the complaint, because he himself had never seen or heard of a patient who had been cured of cancer of the rectum (Raven, 1990).

His contemporary Guy de Chauliac (1300-1368) criticized the limited background knowledge of "chirurgians". He was convinced that a surgeon should be well-read, and should know not only the principles of surgery but also those of

CHAPTER 3

FIGURE 3.1 *The martyrdom of Saint Agatha. According to legend, her breasts were cut off before she was put to death. She is the patron saint of all those suffering from afflictions of the breast (Koninklijke Bibliotheek, The Hague. From the Book of Hours of Philip the Good (1435); Source: De Moulin, 1983; reproduced by courtesy of the editor).*

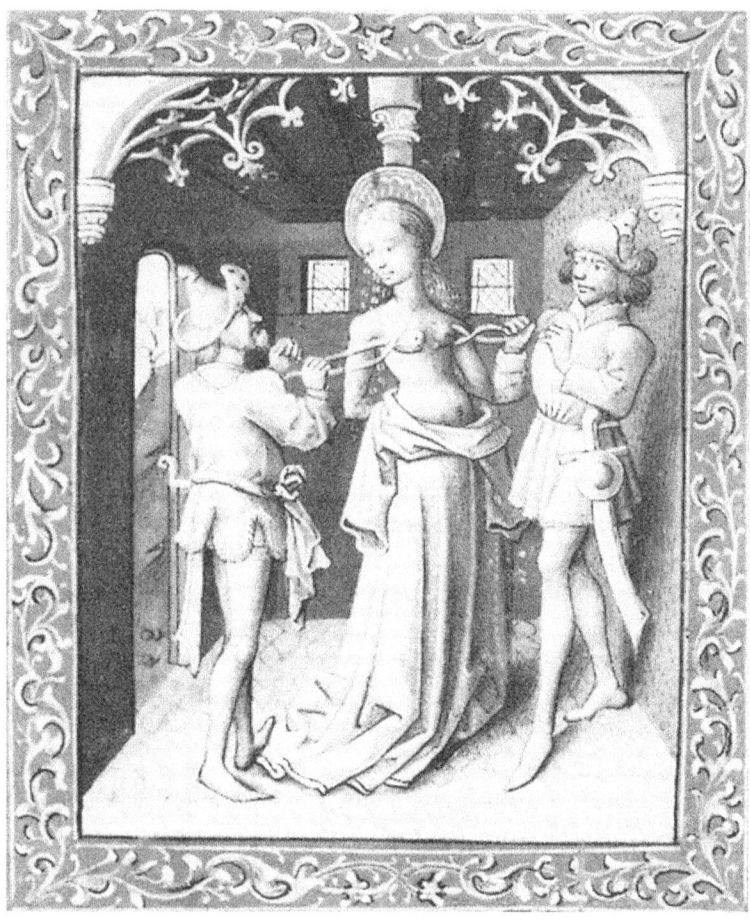

internal medicine, both in theory and in practice. Paracelsus noted that "internal medicine and surgery...must not be separated except in practice; every physician must be learned in both types of medicine" (Hill, 1979).

A great deal of attention was devoted to conservative methods in the Middle Ages. Drawing poultices and a wide variety of plasters were prescribed for the treatment of closed cancers, while many kinds of ointments and powders were used for ulcerating tumors. Internal treatment consisted of all kinds of diets, laxatives and bloodletting to restore the balance of the humors. The rule was not to operate at an early stage.

The first anatomic illustrations, which were important to the work of surgeons, appeared at the end of the Middle Ages. The first examples were published by the German surgeon Hieronymus Brunschwig (1450-1533) from Strasbourg (Hill, 1979). It was more than a century later, in 1543, that Vesalius's beautifully drawn anatomic atlas saw the light of day. The illustrations it contained were so precise that they can still be used as a guide to dissection today.

The fall of Galen as the medical authority par excellence generated not only a host of bizarre theories about how cancer came about but also remarkable recommendations about how to treat it. Today, most of these treatments would be classified as alternative therapies. The Viennese school, for example, recommended the use of rough chervil (*Chaerophyllum temulum*). Stolterforth and Cromp proudly claimed that they were able to cure ulcerating tumors with the aid of mercury. It seems likely however that the lesions they were treating were the result of tertiary lues (Cabanne et al., 1983).

John Muir, a district surgeon from Sterkstroom in South Africa with an MD from Edinburgh, cited two remarkable cures from the past in his article "The Cancer Curer in South Africa" (Muir, 1906?). The first was ascribed to Théophile Bonet (1628-1689) of Geneva. In Muir's words,

_____ *A woman had cancer of the breast, which was already so severe, that eight holes had been eaten into it, and recovered through the following expedient. She took eight frogs applied to the breast in a muslin bag, which attached themselves instantly thereto, as firmly as leeches. When they had sucked to repletion, they dropped off in violent convulsions without the sucking causing pain. This was repeated until 120 frogs were used, which all from time to time sucked until they died. And the breast was not only cured, but returned again to its normal size absolutely.*

The second cure was prescribed by Wilhelmus Fabritius Hildanus (1560-1634), who will be mentioned again in Chapter 4. Muir records this as follows:

_____ *Fabricius asserts from certain experience that the following water is admirable in curing ulcerous Cankers. It is made thus: Take sucking puppies, put them in Wine, and distill it half off in Balneo: then take the Puppies out, and boil them in a sufficient quantity of Golden Rod Water or in*

CHAPTER 3

FIGURE 3.2 Bloodletting. From the Luttrell Psalter (1340). This illustration shows a barber-surgeon bleeding a patient, whose arm rests on a "barber's pole.". Bloodletting was widely used in the treatment of diseases in the past, since it was believed to be effective in restoring the balance of the humors (vital fluids) in the body (Source: Shimkin, 1979, courtesy of the National Institute of Health, Bethesda, MD, USA).

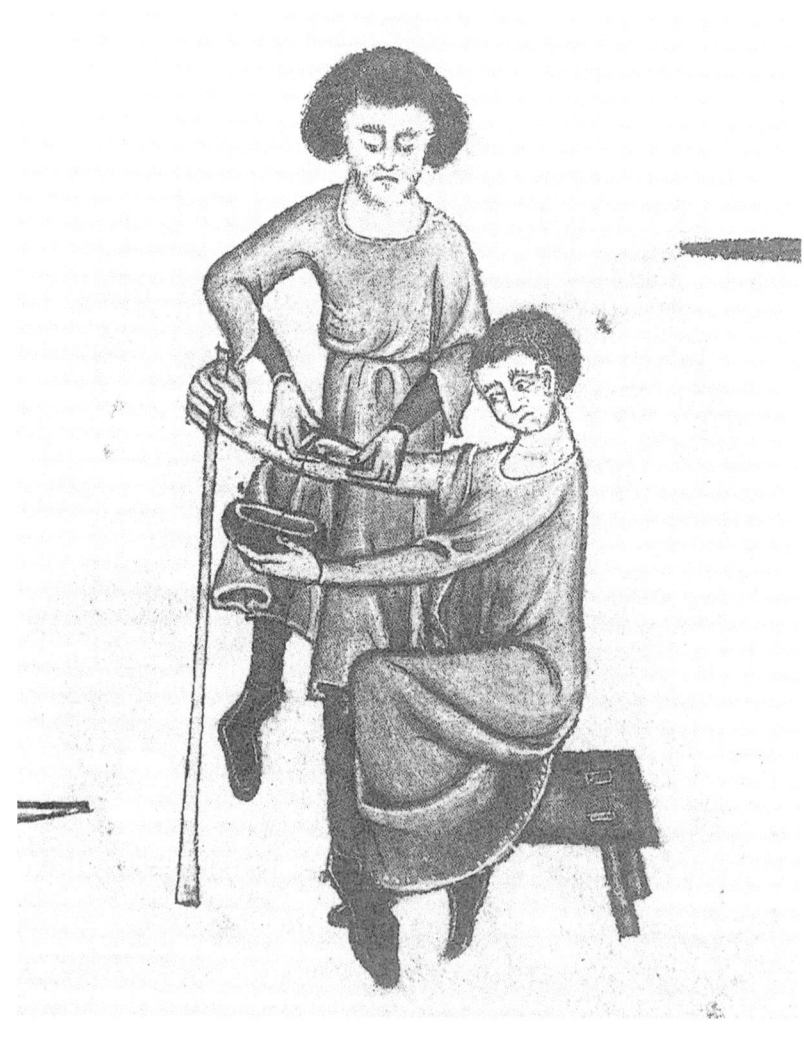

common Water, with Golden Rod in it; when the Decoction is made, add the Water that was distilled off the young Dogs and boil them together till the flesh come from the Bones. Then distill them all in Balneo, Keep the Water for use. Wet dry clothes or rags in this, and apply it to the ulcerous Carcinoma. For from certain Experience it heals the sore by cleansing and drying.

These two cures were also mentioned by Kardinal and Yarbro (1979).

So much for our initial brief overview of the often curious remedies from the past. In the following chapters, we will see in much greater detail how more scientifically based, and more effective, approaches gradually developed in the various fields of cancer treatment.

[4]

The maturing of surgery as a treatment of cancer

Our brief review of the history of cancer treatment in the previous chapter shows that surgery can rightly claim to be the oldest form of therapy for this disease. Before going on to consider how the surgical treatment of cancer has developed over time, it would seem to be appropriate to pay some attention to the position of the surgeon in the healthcare system in the past.

The position of surgery in the medical world in the past

Initially, there seems to have been little distinction made between physicians and surgeons. We saw in Chapter 2 that Galen learned anatomy as well as the curative properties of herbs and minerals. His first job involved providing medical care for gladiators, where he learned a great deal from observation of the wounds they suffered.

There have been other famous surgeons in the distant past, possibly including Imhotep (2650-2600 BC), chancellor to King Djoser and high priest of the god Ra, who is the first practitioner of medicine known by name (he was mentioned in Chapter 2). Two millennia later, Sushruta (c. 6th century BC) was a physician and surgeon in ancient India who wrote an influential book describing 120 surgical instruments and 300 surgical procedures, and who divided surgery into 8 categories. He was known as the "Father of Surgery."

It is well-known that the word 'surgery' is derived from the Greek words *xeir*, meaning hand, and *ergon*, meaning work. This indicates that surgeons were regarded as manual workers by the ancient Greeks. On the other hand, there is another Greek word for a medical practitioner, *iatros*, derived from the verb *iasthai*, to heal. This was used interchangeably to denote a physician and a surgeon.

CHAPTER 4

FIGURE 4.1 Henri de Mondeville (c. 1260- c. 1320), a surgeon and a member of the clergy as was usual at that time. He worked in Montpellier and Paris (from E. Nicaise, 1893; source: Shimkin, 1979, courtesy of the National Institute of Health, Bethesda, MD, USA).

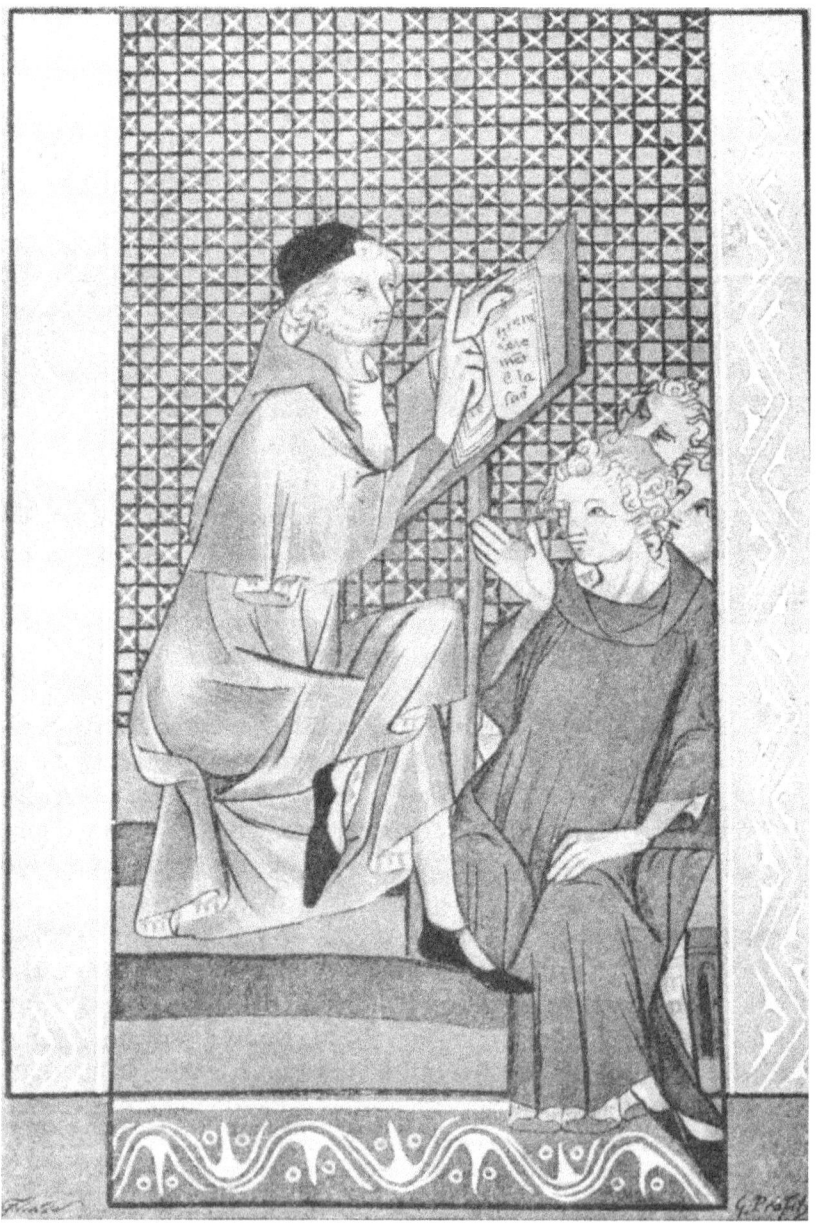

While there may have been little distinction made between a physician and a surgeon in antiquity, the situation gradually changed. Surgeons came to be regarded as craftsmen, who were subordinate to the much more learned physicians. One contributory factor was doubtless the fact that the ancient Greeks and Romans, and the followers of Christianity, Judaism and Islam, were all reluctant for various reasons to cut into the human body, living or dead. This has been discussed at some length in Chapter 2, in connection with the possible ban on autopsies in the past.

Surgeons who had the status of manual workers were generally barbers too, and in fact that was often their main occupation and source of income. Celsus (c. 30 BC-AD 38) had the following to say about the requirements to be met by surgeons:

A chirurgeon must be young, or in any case not advanced in Years; he must have a steady Hand that does not tremble; and he should be able to use the Left Hand as well as the Right. He must have clear, sharp Sight, and must also be brave and intrepid and in no way given to Pity; so that he sets his will on healing the person who is under his Hand; and is not at all moved by his screams; to hurry more than is necessary, or to cut less than the situation calls for. He must behave in all respects and in all cases as if he is completely indifferent to the Patient's weeping and wailing (Platner, 1764).

Since the Middle Ages, surgeons – formerly called 'chirurgeons' – have always done their best to achieve an academic status; but initially without success. They performed a purely practical function: apart from caring for wounds and applying dressings, their tasks included bloodletting, lancing boils and giving enemas (Houtzager, 1981).

The chirurgeons of the Middle Ages were subordinated to *doctores medicinae*, who had received a thorough university education – the best that was available at that time. The medical school of Salerno was renowned for the quality of its courses, as were the medical faculties of the universities of Leuven, Paris, Montpellier, Padua and Bologna. The relationship between the doctors and the chirurgeons was generally far from cordial, as illustrated by the following telling example quoted by Henri de Mondeville (c. 1260 - c. 1320), who was a member of the clergy as well as a surgeon, as was usual at that time. He had studied in Paris, and worked in both Montpellier and Paris (Figure 4.1). He related that when a *doctor medicinae* was consulted in connection with a surgical case other than a wound, dislocation or fracture, he would rarely refer the patient immediately to a surgeon for treatment. Instead he would say, artfully:

My good man, it is well known that surgeons are arrogant and completely ignorant, and that the little store of knowledge they have was obtained from us doctors; moreover, they are both malicious and cruel in their dealing with others. You will be better off with a doctor; it is not for nothing that a doctor charges such a high fee. Since I am well disposed to you, I will treat you to the best of my ability, even though I am no surgeon.

If the patient was cured, that was the end of the matter. If he did not improve, however, at a certain point the doctor would say:

_____ *Sir, I have told you that I am no surgeon. Nevertheless, I have treated you in accordance with the rules of the art. In the meantime, however, I have had such pressing calls upon my time that I am no longer able to provide you with the necessary care. I therefore advise you to take a surgeon from now on, and I can recommend such and such a one (De Moulin, 1988).*

Leiden was added to the list of universities where young men could train to be doctores medicinae in 1575. The university education was largely theoretical, and based on study of the medical classics, such as Hippocrates and Galen. Many universities got their own teaching hospital in the seventeenth and eighteenth centuries, as Leiden did in 1799, where students could gain clinical experience. Before then, the *doctor medicinae* restricted himself to internal medicine, diagnosis and the prescription of diets, medicaments and purgatives (laxatives). He only wielded the scalpel in order to give anatomical demonstrations by dissecting cadavers in the anatomy theatre – though before the mid-sixteenth century he would have considered this to be beneath his dignity and would have left the task of dissection to the chirurgeon. He taught the chirurgeons and their apprentices anatomy in the form of autopsies. These anatomical dissections were mainly carried out in the winter, to avoid decomposition of the cadavers. During such demonstrations, the *doctor medicinae* would read aloud from the works of Galen. If the written description did not agree with what was demonstrated, because Galen's anatomy was mainly based on investigations of animals, a student who dared to raise a question would be told to look more closely. The popularity of the anatomical demonstrations may be judged by the large number of "anatomy lessons" painted by Dutch masters like Van Mierevelt, Rembrandt and Cornelius Troost in the sixteenth, seventeenth and eighteenth centuries (Houtzager, 1981).

A middle class of medical practitioners gradually grew up between the upper stratum of *doctores medicinae* with their university degrees and the barber-surgeons at the bottom. This group consisted partly of doctors who wanted to get out of their ivory tower, and partly of barber-surgeons with a certain knowledge of medicine. Some of these surgeons may have taken basic academic courses in the faculty of Arts, which means that they had acquired a rudimentary mastery of Latin. The existence of these various professional groups was effectively illustrated in the Dutch edition of Lanfranc's *Chirurgie*, which was recommended on the title-page to "all Physicians and Masters of Medicine, both learned and simple, and all barbers" (De Moulin, 1988). Various other new medical ideas arose during the Ming dynasty (1368-1644) in China. The concept that internal and external treatment should be combined to tackle illness was shared by several physicians and surgeons. The theory was extended to the treatment of cancer by a number of practitioners who recognized contributory causative factors, such as depression and the eating of fried, spicy or charred food.

Chen Shigong (1555-1636) was one of the outstanding surgical figures of this time. He dedicated himself to external medicine for over 40 years. His *Waike Zhengzong* (*The Genuine External Medicine*), first published in 1617, covered a series of surgically treatable diseases and many effective prescriptions. The book outlined the surgical procedure for the repair of a slashed throat, the use of copper wire to excise nasal polyps under local anesthesia, and described in detail cancer of the lip and breast. Chen Shigong is quoted as saying that breast cancer "results from anxiety, emotional depression, and overthinking which impairs the liver, spleen, and heart and causes the obstruction of the channels (through which the hypothetical energy qi flows)."

In Western Europe in the sixteenth century, surgeons tried to raise their social standing and their academic status by forming guilds (Forgue and Bouchet, 1980). An apprentice surgeon who wished to join the guild first had to be examined by a committee of master surgeons belonging to the guild; in the Netherlands, an alderman of the city concerned was generally added in an ad hoc capacity. Candidates who passed the examination were then entitled to practice in the city where the examination was taken, and to open a chirurgeon's shop. Some chirurgeons specialized in certain operations, such as those required in the treatment of cancer. These were generally travelling chirurgeons, who received a fee for their work from the city. They were only allowed to perform an operation after they had received permission from the city council, and had deposited a certain amount in the chirurgeons' coffers (Houtzager, 1981).

The development of surgery

In the thirteenth century, Italy was the only place where surgery flourished. Apart from barber-surgeons and traveling mountebanks, there was a relatively high proportion of trained doctors there who also practiced surgery. In addition, all Italian universities had a combined chair of surgery and anatomy. A hundred years later, surgery also gained greater importance in France, where Montpellier and Paris achieved prominence as European centers of medical innovation. As a result, greater weight was attached to surgery in the medical curriculum at the University of Montpellier and cancer surgery was no longer performed by barber surgeons but by academically trained physicians who were also surgeons.

The University of Paris had had a medical faculty since the beginning of the thirteenth century, but unlike the Italian universities it did not give surgery a structural place in the curriculum. The gap between the Italian and Parisian approaches to surgery was bridged by Guido Lanfranchi, who was born in Milan about 1250 but banished by the ruling Viscontis in 1290 and went to live in France. He initially practiced medicine in Lyon and then in other French cities, but in 1295 he settled in Paris where he was known as Lanfranc. He described surgery as being in a deplorable state when he arrived in Paris. He joined the *Confrérie de Saint-Côme et Saint Damien*, a guild set up to promote the interests of surgeons and to advance the status of surgery. While its members were no longer barbers, they were not yet admitted to the medical faculty. The art of surgery was still learned through an apprenticeship to a master surgeon; however, the *Confrérie* organized regular demonstrations in the *theatrum anatomicum* in Paris, also known as the "School of Surgeons" – a magnificent building that can still be seen in the Rue des Ecoles – which could hold an audience of 750. Lanfranc gave lectures and clinical demonstrations, and published a masterly book on surgery entitled *Chirurgia magna*. This included the stringent requirements to be met by a surgeon:

_____ His temperament should be well balanced, His hands well formed with long slender fingers and he should be free from bodily tremors. He should be modest with a strong but not reckless spirit. He should have a mastery of all sciences, not only of physic but also of all branches of philosophy, logic, grammar and rhetoric. He should moreover have a knowledge of ethics and should lead a blameless life without greed or lechery, jealousy or miserliness. In the patient's house, he should not look on any woman or enter into conflict with the patient's family; he should put the patient at his ease with all due deference, but should inform the relatives if the disease is serious. He shall not treat hopeless cases. He shall offer the poor help for whatever they can pay, but is free to demand a "bona salaria" from the rich.

Lanfranc is known as the father of French surgery. He died in 1315 (De Moulin, 1988).

The famous Renaissance French surgeon Ambroise Paré (1510-1590) was still an old-fashioned barber-surgeon. He served in the King's military campaigns, where he gained much experience in surgery. The battlefield has an age-old reputation as a school for surgeons. Paré wrote a series of books on medical matters. Tumors were dealt with in the seventh book. Paré classified cancers into a number of groups, depending on the fluid from which he believed them to be derived. In other words, he still relied on the old humoral theory according to which the balance between the sanguine, choleric, phlegmatic and melancholic humors determined sickness and health. This is not surprising, given the times in which he lived; but the therapies he devised on the basis of these considerations may be characterized as highly unusual. He recommended bloodletting to get rid of an excess of melancholic humors. More specifically, he suggested that menstruation should be induced in women to correct the nature of the source of the disease, while for men he prescribed hemorrhoidal bleeding. Paré further recommended surgical removal of small cancers, but the use of vesicants for large tumors where operation would no longer be effective (Kardinal and Yarbro, 1979). He introduced the idea – which still makes very good sense today – of sparing the tissues as much as possible in the course of medical treatment. His well-known saying, 'Je le pansai, Dieu le guérit' ('I dressed the wound, but God healed it'), shows not only his religious belief but also his practical understanding that a physician has very little control over the healing process (Hill, 1979).

Another characteristic saying by Paré was reported as follows: when Charles IX, one of the four French kings to whom Paré was official royal surgeon, was ill he is supposed to have said, "I hope that you will treat your King better than the poor in the hospice," to which Paré replied: "No, Your Majesty, that is impossible." "And why?" asked the King. "Because I treat them all like kings, Sire" (Forgue and Bouchet, 1980).

Paris still had two surgeons' guilds at that time, one for those with academic training and one for the barber-surgeons. The two guilds merged in 1655.

The chirurgeons – at least those in France – managed to gain a higher standing in the medical world at the end of the sixteenth century. Paré was the first surgeon from the *Collège de Saint-Côme* in Paris – the successor of the old *Confrérie de Saint-Côme et Saint Damien* – to be awarded academic status.

Although the combined surgeons' guild of Saint-Côme remained subordinate to the medical faculty, it became more and more independent. Moreover, the reputation of surgery was considerably enhanced by the successful operation by Charles-François Félix (1653-1703) on an anal fistula of King Louis XIV in 1687. Félix was the King's first surgeon, and was raised to the ranks of the nobility by him (De Moulin, 1988). But despite the excellent reputation of surgery, there continued to be regular friction between the surgeons and the *doctores medicinae* – and that remains the case up to the present day, although currently the troubles are less frequent.

Barber-surgeons continued to exercise their profession for many years. Even as late as the mid-nineteenth century, it was not uncommon to see a barber's shop in some countries with a sign outside depicting a muscled arm with blood gushing out of it, rather like a spouting whale, as may be seen in old illustrations. The old barber's pole that used to be common in English-speaking countries is also reminiscent of the bloodletting that used to be practiced by barber-surgeons. No high level of surgical skills was expected of these surgeons (De Moulin, 1988).

The surgeon and the treatment of cancer

It is time to return to our discussion of the contribution surgery has made to the treatment of cancer. The history of surgery contains a strikingly large number of descriptions of breast cancer operations. This is probably because it is the most common form of visible cancers, and also because hardly any operations on

FIGURE 4.2 Illustration of a mastectomy from the book Armentarium Chirurgicum by Johann Schultes, published in 1666 (source: Shimkin, 1979, courtesy of the National Institute of Health, Bethesda, MD, USA).

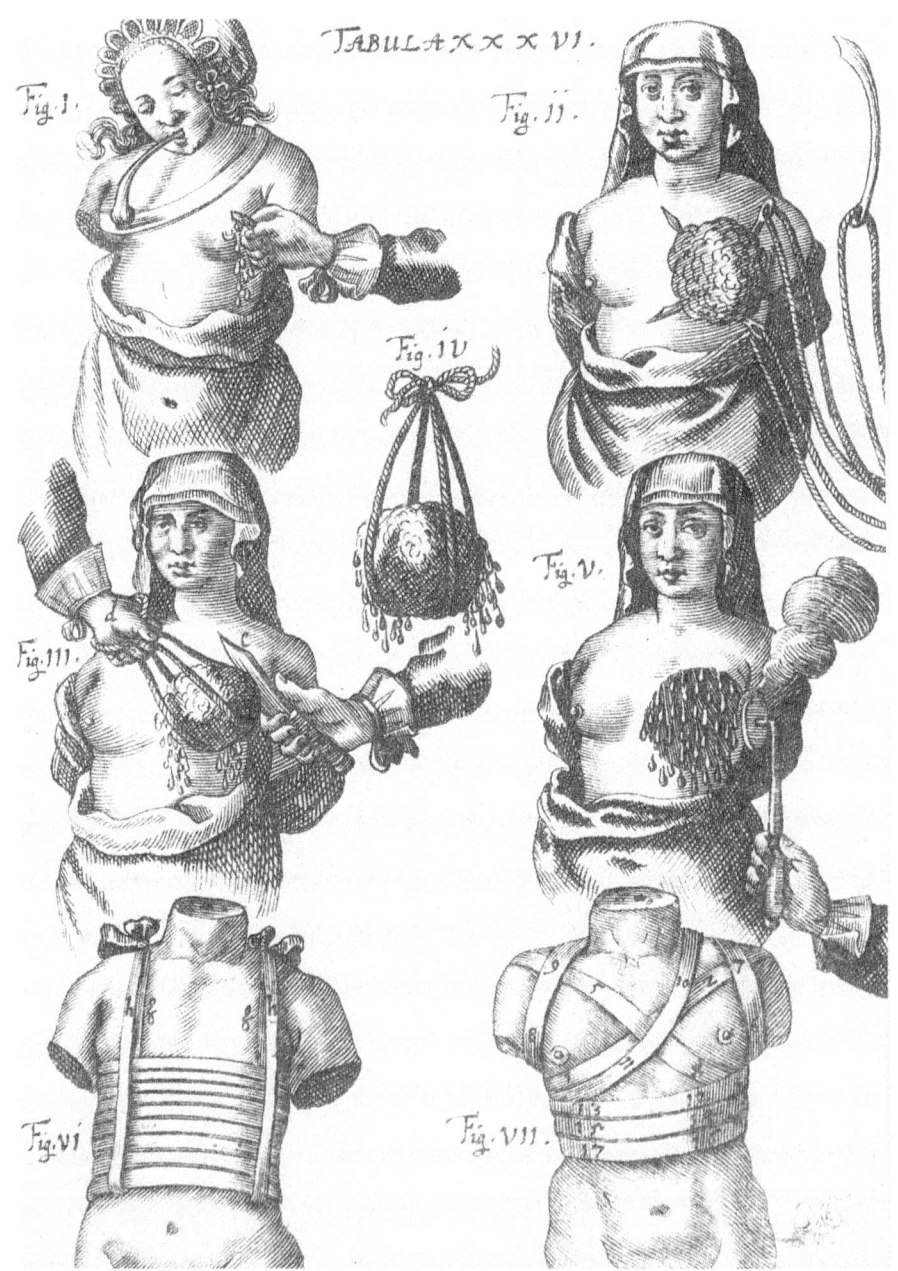

internal tumors were performed in the past. The approach taken to breast cancer has already been dealt with several times in previous chapters, but this topic has been described by many other authors. For example, Johann Schultes (often known by his Latinized name Scultetus, 1595-1645), a surgeon who practiced in Ulm in southeast Germany, illustrated the various steps in a simple mastectomy in his well-known book, *Armentarium Chirurgicum*, published in 1655 (Figure 4.2) (Hill, 1979). De Moulin goes into the surgery of breast cancer in those days in much greater detail. According to him, most surgeons and medical authors considered an operation to be the preferred form of treatment though a large number of contraindications were also mentioned. A difference of opinion also existed about whether an ulcerating cancer should be operated on. Cornelis van de Voorde (c. 1630-1678), a Dutch *doctor medicinae* and surgeon who practiced in Middelburg and who was known for his textbook *Lichtende fakkel der chirurgie, of hedendaagse Heelkonst* (The Flaming Torch of Chirurgy, or Modern Surgery, published in 1664) agreed with others in believing that ulceration led to spontaneous, natural secretion of black bile and should therefore be left undisturbed.

If however the tumor had not yet grown through the skin, simple ablation (removal of the breast only) without closure of the wound was the method of choice. To this end, the patient was placed in a semirecumbent position and the arm on the affected side was raised to tense the muscles situated under the breast. The breast was then cut off with a rapid movement of a large razor. Hot irons or styptic substances in combination with a compression bandage were used to halt the flow of blood. Such an operation only lasted a few minutes. To get a good purchase on the breast during the operation, many surgeons passed one or two traction threads through the base of the breast. Others used a large two-pronged fork to lift the breast off the wall of the torso. Hendrik Ulhoorn (1687-1746), a surgeon from Amsterdam, designed a breast removal clamp that bore a close resemblance to a large cigar cutter. In Diderot and d'Alembert's famous *Encyclopédie*, the monument of the Enlightenment, however, the use of these aids was rejected (Figure 4.3) (De Moulin, 1988).

Wilhelmus Fabritius Hildanus, regarded as the father of German surgery, whose unusual treatment of ulcerating breast cancers was mentioned in Chapter 3, was the first to perform an axillary dissection (removal of the lymph nodes in the armpit) in breast cancer cases (Cabanne et al., 1983). Johann van Horne (1621-1670), professor of anatomy and surgery at Leiden, advised that breast cancer should not be operated on if there were swellings in the armpit, but some surgeons were prepared to remove the enlarged glands along with the affected breast (De Moulin, 1988).

Guillaume de Houppeville, a surgeon in Rouen, published an interesting book in 1693, entitled *The cure of breast cancer*, in which he gave a remarkable defense of mastectomy in cases of cancer. He claimed that the affected breast could be amputated without much pain. The reason he gave for this assertion was that the Ama-

CHAPTER 4

FIGURE 4.3 Instruments used in breast operations in the eighteenth century, as shown in Diderot and d'Alembert's Encyclopédie.

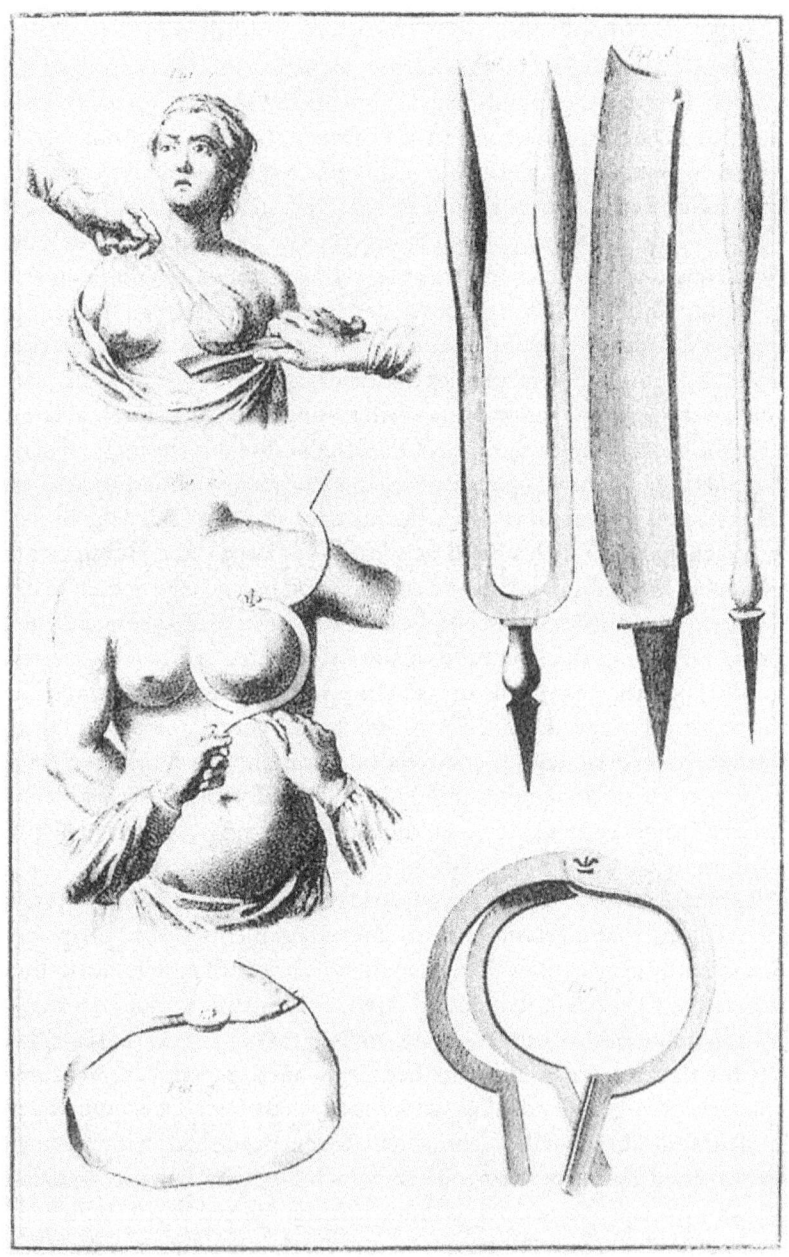

zons spoken of by the ancient Greeks were supposed to have the right breast removed in their youth. He stated that the pain due to the operation was much more bearable than that caused by the chronic cancer, supporting these views with the aid of six studies of cases that had been treated according to his method – including one woman who had been cured for five years (Cabanne et al., 1983).

It is noteworthy that Jean-Louis Petit (1674-1750) described the removal of the entire breast together with the pectoral fascia (the thin layer of connective tissue covering the pectoralis major, the main muscle of the chest wall) and the axillary glands (the lymph nodes of the armpit) in his handbook, published posthumously in 1774, while in the same year Bernard Peyrilhe recommended removal of the pectoral muscles as well. This shows that the principles of what would later be known as Halsted's operation had already been formulated in the second half of the eighteenth century (De Moulin, 1988).

Henri François Le Dran, the Parisian surgeon who finally demolished the black bile theory in 1757, regarded cancer – as we have seen – as a topical (local) disease in its early stages. It follows logically from this premise that cancers should be treated locally while they are still of limited extent. The only chance of cure, according to Le Dran, was thus early surgical removal of the tumor (Bett, 1954). This line of thought represented a major change in the approach to cancer since the time of Galen, who as we have seen believed in systemic treatment.

The work of surgeons gradually became more important. The major increase in surgical activity in the nineteenth century was largely due to two main developments: the introduction of general anesthesia and of antisepsis. These two advances had such an effect in increasing the possible scope of surgery that a separate section will now be devoted to each one in turn.

Anesthesia

Effective pain control was achieved very late on a historical time scale. This was one of the reasons why operations were feared in the pre-anesthesia era. It also contributed to the poor image surgery had in general. No real advances could be made in surgery until adequate methods of stilling pain were available. It is therefore appropriate to pause at this point to review the history of anesthesia, which has made such great contributions to the discipline of surgery.

Little data is available on the methods used to combat pain in antiquity, and even less is known about the effectiveness of the substances that were used for this purpose. The Ebers papyrus mentions the use of opium as an anesthetic, while Galen similarly recommended poppy extracts as a means of controlling the pain due to cancer (Cabanne et al., 1983). Henbane or stinking nightshade (Hyoscyamus niger), known for its hallucinogenic properties, and hemp (cannabis) were used as narcotics in India (Forgue and Bouchet, 1980).

It is known that large amounts of alcohol were often given to produce sedation. Forgue and Bouchet describe an abdominal operation in Uganda where the woman was given banana wine to drink until she was insensible, after which the operation could take place. Another member of the nightshade family, mandragora (mandrake) has been credited since time immemorial with pain-stilling properties among its many other alleged mystical and magical powers. There are many references to the mandrake in literature, including the Bible. Shakespeare refers four times to "mandrake" in his plays, and twice to mandragora. Furthermore, folk tales are full of references to magic sleep potions and the like, such as the poisoned apple that put Snow White into a death-like sleep until she was revived by the handsome prince (Rushman et al., 1996).

The first real step in the conquest of pain was the introduction of "laughing gas" or nitrous oxide. This compound was discovered in 1772 by the English chemist Joseph Priestley; P.C. Barton (1786-1828) from Philadelphia described its euphoric effects in 1808. The renowned English chemist Sir Humphry Davy (1778-1829) was the first to subject the physical properties of laughing gas, including its anesthetic effect, to scientific investigation. His report on this study, published in 1800, made his reputation. On this basis, he should be regarded as the father of anesthesia. Davy performed experiments on goldfish, cats and rabbits and then on himself and his friends. He described how inhalation of large quantities of the gas made a headache disappear immediately. On another occasion, he had a headache together with pain from an inflammation caused by dental treatment of a wisdom tooth; and inhalation of the gas once again cleared up the pain. On the basis of these observations, he proposed that the gas should be used to control pain during surgical operations. No heed was paid to his advice, however, and laughing gas was given no medical applications at that time. Despite Davy's findings, the gas continued to be used for entertainment purposes only. Inhalation of the gas at fairs and in domestic "laughing-gas parties" brought those involved into a state of utmost hilarity and promoted highly uninhibited behavior.

Knowledge of the ability of laughing gas to relieve pain and its other advantageous properties might have been lost forever but for the curious chain of events described below (Bouchet, 1983). "Professor" Gardner Quincy Colton (1814-1898) was an American showman, lecturer and former medical student who left medical school and travelled the country giving lectures and presentations after making $535 from his first public demonstration of the effects of nitrous oxide. On 10 December 1844, his travels took him to Hartford, Connecticut. A day after his public presentation there, he gave a private demonstration of the powers of laughing gas. Horace Wells (1815-1848), a local dentist, was one of those present. Wells saw how a young assistant apothecary, Samuel Cooley, cut his shin while under the influence of the gas, and related later that he had felt no pain during the incident.

Since Wells himself was in considerable pain at the time from a wisdom tooth, he asked Colton to administer the gas to him in his dental practice, after which another dentist of his acquaintance, John M. Riggs, could extract the offending tooth. When Wells came around from the narcosis he exclaimed, "this is the start of a new era for dental extraction!" Wells learned how to make nitrous oxide from Colton, and subsequently used this method of narcosis in his dental practice. The gas was administered by holding the patient's nostrils closed while blowing the gas (contained in an animal's bladder) via a wooden tube into the patient's mouth until he fell asleep.

After Wells had used this method successfully in his own practice for some time, he went to Boston to demonstrate it to a wider medical audience. Boston was the center of medical science in North America at that time. William Thomas Green Morton (1819-1868), a former colleague of Wells's, introduced him to a number of surgeons at Massachusetts General Hospital, including Dr. John Collins Warren (1778-1856). These two men will be making a repeat appearance in our story shortly. Warren invited Wells to demonstrate a dental extraction with nitrous oxide anesthesia to Warren's students at Harvard Medical School. Unfortunately, Wells did not give the patient enough laughing gas during the demonstration, and the patient complained of pain. The whole session turned into a fiasco, and Wells was booed out of the lecture theatre and accused of fraud. This event occurred in 1845. Despite this setback, Wells carried on using laughing gas in his own practice, but there was no question of its general application. In 1863, Colton introduced laughing gas in another dental practice, this time in New Haven, Connecticut (Rushman et al., 1996).

In the meantime, interest had focused on ether as a possible anesthetic. Diethyl ether was first synthesized in 1540 by Valerius Cordus (1515-1540), pharmacologist and botanist from Erfurt in Germany. He called it *oleum dulci vitrioli* or "vitriol." August Sigmund Frobenius, a German chemist, coined the name "ether." At that time, ether – like laughing gas – was used for recreational purposes in both America and Europe; "ether parties" were a common occurrence. It has been suggested in an article by Walter Channing that the analgesic effect of ether was discovered by chance in 1833 when an unknown chemist wiped it over his wife's face to cool her brow while she was in prolonged labor during the birth of their child, and noticed that she no longer complained of pain. Another name that crops up in the history of ether is that of Crawford Willamson Long (1819-1878), a general practitioner in Jefferson, Georgia, who had often inhaled ether and had observed that when he was hit while under narcosis – even if the blows were so hard that they left bruises – he could not remember being hit at all. This led him to believe that ether might be useful in surgery. After small-scale trials had proved its utility, he used it in his practice but did not publish his results until 1849.

The main contribution to the introduction of ether as an anesthetic was however once again made by a dentist, the above-mentioned William Morton, because he published his findings before Long. As we have seen, Morton had attended the failed laughing gas demonstration given by Wells at Massachusetts General Hospital. He regarded ether as an alternative. He had observed the favorable effect produced in patients who had inhaled ether vapor after he placed liquid ether in the painful cavities left after tooth extraction. Morton then tested the ether on himself, a dog and two young assistants. Although these trials were a success, he felt that he needed more chemical advice before he took the matter further. He therefore consulted Charles Thomas Jackson (1805-1880), a chemist from whom he had previously received lessons in Boston. It may be mentioned, incidentally, that these two were later involved in a bitter controversy about who deserved the credit for the introduction of ether anesthesia. After he had received the information he needed, Morton tried out the ether on his patients. When this worked well, he asked John Warren, the above-mentioned senior surgeon at Massachusetts General Hospital, for permission to administer ether to a patient who had to be operated on. This historic event occurred on 16 October 1846. The operation involved the removal of a vascular tumor under the mandible together with part of the tongue, and took place in what is now called the Ether Dome of Massachusetts General Hospital. The patient was the printer and journalist Edward Gilbert Abbott, and the operation was performed by John Warren himself. The patient felt no pain throughout the whole procedure. The news of the successful operation spread like wildfire through the hospital (Figure 4.4).

Oliver Wendell Holmes (1809-1894), gynecologist and professor of anatomy and physiology at Harvard Medical School in Boston, but better known to the general public as an author and poet, also heard of this event. It was he who coined the name "anesthesia" for the effect produced by the ether. He wrote a letter to Morton, including the following passages:

_____ *Dear Sir, Every one wants to have a hand in a great discovery. All I will do is to give you a hint or two as to names....The state should, I think, be called 'Anaesthesia.' This signifies insensibility, more particularly (as used by Linnaeus and Cullen) to objects of touch... The adjective will be 'Anaesthetic'....the term will be repeated by the tongue of every civilised race of mankind....You could mention these words which I suggest for their consideration.*

After the news of this operation was reported in a publication dated 18 November 1846 by Henry Jacob Bigelow (1818-1890), one of the surgeons at Massachusetts General Hospital, it spread rapidly throughout the world. It should be remembered that "rapidly" had a different meaning in the mid-nineteenth century to that taken for granted nowadays – even though Samuel F.B. Morse, the inventor of the Morse code, had actually developed and patented an electric telegraph in the United States in 1837, less than a decade before the above-mentioned operation. Morse sent America's first telegram on 6 January 1838, with the message "A patient waiter is no loser," a distance of 2 miles (3 kilometers) in the state of

FIGURE 4.4 Fragment of a painting (1882) entitled 'The First Operation Under Ether' by Robert Hinckley, which hangs in the Francis A. Countway Library of Medicine in Boston. It depicts the first successful operation under general ether anesthesia, performed by John Collins Warren at Massachusetts General Hospital in Boston on October 16, 1846.

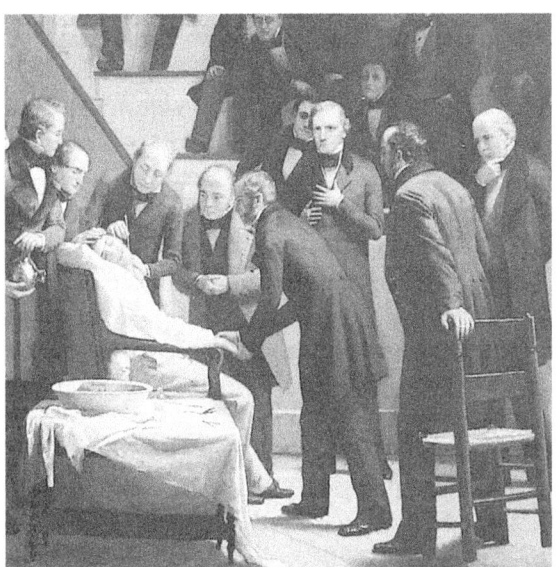

New Jersey, while on 24 May 1844 he sent the historic message "What hath God wrought" (quoting from the Book of Numbers 23:23) from the Capitol building in Washington, DC, to a railroad depot in Baltimore. The first commercially successful transatlantic telegraph cable was completed on 18 July 1866, and by the 1870s appreciable amounts of news were being telegraphed at the speed of light all around the world. Be this as it may, in 1846 all news between America and the rest of the world still had to be carried by boat. The Cunard steamship Acadia left Boston on 3 December 1846, carrying a letter written on 28 November of the same year by Jacob Bigelow, the father of the surgeon Henry Jacob Bigelow, to his friend Dr. Francis Boott in London. The letter took three weeks to reach its destination. Boott told the news to his neighbor James Robinson, who happened to be a dentist. On 19 December 1846, Robinson extracted an impacted molar from a Miss Lonsdale under ether anesthesia in Boott's house at 24 Gower Street. This is commemorated by a blue plaque on the wall of the London School of Hygiene and Tropical Medicine, which now stands on the site. The patient felt no pain, and did not move a muscle during the entire procedure, which was witnessed by Robinson's wife, two of his children and by Dr. Boott himself. The subsequent trials were unsuccessful, due to a defect in the inhalation device. Operations performed after the device had been repaired were a success, however, and the technique was adopted by many dentists throughout the country (Rushman et al., 1996).

Less than a year after the successful results obtained with ether, a new substance was added to the anesthetic arsenal. The American chemist Dr. Samuel Guthrie synthesized chloroform in 1831 in the village of Sackets Harbor, NY on the shores of Lake Ontario, using chlorinated lime and whiskey as his starting materials. The German chemist Justus von Liebig and the French chemist Eugène Soubeiran also succeeded in making chloroform independently, at practically the same time. The French chemist Jean-Baptiste Dumas analyzed the new compound, and named it chloroform, in 1834 (Thorwald). James Young Simpson (1811-1870), professor of obstetrics at Edinburgh University and Queen Victoria's gynecologist, published a report on 10 November 1847 of the good results he had obtained by giving women chloroform to inhale during childbirth. This volatile liquid, much more pleasant to use than ether, rapidly displaced the latter as an anesthetic (Bouchet, 1983). Chloroform anesthesia came of age in England after John Snow, the leading anesthetist in London at the time, administered it to Queen Victoria at her request and that of her consort Prince Albert when she gave birth to her eighth child, Prince Leopold. The delivery was painless and free from complications. From that moment, *narcose à la reine* was all the fashion (Thorwald). Chloroform was widely used in short operations during the next few decades. It was, however, quickly replaced by ether again when it was discovered to have some highly toxic properties, in particular a tendency to cause fatal cardiac arrhythmia.

Looking back on our review of the history of anesthesia we see that three important anesthetics were introduced in the course of a three-year period: nitrous oxide (laughing gas) in 1844, ether in 1846 and chloroform in 1847. The time must have been ripe for it.

In fact, however, an effective method of anesthesia had already been developed in Japan nearly half a century earlier. The surgeon Seishu Hanaoka (1760-1835) managed to produce general anesthesia as early as 1805, with the aid of a herbal mixture he called tsusensan[1] that he had formulated himself. The herbs he used were all known in East Asia for their medicinal properties, but also for the toxicity of certain components, which meant that they had to be used with great care. After twenty years of experimentation, mainly on cats, he arrived at the right formulation that proved capable of putting a cat to sleep for a twenty-four-hour period. He then tried the mixture on his wife, who was glad to play the part of a human guinea pig. She was unconscious for three whole days. After a few more experiments on his wife – who ultimately lost her sight as a result of the experiments – he was confident that he had the right combination of ingredients. Patients who took his tsusensan became insensitive to pain and lost consciousness for a period ranging from a half day to an entire day, depending on the dosage. The first patient that Hanaoka anesthetized in this way was a sixty-year-old woman with breast cancer. He removed the growth, and the anesthesia wore off after five hours. He subsequently operated on another 156 women for breast cancer. His success allowed him to raise his fees, and to attract a large number of students. It might be asked why this technique did not quickly achieve worldwide popularity. The reason was that the students had to swear a solemn oath, sealed in their own blood, never to pass on information about the knowledge and techniques they had learned at the school to outsiders – even their closest friends – since as indicated above failure to stick to the correct procedure precisely could be deadly dangerous, and Hanaoka wanted to avoid accidents. It should be remembered that such secrecy and the protection of professional know-how was in line with Japan's centuries-long tradition of living in isolation from the outside world. It was not until this isolation was broken in the 1850s – largely under pressure from the United States – that professional secrets like that of Hanaoka's were made public. But by that time laughing gas, ether and chloroform were already well-established in the medical world and there was no longer any place for tsusensan (Van Dierendonck 2008, Sawako Ariyoshi 1994).

---

1 Tsusensan consisted of 8 parts of Datura alba (white Angel's trumpet or thorn apple), 2 parts of Aconitum japonicum (Japanse Monkshood), 2 parts of Angelica dahurica (Angelica root), 2 parts of Angelica decursiva, 2 parts of Ligusticum wallichii (Szechuan lovage) and 2 parts of Arisaema japonica (related to Jack-in-the pulpit).

Antisepsis

A second advance that was crucial for the further development of surgery was the introduction of antisepsis, largely thanks to the efforts of one man: Joseph Lister (1827-1912). He was made Lord Lister and a member of the Order of Merit (a distinction personally awarded by the British monarch to a select group of individuals for outstanding services to the armed forces, science, the arts and the promotion of culture) for his work on this and other important medical issues. Before antisepsis, many operations failed due to the development of gangrene (necrosis of parts of the body, starting from the operation wound) and sepsis (general infection, spreading throughout the body). This was the other main reason for the poor repute of surgery. A number of scientific developments encouraged Lister to do something about this serious problem.

Oliver Wendell Holmes in Boston in 1843 and Ignaz Philip Semmelweis (1818-1865) in Vienna in 1847 reported that puerperal fever (also known as childbed fever, a frequent cause of death at that time) was infectious, and was due to poor hygiene. On the basis of these warnings and of the work of Louis Pasteur (1822-1895), the French chemist and microbiologist who formulated the germ theory of disease, Lister introduced the use of phenol (or carbolic acid, as he called it) as a disinfectant in operations in 1867 at Glasgow Royal Infirmary, where he worked in addition to his position as professor of surgery at Glasgow University. He described his findings in a series of historic articles in *The Lancet* that same year.

When he made his clinical rounds at the Glasgow Royal Infirmary, Lister could not avoid seeing many patients in the crowded wards dying of infection after their operations. Moreover, the ward stank of putrefaction. After making acquaintance with the experiments of Louis Pasteur and his germ theory, he became convinced that the suppuration of the patients' wounds was caused not by the "miasmas" (unhealthy air) in the wards but by the presence of microbes or germs. Lister was determined to clean not only the air but everything to do with the operations – from the surgical instruments and dressings to the surgeons' hands. After a number of failed experiments, Lister chose carbolic acid as his disinfectant and decided to test its effect on open fractures of the leg, which were particularly liable to suppuration. He placed large pieces of gauze soaked in carbolic acid on the wounds. When this gave good results, he decided to extend the approach by sterilizing the operation wound and the surgical instruments with a carbolic acid spray. The vaporizers spread the carbolic acid around so plentifully that the patient, the operating surgeon and his assistants were literally drenched in phenol. The reduction in the number of infections was astounding, and one might expect that his approach would immediately be copied on a very wide scale. That was not the case, however, since Lister's prescriptions for antisepsis meant that people had to break with long-standing procedures. His suggestions were initially greeted with a great deal of prejudice. Nevertheless, antiseptic surgery gradually spread. Karl

Thiersch was the first German surgeon to introduce this new approach, and many others in that country quickly followed his example. It took longer for antisepsis to gain ground among French surgeons, but after evidence accumulated that the use of carbolic acid led to a spectacular drop in blood poisoning and suppurating wounds their resistance to the new method fell away quite suddenly and it became generally introduced in France.

When antisepsis had convincingly proved its worth, surgeons tried to go a step further and keep germs out of the operating environment altogether. This led to the development of asepsis, which gradually reduced the dependency on Lister's brilliant discovery. Asepsis was made possible by the steam sterilization of surgical dressings, a technique developed by the Baltic German surgeon Ernst von Bergmann (1836-1907) in 1886, and the introduction of the sterilization of surgical instruments in autoclaves by the French surgeon Félix Terrier (1837-1908) in Paris in 1883.

Finally, William Steward Halsted (1852-1922), of The Johns Hopkins Hospital in Baltimore – considered by many to be the most innovative and influential American surgeon of all time – recommended the use of rubber gloves during operations. Halsted will reappear in this narrative later, in different roles. His original intention had not been to improve hygiene, but to make life easier for his outstanding theatre nurse Caroline Hampton, who suffered from rashes on the hands and arms brought on by the mercuric chloride used at the time to sterilize surgical instruments. He therefore asked the Goodyear Rubber Company to make a pair of thin rubber gloves for her. The surgeon and the nurse fell in love over the operating table, and married. History does not relate whether love or concern for the well-being of a valued member of staff was the real motive behind this request to Goodyear. As it happens, a trainee assistant in gynecology named Hunter Robb, who was working in the same hospital around the same time, also asked the Goodyear Rubber Company to make rubber gloves for him in order to protect women against puerperal fever. He published his findings in 1894, ten years before Halsted (Van Maanen et al., 1998). The white coat worn by doctors as a symbol of purity also came into use at the end of the nineteenth century. Until then, doctors always wore red or black academic robes.

Surgery became fully aseptic at this time, leading to a massive drop in rates of infection. It may be mentioned, for example, that the French surgeon Leopold Ollier (1830-1900), called the father of orthopedic surgery, who was professor of clinical surgery at Lyon Medical School and surgeon at the Hôtel-Dieu Hospital in Lyon, reported that the death rate after amputation among his patients fell from a terrible 48% before asepsis to 10% after the introduction of asepsis, other operative conditions remaining equal. In the last series of 49 amputations he recorded, in fact, the postoperative death rate actually fell to zero.

The introduction of anesthesia and antisepsis finally brought operations on the internal organs within the bounds of possibility (Bouchet, 1983).

CHAPTER 4

Modern oncological surgery

Modern surgical treatment of cancer dates from the beginning of the nineteenth century. On Christmas Day 1809, the rural doctor Ephraim McDowell (1771-1830) from Danville, Kentucky, operated on Jane Todd Crawford in the kitchen of his house to remove a gelatinous ovarian tumor weighing 11 kg. The patient sang hymns during the operation, which lasted twenty-five minutes, while her relatives stood on guard outside to deal with the surgeon in the event that Mrs. Crawford should die from the operation. It is claimed that they even had a noose ready for him and hanging from a nearby tree. Fortunately, however, the patient made an uncomplicated recovery and survived the operation for more than thirty years. In view of the primitive conditions prevailing at that time, this operation might be judged to be a foolhardy act on the part of McDowell, but it was not. He had had excellent medical training, from the renowned surgeon, gynecologist and anatomist John Bell (1763-1820) in Edinburgh, among others, and had taken ten days to prepare very thoroughly for this epoch-making venture (Figure 4.5). Until that time, ovarian cancer had been considered to be an incurable condition, eventually leading to the patient's death due to complete exhaustion. The Scottish doctor Alexander Hamilton had stated in his treatise on *The management of female complaints*, which went through several editions between 1792 and 1818, that opening the peritoneum and exposing the human internal organs to the cold air led immediately to infection with fatal results, and that tumors of the ovaries should therefore "be left to nature." Professors of surgery in those days proclaimed:

_____ *It will never be possible to excise internal tumors, be they of the womb, the stomach, the liver, the spleen or the intestines. God has set a limit to surgeons' abilities here. Those who exceed this limit commit an act of murder....*

McDowell's bravery in undertaking this operation was equaled only by that of his patient, who begged him to perform it. She rode 60 miles to get to Danville, tied on to her horse, with her tumor resting on the horn of her saddle. She said that she would rather die under the surgeon's knife than endure a lingering death without surgery. Her resolute attitude encouraged McDowell to perform the operation (Thorwald). This was the first of thirteen elective procedures carried out by McDowell; eight of his patients survived. A bronze statue of McDowell stands in the Capitol building in Washington, DC, a United States stamp was issued in his honor in 1959, and several paintings depicting this historic operation have been made (Figure 4.5, Hill, 1979).

As mentioned above in the section on anesthesia, the American surgeon John Collins Warren was the first to remove a cancerous tumor under ether anesthesia. However, Europe was at the forefront of advances in the field of surgery at the end of the nineteenth century. The two surgical giants at that time were the German-

FIGURE 4.5 Painting (1877-78) by George Kasson Knapp of the first successful surgical removal of a large ovarian cyst, performed by Dr. Ephraim McDowell in 1809.

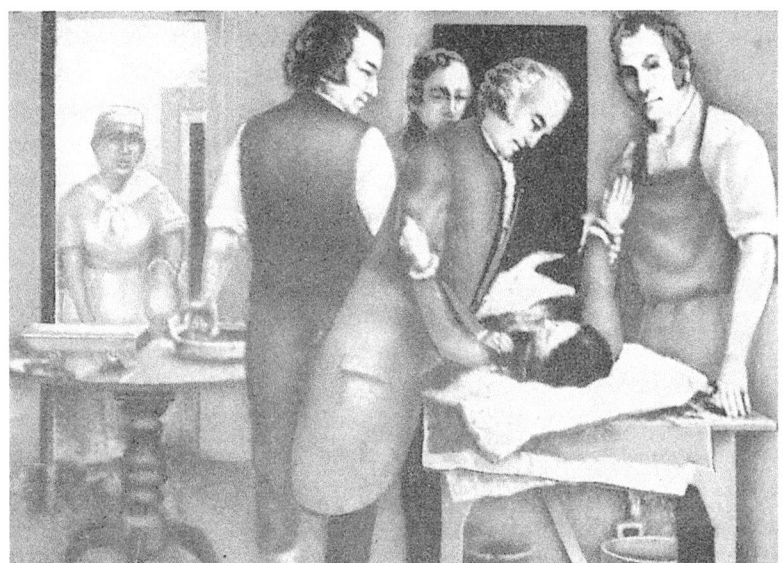

born Austrian surgeon Albert Christian Theodor Billroth (1829-1894) and Emil Theodor Kocher (1841-1917).

Billroth, the older and more resolute of the two, was professor of surgery in Vienna. He is regarded as the father of abdominal surgery. After he had tried out his gastric resection techniques on dogs, he achieved fame by being the first to remove the pylorus (the valve-like structure at the end of the stomach) as part of the treatment for cancer on 22 January 1881. The patient was Therèse Heller, a 43-year-old mother of eight childern who was suffering from gastric obstruction caused by a tumor of the pylorus that had been causing her to vomit for the preceding six weeks. The tumor was palpable in the upper abdomen. The day before the operation, the patient's stomach was washed out with 14 liters of water. The patient was sedated with a mixture of chloroform, ether and alcohol by one of Billroth's experienced private assistants, Dr. Barbieri (Santoro, 2005). The operation comprised resection of the affected parts followed by an end-to-end anastomosis (joining up of the remaining ends of tissue); this technique is still known as the Billroth-I operation. A few years later, in 1885, Billroth described another reconstructive technique known as gastrojejunostomy or the Billroth-II operation, involving resection of the pylorus and joining a length of the small bowel (jejunum) side-to-side to the bottom of the stomach for drainage.

Billroth had an excellent reputation in the medical world, thanks to his introduction of new gastric surgery techniques and his many other original contributions, such as the first resection of the esophagus and laryngectomy (surgical removal of the voicebox). He was also renowned for the introduction of the concept of the clinical audit: he gave an honest and detailed account not only of the successes but also the failures of his clinic, thus providing a basis for improvement of the performance. Apart from his medical skills, Billroth was a talented amateur musician and lover of music. He was a close personal friend of Brahms, and was a frequent guest conductor of the Zurich Symphony Orchestra during his period as professor of surgery at Zurich in the 1860s.

Theodor Kocher was a surgeon in Bern, Switzerland who was awarded the Nobel Prize in 1909 for his work on thyroid surgery and his analysis of the problems due to underproduction of thyroid hormones arising after resection of the thyroid gland. He observed that surgically successful resection of the thyroid gland led to cretinism (severe impairment of physical and mental development). After describing this problem, he proposed a solution: the surgeon should not remove the thyroid tissue completely but should leave a fragment in situ thus permitting sufficient production of thyroid hormones. Kocher's meticulous operating technique resulted in an extremely low rate of postoperative mortality: in one series of six-hundred patients, only one died.

Both Billroth and Kocher did however encounter another problem after thyroid surgery, for which William Steward Halsted was able to offer an explanation. Billroth, noted for his quick but not exactly meticulous surgical technique, was concerned to observe the frequent occurrence of postoperative tetany (painful muscle cramp) in his patients; however, they never developed myxedema (poor condition marked by lethargy and dry, yellow skin, due to inadequate or absent thyroid function). Kocher's patients, on the other hand, did not get tetany but often suffered from myxedema. Halsted suggested that Billroth often accidentally performed a parathyroidectomy (resection of the parathyroid gland) on his patients, while this never happened to Kocher's patients thanks to his very careful operating technique. This was later confirmed by further study (Hill, 1979). It may be mentioned in passing that we also owe the Kocher clip or hemostatic forceps (used to control the bleeding from blood vessels) to Kocher.

Surveys of advances in surgery generally limit themselves to the big events such as the first gastrectomy (surgical removal of the stomach) and the first esophagus resection, but due attention should also be paid to the smaller advances, without which the big ones could never be made. A good example is the Lembert stitch (or Lembert suture) first described in 1826 by Anton Lembert (1802-1851) as a means of providing secure serosa-to-serosa connections. (Serosa is the medical name for the thin membrane lining most body cavities.) This is still the standard procedure for making gastrointestinal anastomoses, and medical students still have to learn how to make Lembert stitches (among many other things) in preparation for surgical practice.

Surgery of the stomach would not have been able to develop to its present level without a deep understanding of the physiology of the gastrointestinal system. William Beaumont (1785-1853) made a significant contribution to our knowledge in this field. He was a surgeon in the US Army who was called on in 1822 to treat a young man named Alexis St. Martin, a French-Canadian employee of the American Fur Company on Mackinac Island, for accidental gunshot wounds that were so severe that it was not thought that he would survive: the buckshot had ripped open the lower part of his torso and his abdomen, and pierced his left lung, diaphragm and stomach. Thanks to the excellent care he received from Dr. Beaumont, the young man recovered but he was left with a permanent hole (fistula) in his stomach. Over the years, Beaumont made use of the fistula to study the production of gastric juices and the physiology of the digestive process directly. He published his findings in 1833 in the classic book *Experiments and Observations on the Gastric Juice and the Physiology of Digestion*.

The French physician and physiologist Claude Bernard (1813-1878), whose illustrated manual of operative surgery and surgical anatomy (co-authored with Charles Huette) from 1848 was reprinted as late as 1873 and translated into English, German, Dutch, Italian and Spanish, is generally recognized as the father of experimental medicine, following his teacher François Magendie (1783-1855). His wide-ranging research into the physiology of the gastrointestinal tract, the pancreas and the liver helped to provide a firm basis for the assessment of the consequences of surgical operations.

Various developments in the field of general surgery also had an important impact on cancer surgery. For example, Karl Thiersch, professor of surgery at Erlangen who described the epithelial nature of cancer, also introduced a radically improved method of split-skin grafting in 1886. The Thiersch graft (also known as the Ollier-Thiersch graft) is still used today to repair skin defects left by cancer surgery. In 1873, Friedrich von Esmarch (1823-1908) from Kiel, Germany described the development of a rubber tourniquet that could be used to deprive the extremities of blood before operating on them. This principle is still used to facilitate the excision of tumors of the extremities, or the perfusion of tumors of the limbs with cytostatics, but the necessary constriction is now produced by inflating a cuff around the limb rather than by tightening a tourniquet (Hill, 1979).

To give a clearer overview of the developments in the various fields of cancer surgery, we will now describe them with reference to the type of cancer involved.

Gastrointestinal tumors

Jules Emile Pean, a renowned French surgeon, performed the first gastric resection for cancer of the stomach on 9 April 1879. Sadly, the patient died on the fifth postoperative day. About a year and a half later, on 5 November 1880, Ludwig von Rydygier, later professor of surgery at the University of Cracow, performed a similar operation at his private surgical clinic in Culm (now Chelmno); this patient survived nine days. The first successful gastric resection was performed by Billroth on Thérèse Heller in 1881, as described above. The first total gastric resection was performed by the Swiss physician Carl B. Schlatter (1864-1934) in 1897 (Raven, 1990).

Well-known people who have died of stomach cancer include Napoleon, the Irish writer James Joyce and Pope John XXIII – known to many as "the most loved pope in history" (Santoro, 2005).

The first successful operation on the esophagus, by Billroth, was also mentioned above. Henri Pillore, a surgeon in Rouen, performed the first elective colostomy in 1776, for cancer of the rectum. According to Pillore's own account, translated much later by Tilson Dinnick, the patient, whose name was Morel, was a wine merchant and posting master (that is, he was probably in charge of a staging post where stagecoaches could change horses and passengers could rest) from Vert-Gallant in the district of Brai. (The modern names are Vert-Galant, in the Pays de Bray; this little hamlet is about 15 km northeast of Rouen.) He had been suffering from constipation, and went to Rouen for medical assistance. He was prescribed laxatives, and when they did not help he was advised to swallow two pounds of mercury in the hope that that might clear the obstruction; but that was no help either. He then consulted Dr. Pillore, who on digital examination found a rectal carcinoma that was completely obstructing the lumen. Pillore suggested that a colostomy should be performed, and the patient agreed. To be on the safe side, Pillore requested a second opinion from five of his colleagues. They all rejected Pillore's proposal, but when the patient asked whether they had any alternative they said they did not. He also asked whether his condition was fatal. When they all confirmed that it was, Morel urged Dr. Pillore to perform the operation. Immediately after the operation, the patient's bowels discharged and his abdomen became much less distended. Fourteen days layer, the stoma had healed sufficiently for the stitches to be removed. The patient felt very well. From postoperative day 20, however, his abdomen started swelling again and the patient finally died on day 28. Pillore suggested that the cause of death was actually the massive dose of mercury the patient had ingested, which appears to have led to gangrenous inflammation and perforation of the intestines (Corman, 2000).

The first surgical removal of the rectum as a treatment for cancer was performed by Richard von Volkmann (1830-1889) from Halle in Germany, who published an account of it in 1887. The same year saw a publication by the German surgeon Paul Kraske (1851-1930), describing his approach to resection of the rectum that involved removing the coccyx and part of the sacrum; this technique is still known as Kraske's operation. Abdominoperineal resection (involving a combined approach to the rectum via the abdomen and the perineum) is generally associated with the name of the English surgeon Sir Ernest Miles (1869-1947), who published his reasoned arguments for this technique in 1908. Vincenz Czerny (1842-1916), a Czech surgeon who worked in Germany and Austria, had however already performed an operation of this type as early as 1884. Another early worker in this field was H. Widenham Maunsell from New Zealand, who is claimed to have performed the first planned abdominoperineal resection in 1894 (Hill, 1979).

Operations on the colon (large intestine) were long considered too risky, because of the danger of bacterial infection from the intestinal flora. However, the French surgeon Jean-François Reybard (1795-1863) from Lyon reported in 1844 on an operation he had performed in 1833, which involved removing a tumor the size of an orange from the flexure of the sigmoid and joining up the free ends of the intestine. The patient had survived the operation for ten months before succumbing to a recurrence of the cancer (Nordenstam et al., 2007).

The Royal Academy of Medicine in Paris appointed a committee on March 7, 1843, to investigate Reybard's claim to have cured a cancer of the sigmoid. The report of this committee (probably the first on new and unproved methods of cancer treatment) contains Reybard's detailed description of the complicated, double, interrupted intestinal suture, with all its needles, threads, loose ends, knots and tufts, that still bears his name. The chairman of the committee reported to the Academy on July 30, 1844, that his committee had studied Reybard's technique as demonstrated unsuccessfully on seven dogs, and had obtained clinical data concerning the patient, Joseph Valernaud, who lived until March 16, 1834, nearly a year after the operation. The surgical specimen had been discarded and there had been no autopsy. It was, therefore, impossible for the committee to learn anything of value to science from this case. Reybard was thanked and complimented upon his enthusiasm and the commitee's report was filed in the archives of the Academy (Reybard et al. 1844).

Professor W. Körte, surgical director of the still existing Krankenhaus am Urban in Berlin, reported in 1883 that the Austrian surgeon Karl Maydl (1853-1903) had described eighteen colostomy operations carried out in Germany by various surgeons, including one performed by himself. Eight of the patients involved recovered. Even though Maydl's patient was among those who responded well, Maydl still expressed his doubts about the advisability of this operation (Körte, 1900). The first truly successful colectomy was not performed until 1914, by the French surgeon René Leriche (1879-1955) in Lyon (De Moulin, 1988).

Surgery of the pancreas has also had a difficult history, though the existence of tumors in this organ has long been known. Giovanni Battista Morgagni (1682-1771), professor of pathologic anatomy at Padua, was the first to describe cancer of the pancreas, which he did in 1761 (Tsuchiya and Fuhsawa, 1999). Sir Frederick Grant Banting (1891-1941), a Canadian physiologist and biochemist, his student Charles Herbert Best and the Scottish physiologist John James Richard Macleod (1876-1935), working at the University of Toronto, isolated insulin and proved its importance for the treatment of diabetes. Banting and Macleod won the Nobel Prize in 1923 for this discovery, though there was some controversy about this award since it was claimed by some that Macleod played only a nominal role and that Best should have received the prize instead of him. One of the spin-offs of this research was the discovery that insulin also had an important impact on surgery of the pancreas for the treatment of cancer of that organ.

Allen Oldfather Whipple (1881-1963) was an American surgeon who was born in Persia (present-day Iran). When he described a technique for pancreaticoduodenectomy (surgical removal of the pancreas and the duodenum) in 1935, pancreas surgery was a shambles. Whipple's original approach was to perform a two-stage operation, the first stage comprising displacement of the bile duct together with gastrojejunostomy. In the second stage, about three weeks later, the duodenum and the head of the pancreas were removed. The procedure was quite soon modified, however, so that the entire operation could be performed at one time (Figure 4.6). Unfortunately, Whipple's operation is still considered only for a limited number of patients with cancer of the pancreas, since by the time the carcinoma is discovered the tumor is often too big to be operable, or has metastasized. It can however often also be of use in treatment of carcinomas of the papilla of Vater and the duodenum. Whipple received many awards during his lifetime. There was one he was definitely not proud of, and he never showed it to anyone. This was a medal he received from Adolph Hitler for his care of four victims of the Hindenburg disaster, who received severe burns when the German zeppelin *Hindenburg* caught fire and was completely destroyed while attempting to dock in New Jersey on 6 May 1937, after a transatlantic flight. Whipple had received instructions from

FIGURE 4.6 a and b Schematic representation of the resection (a) and reconstruction (b) phases of the Whipple operation for carcinoma of the pancreas (from C.J.H. van de Velde, J.H.J.M. van Krieken, P.H.M. De Mulder and J.B. Vermorken (eds.), Oncologie, Bohn, Stafleu van Loghum, 2005).

a

Resection: removal of the duodenum and the head of the pancreas

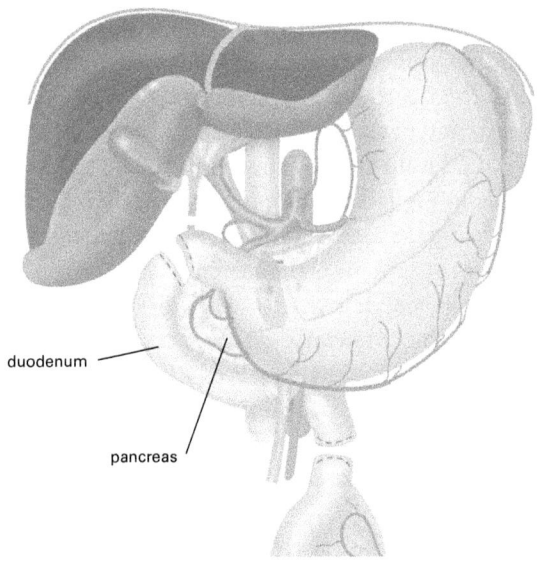

b

Reconstruction: diversion of biliary duct; attachment of stomach opening and pancreas remnant to the jejunum

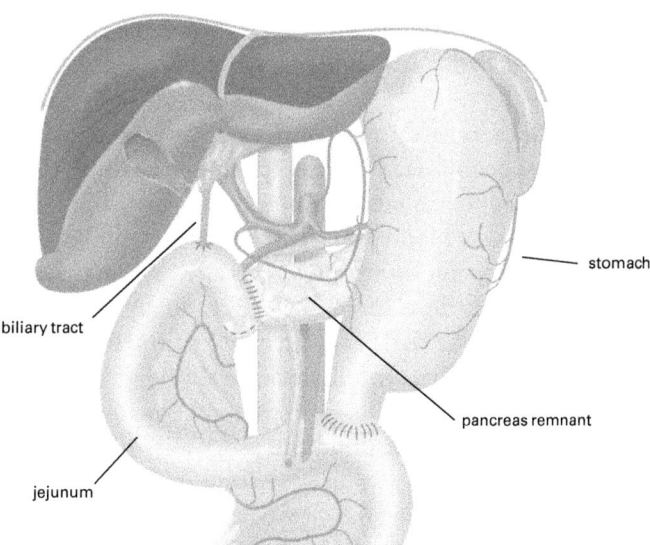

Berlin to make sure that the four patients – all officers of the Hindenburg – did not receive any Jewish blood. The four men survived thanks to transfusions of blood from the blood bank–which did not provide a certificate guaranteeing the Aryan antecedents of the blood (Fuhrman, 2005).

Elective surgery for bile-duct cancer was made possible when Evarts Graham (1883-1957), Glover Copher and Warren Henry Cole developed the technique for oral cholecystography in 1924.

It would take us beyond the scope of this book to describe all the subsequent advances in gastrointestinal surgery in detail, but a couple of points stand out. Firstly, the possibility of removing metastases from the liver. Another fairly recent advance in the treatment of rectal carcinoma deserves further mention, namely the introduction of total mesorectal excision (the TME procedure), which was reported by R.J. Heald and co-workers in 1982. Heald was a surgeon at the Basingstoke Clinic in England. In response to the high local recurrence rate after rectal resection, he introduced *en bloc* resection of the rectum together with the mesorectum since the latter was the region where the initial metastases were typically found (Heald, 1998). His results were initially greeted with skepticism, since he claimed a recurrence rate of 4% as compared with values ranging from 20% to 60% achieved by other surgeons. However, a large-scale multidisciplinary randomized study involving many Dutch clinics, headed by Cornelis van de Velde, professor of surgery at Leiden, confirmed his conclusions.

Breast cancer

Sir James Paget (1814-1899) made an important clinical observation in the field of breast cancer when in 1874 he described "Paget's disease of the nipple," an eczematous condition of the nipple and its immediate surroundings. This condition is still regarded as a warning signal for breast cancer, and if found is always followed by a biopsy.

Breast cancer treatment strategy underwent a major change of direction after the introduction of radical mastectomy in 1890 by William Stewart Halsted (Figure 4.7). This approach was developed in response to criticism published in 1867 by Charles Hewitt Moore (1821-1870) from the Middlesex Hospital in London of the inadequate operating technique prevalent at that time. Starting from the idea that cancer initially develops locally and gradually spreads to the surrounding tissue, Halsted thought that radical removal of the breast together with the underlying muscles and the lymph nodes in the neighboring armpit would provide the best chance of cure. This line of thought is no longer considered valid, since if the cancer is locally widespread the prognosis will almost certainly be determined by micrometastases at a distance from the original source. Nevertheless, radical mastectomy remained the method of choice for nearly a century. In the long run, the mutilating nature of this procedure led to a search for other, equally effective

FIGURE 4.7 Illustration of radical mastectomy (a) as proposed by the surgeon William Stewart Halsted, together with a photograph of Halsted (b). (source: Shimkin, 1979, courtesy of the National Institute of Health, Bethesda, MD, USA).

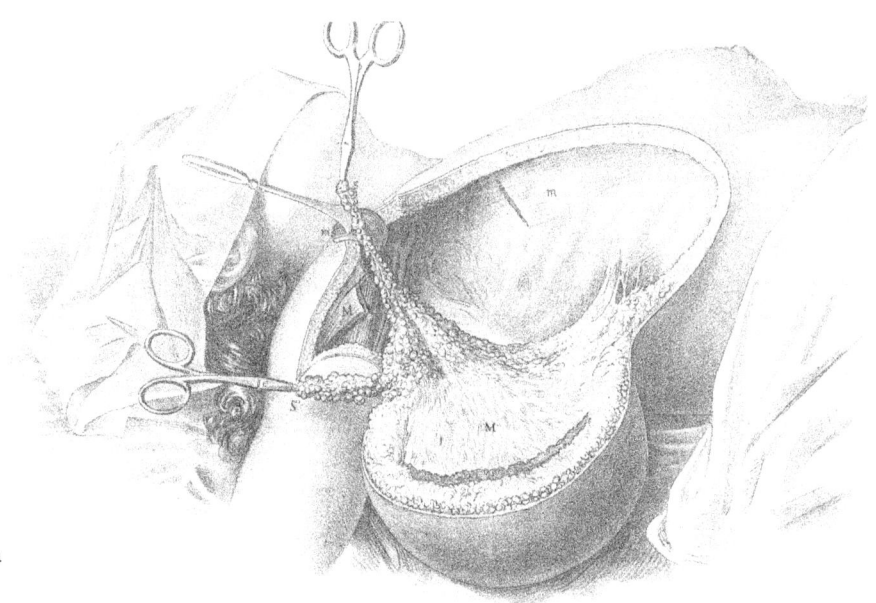

a

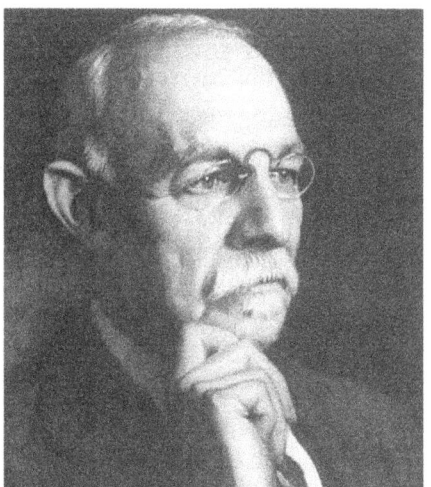

b

methods that did not attack the integrity of the patient's body in such an extreme way (Hill, 1979). One of the leading figures in the campaign against radical mastectomy in the United States was George Crile Jr. (1908-1992), son of the George Crile mentioned in the section on tumors of the head and neck.

Robert McWhirter (1904-1994), professor of medical radiology at the University of Edinburgh, came up with an alternative to radical mastectomy in 1948. This comprised simple removal of the breast, followed by irradiation of the breast and regional lymph nodes. He believed that this approach would not only reduce the operational trauma but also lead to a lower risk of dissemination of the cancer cells (McWhirter, 1948). A randomized trial carried out by the Danes Sigvard Kaae and Helge Johansen showed that McWhirter's approach led to results that were just as good as the more aggressive radical mastectomy (Kaae and Johansen, 1977).

In the US, the National Surgical Adjuvant Breast and Bowel Project (NSABP) Group, headed by Bernard Fisher, professor of surgery at the University of Pittsburgh, went a step further by initiating a large-scale study of the value of breast-conserving surgery. Patients were assigned at random to a group scheduled for total mastectomy, a group that underwent lumpectomy (removal of the tumor alone) if the tumor did not exceed 4 cm in size, and a group that underwent lumpectomy followed by irradiation of the breast. The axillary lymph nodes were removed in all patients. This study showed no significant differences in survival rates between the three groups (Fisher et al., 2002).

The trend towards early detection of breast cancer means that such breast-conserving operations are possible in many cases; this must be regarded as a significant advance in the treatment of this disease.

The introduction of the sentinel lymph node biopsy technique was another important step toward as more patient-friendly treatment of breast cancer. This technique is based on identification of the lymph node first reached by metastasizing cancer cells from the region of the tumor, which is known as the sentinel node. To this end, a tiny amount of radioactive technetium albumin colloid is injected at the site of the primary tumor, if necessary with a small amount of a blue dye; these substances are then transported via the lymph ducts to the nearest lymph node. The sentinel node, which is identified by detecting the radioactivity with a Geiger counter or by visual inspection of the blue dye, can then be removed for pathological investigation. If it is found to be affected by the cancer there is no need to remove the other nodes; this procedure thus avoids unnecessary postoperative lymphedema (accumulation of lymph) in the arm that is often a consequence of biopsies. The sentinel node technique was based on animal experiments by R.K. Gilchrist in 1940 and I. Zeidman and J.M. Buss in 1954. The term "sentinel node" was first used by Gould et al. in 1954, who used the identification of a sentinel node as an indication for parotidectomy (resection of the salivary gland next to the ear). The patient they were treating had a tumor of the parotid gland; a normal-looking lymph node in the drainage area of this gland was selected as a possible sentinel node and sent to the pathologist for examination. When this turned out to be positive, it was decided that the patient required parotidectomy combined with radical neck dissection to remove as much of the affected areas as possible; further details of this type of surgery are given below in the section on tumors of the head and neck. Nearly two decades later, in 1977, Ramon M. Cabanas from the Victory Memorial Hospital in Brooklyn, New York, observed a sentinel node in the lymph drainage area of the penis. K. Kett from the University of Oslo, B. Christensen from Copenhagen and C.D. Haagensen, professor of clinical surgery at Columbia University, independently pioneered the introduction of the sentinel node technique for breast cancer patients (Tanis et al., 2001).

Lung cancer

Modern thoracic surgery was impossible before the introduction of endotracheal anesthesia with positive ventilation pressure, which avoided the risk of lung collapse under the pressure of the atmosphere. The German surgeon Ernst Ferdinand Sauerbruch (1875-1951) sought a solution to this problem through the use of a hypobaric chamber (a chamber where the air pressure is less than the atmospheric air pressure). He designed this chamber – which came to be known as the Sauerbruch chamber – in 1904, while he was still an assistant in the clinic led by Johannes von Mikulicz (1850-1905) in Breslau. Sauerbruch performed the first open-lung operation in this hypobaric chamber in 1908. The patient's head was left outside the chamber, so the anesthetist could monitor his condition. This rather cumbersome solution was technically feasible, but gave rise to so many problems of patient management and coordination of the surgical team in the big chamber while making it impossible to deal easily with complications that the method was deemed impractical and was little used. Sauerbruch did use the method for many years, and continued to defend its use. Sauerbruch was a towering figure in the world of thoracic surgery, and made many other contributions in this field. Sadly, increasing dementia towards the end of his life led him to carry out many absurd operations, often with fatal results. While his position of authority allowed him to continue this practice for some time despite concerns expressed by colleagues, he was finally dismissed from his position in 1949.

Almost immediately after the introduction of Sauerbruch's hypobaric chamber, a much simpler and potentially more effective method came on the scene, that of intratracheal positive-pressure ventilation which involves blowing a constant stream of air mixed with an anesthetic into the lungs through a tube inserted into the windpipe. The modern tube with inflatable cuff was developed in 1909 by Samuel James Meltzer (1851-1920) and his son-in-law John Auer (1875-1948) at the Rockefeller Institute in New York. This method was thus known before the First World War and was used to a certain extent during that war, but was not employed on a large scale until after the Second World War (Hill, 1979). It enabled G. Divis to remove pulmonary metastases in 1927 (Rosenberg, 2001), and Evarts Graham to perform the first successful pneumonectomy for lung cancer in 1933. The patient lived for thirty years after the operation, without any sign of a recurrence. Edward Churchill (1895-1972), professor of surgery at Harvard Medical School, introduced pulmonary lobectomy in 1931. During the late 1930s he worked with the English surgeon Ronald Belsey (1910-2007), then in Harvard as a visiting scholar, to refine lung resection with their technique of segmental resection. They published their results in 1939 (Hill, 1979). Belsey later worked as a surgeon at St. Thomas' Hospital in London and then in Bristol, where he made the thoracic unit at the Frenchay Hospital an internationally renowned center of excellence.

Neurologic tumors

Sir Victor Horsley (1857-1916) was the first to venture into the domain of modern neurosurgery. He died at the early age of 59 in Mesopotamia (present-day Iraq) from heat stroke while performing field surgery duty in the English expeditionary force during the First World War. He is known as the first surgeon to remove a spinal tumor, in 1887. He also performed important animal experiments and cranial surgery in humans, and is sometimes called the father of neurosurgery (Lyons, 1987). His work was continued by Harvey Cushing (1869-1939) from The Johns Hopkins Hospital in Baltimore and the Peter Bent Brigham Hospital in Boston, and by Walter Edward Dandy (1886-1946), also from Johns Hopkins. While both Cushing and his pupil Dandy were outstanding surgeons, powerful personalities and gifted authors, it is Cushing who is generally seen as the great pioneer of neurosurgery. Cushing's hypophysis operation from 1912 and Dandy's operations on the trigeminus and acoustic nerves are still regarded as models of perfection by present-day neurosurgeons. Cushing operated on more than 2000 brain tumors, in particular primary gliomas and meningeomas. He was however very hesitant to operate on metastases. He introduced the vascular clip (also known as the "silver clip" or Cushing's clip), designed to reduce blood loss during operations, in 1911 and in 1928 he pioneered electrocauterization for control of bleeding in cooperation with W.T. Bovie. He also demonstrated how elevated intracranial pressure should be treated.

Alongside the brain, the spinal cord is the second field of interest to the neurosurgeon. Many have contributed to the development of spinal surgery, including Gilbert Horrax (1887-1957) of the Lahey Clinic near Boston, who described the advances made in this field throughout the ages in the book *Neurosurgery. An historical sketch*, published by Charles C. Thomas in Springfield, Illinois in 1952.

The third application of neurosurgery in the field of cancer was for pain relief. The Portuguese neurologist Antonio Egas Moniz (1874-1955) was a pioneer in this domain. He won the Nobel Prize in 1949 for his controversial introduction of the surgical operation of prefrontal lobotomy (cutting through the connections between the prefrontal cortex and the rest of the brain to limit the flow of sensory information). This operation became quite popular throughout the world in the 1940s, mainly for the treatment of mental illnesses such as schizophrenia. Moniz pointed out that it could also be highly effective in reducing extreme pain. The arrival of psychotropic drugs (of which chlorpromazine was the first, in 1952) soon led to a rapid decline in the use of this operation, and it is now generally regarded as a barbaric mistake except in certain very rare cases. In the 1950s, it was sometimes used in combination with hypophysectomy in the treatment of metastasized breast cancer.

Other important pain control measures were chordotomy (selective severing of the sensory nerves in the spinal column), introduced in 1912 by W.G. Spiller and E. Martin (Rosenberg, 2001), and rhizotomy (selective severing of the dorsal nerve roots in the spinal cord) (Hill, 1979).

Finally, it may be mentioned that George Crile, who will reappear in the next section, was the first to perform major operations under anesthesia with intraneural injections of cocaine, in 1887.

TUMORS OF THE HEAD AND NECK

Surgeons were initially very reluctant to operate on tumors of the head and neck, especially because of the risk that the patient would be left massively mutilated and the more immediate risk of uncontrollable bleeding during the operation. Pietro de Marchetti (1589-1673), professor of surgery at Padua and author of the *Observationum Medico-Chirurgicarum Sylloge*, was one of the first to remove a tumor of the tongue. He performed this operation in 1664, with the aid of cauterization. Cautery was replaced by use of the scalpel around 1800. Antoine Louis (1723-1792) introduced the use of a ligature to cut off the arterial blood supply to the tumor in 1759, but the continued risk of hemorrhage stimulated the search for other methods. Home in 1805 described a procedure for glossectomy by means of a ring of sutures, while Bell in the second half of the nineteenth century introduced an instrument known as a "chain ecraseur," which incorporated a screw-operated tightening device that allowed a chain to be gradually pulled tight around the tumor until it was pinched off. The ecraseur was also used for other surgical purposes, such as the removal of uterine and ovarian tumors. Examples produced by different makers may be found in many medical museums and among the stock of many medical antique dealers.

Sir Henry Trentham Butlin (1845-1912) is generally regarded as the father of British head and neck surgery. He was appointed Surgical Registrar at St. Bartholomew's Hospital in London in 1872, and elected to the position of Assistant Surgeon in 1880. As the junior surgeon, he was allotted the most unpopular task, the treatment of tumors of the head and neck. When this position became vacant, the senior surgeon (who was also chairman of the Appointments Committee) said,

CHAPTER 4

"Well, Butlin is the youngest. He will have to do it." As Butlin himself said later, this meant that he was given a job for which he had not the slightest qualifications. He did it so well, however, that he was knighted in 1911 – just a year before his death. He achieved renown for his contributions to the treatment of cancer of the mouth in general and cancer of the tongue in particular. He recommended removal of the regional lymph nodes as early as 1898. Before he started his work, the cure rate for carcinoma of the tongue was 5%, while later on in his career it had risen to 41.5% (McGurk and Goodger, 2000).

Radical surgery of tumors of the head and neck was developed by a number of innovative surgeons, including John Collins Warren from Boston (already mentioned in the section on anesthesia). One epic incident in this history was the operation performed by William Williams Keen (1837-1932) and a team of other surgeons in 1893, to remove a sarcoma from the hard palate of Grover Cleveland, who was then President of the United States. At that time, the country was in the grip of a depression and the general atmosphere of financial panic threatened to disrupt the national economy. If news of the President's illness had leaked out, it could have destroyed public confidence in the country's currency, leading to an economic disaster. The operation was therefore carried out in the deepest secrecy, on board the presidential yacht. It lasted an hour and a half and was a real ordeal for the President, who later told a friend, "My God, they nearly killed me!" But he recovered well, and since the surgical incision was inside his mouth the operation left no visible scars. The operation was a success, as was the campaign to keep it secret. It was not until 1917, nine years after Cleveland's death and 24 years after the operation, that William Keen revealed details of the operation in an article (Patterson, 1987). The tumor was preserved, and is now on display at the Mutter Museum in Philadelphia. News of the operation raised medical confidence in the feasibility of radical extirpation of cancers of the face and oral cavity. Despite his involvement in the above incident, Keen was best known as the first American brain surgeon. He was an eminent physician, with a wide range of activities, and served six American presidents as medical adviser. It was he who diagnosed Franklin D. Roosevelt's paralysis as polio in 1921 (though it is currently believed that the President's ailment was in fact probably Guillain-Barré syndrome). This was another presidential complaint that had to be carefully concealed from the public.

The American surgeon George Crile (1864-1943) described the classical method of radical neck gland dissection in 1906, on the basis of his own experience of 132 operations. He made many other contributions to medical science and practice. In addition to his long-standing interest in the mechanism and treatment of shock, he performed the first successful blood transplantation from one human to another, also in 1906.

The problem faced by surgeons wishing to operate on tumors of the larynx was that they are so difficult to see and that any attempt to insert a laryngoscope into the patient's throat while the patient was conscious was met by powerful gag reflexes. A solution was found in indirect laryngoscopy, in which the physician shines a bright light into the patient's mouth via a concave mirror held between the physician's teeth and views the image. An improved construction was proposed in 1864 by Dr. Thomas J. Walker, a surgeon at Peterborough Infirmary in England: he mounted the mirror on a headband that could be worn on the physician's head, thus leaving his hands free to manipulate. There is disagreement about who invented the first indirect laryngoscope. Some give the credit to the world-famous German physician and physicist Hermann von Helmholz (1821-1894) whose first important invention (in 1851) was the ophthalmoscope, which revolutionized medical examination of the eye. Others cite the Spaniard Manuel Garcia (1805-1906), equally famous in his own field as a professor of music in Paris and London, whose pupils included Jenny Lind, the "Swedish Nightingale." Garcia is said to have developed this instrument to help him to analyze the singing technique of his pupils. Indirect laryngoscopy became better known to the medical world through the publications of the Austrian neurologist Ludwig Türck (1810-1868) in Vienna and Johann Nepomuk Czermak (1828-1873). However, the most powerful advocate of indirect laryngoscopy was Sir Morrell Mackenzie (1837-1892), known as the father of laryngology, an English laryngologist of Scottish descent who became the personal physician of both the English and German royal families. He learned the technique of indirect laryngoscopy in Vienna and introduced it to London. He also founded the London Hospital for Diseases of the Throat in Soho, which prompted Sir James Paget (mentioned in the section on breast cancer) to joke, "Someone should found a hospital for diseases of the big toe" (McGurk and Goodger, 2000). The use of indirect laryngoscopy declined following the introduction of fiber-optic flexible laryngoscopes in the 1970s and their perfection in the 1980s, as described for example in the book *Endoscopic Evaluation and Treatment of Swallowing Disorders* by Susan E. Langmore.

The American head and neck surgeon Jacob da Silva Solis-Cohen (1838-1927) was the first to perform a partial laryngectomy, while Billroth performed the first full laryngectomy for cancer on New Year's eve 1873 (Shah, 1998). The treatment was effective in curing the cancer, but as is inevitable in such cases the patient was no longer able to speak since the vocal cords had been removed. At that time, the only way patients could regain their voice was by learning how to swallow air and modulating the burps they produced. Nowadays, more sophisticated (electronic) methods of voice replacement are available that give a more natural-sounding result.

Sir Morell Mackenzie also treated the German Kaiser Frederick III. The Dutch ENT specialist R. Wentges from Nijmegen reviewed this case in his article *Een keizer zonder stem* (A Voiceless Kaiser) (Wentges, 1995), and much of the following account is translated from that article. Frederick complained of increasing hoarseness in January 1887, when he was 56 years old and still Crown Prince. His personal physician Dr. Wegner prescribed inhalations, but when a six-week course of these did not help Carl Gerhardt, professor of internal medicine at the University of Berlin, was consulted. He was able to examine the Crown Prince's vocal cords with the aid of a mirror, and observed a swelling at the rear of the left true vocal cord. This was surgically removed in a number of sittings, but the hoarseness persisted. Six weeks later, moreover, the mobility of the left vocal cord was found to be reduced, which was considered to be a possible sign of cancer. Gerhardt therefore called in a number of other specialists, of whom Professor Ernst von Bergmann (mentioned above in connection with the sterilization of surgical dressings) was the chief. On the basis of Gerhardt's suspicion of cancer, von Bergmann decided that the best approach was a laryngofissure – that is, surgical opening of the larynx to reveal the tumor and thus facilitate its removal. This was however an operation associated with high mortality at that time. Possibly at the urging of Princess Victoria, wife of Frederick and eldest child of Queen Victoria of England, it was decided to consult Sir Morell Mackenzie before proceeding further. On arrival in Berlin, Mackenzie went straight to the Neue Palast and got to work. He observed a swelling the size of a split pea at the rear of the Crown Prince's left vocal cord. The German specialists continued to believe that an operation was called for, but Mackenzie thought it necessary to have microscopic confirmation of the existence of a cancer first. He performed the biopsy himself, and sent the material for assessment to the greatest pathologist of that time, Professor Rudolf Virchow. Two days later, Virchow reported that he had been unable to confirm the presence of a cancer, and needed a bigger sample. The new biopsy meant that more than half of the tumor had been removed, but Virchow still found no signs of cancer. It was decided that Mackenzie should take over the treatment. The Crown Prince went to London, where Mackenzie removed the rest of the tumor. Once again, Virchow found no evidence of cancer. Mackenzie advised Frederick to winter on the Mediterranean, to get away from Berlin's cold winter climate. But there his condition deteriorated. Various specialists were consulted, and all concluded that the Crown Prince was suffering from a malignant growth. Dr. Krause of Berlin proposed treatment with potassium iodide, for the Crown Prince's suspected syphilis. Since this was a low-risk treatment, the advice was followed. The suggestion was also made to the Crown Prince that he should undergo a laryngectomy (total removal of his voicebox). He refused this, but agreed to tracheotomy (cutting a hole in his windpipe). Frederick's condition became so serious that the tracheotomy was performed on 9 February 1888, and a silver canula was inserted. At the same time, samples of the Crown Prince's sputum were prepared for microscopic examination. Professor von Waldeyer from Berlin found large numbers of cancer cells in these samples. Kaiser William I died on 9 March 1888, and Frederick became the new Kaiser. He died three months later, on 15 June, of bronchopneumonia. Postmortem examination provided histologic confirmation of cancer of the larynx. An official report entitled *Die Krankheit Kaiser Friedrich des Dritten*, signed by von Bergmann, Gerhardt and von Waldeyer among others, appeared on 11 July; it accused Mackenzie of incompetence and malpractice. Mackenzie's response on 15 October took the form of a book entitled *The fatal illness of Frederick the Noble*, in which he depicted von Bergmann as an incompetent, unreliable figure. This publication caused Mackenzie to be censured by the Royal College of Surgeons.

In his article, Wentges concluded that Frederick's syphilis had led to a subglottal carcinoma (a cancerous growth under the tongue). The tragedy for Mackenzie was that the German doctors had reached the right diagnosis on the basis of the wrong arguments while he, with his "modern" approach to the problem, had not arrived at the proper diagnosis. One result of this comedy of errors was that confidence in the diagnostic relevance of a biopsy was badly shaken, and took a long time to recover.

The first trachea resections were performed in the 1960s by Hermes Grillo (1933-2006) at Massachusetts General Hospital in Boston. Twenty years earlier, in the 1940s, Hayes Martin (1892-1977), radiotherapist and general surgeon at Memorial Hospital for Cancer and Allied Diseases in New York City, had introduced radical en bloc resection of the neck glands together with the related mandibular tumor. This is often called the commando operation or commando resection, as a comparison with the dedicated teamwork that underlay the allied commando raids during the Second World War (Hill, 1979). More straightforwardly, the term can be seen as a contraction of *combined mandibular* resection. This operation gives rise to a major defect, which needs to be corrected by reconstructive surgery.

The reintroduction of reconstructive surgery can be regarded as a direct result of the Second World War and of the many terrible wounds it generated in combatants and the civilian population alike. This technique was already known in antiquity. The Ayurveda system of medicine, which is thought to have arisen in India between 1200 and 700 BC, contains descriptions of operations like rhinoplasty (plastic surgery of the nose). Sushruta, a surgeon from the Dhanvantari school of Ayurveda who flourished around the 6th century BC, was mentioned at the beginning of this chapter. He is known as the father of plastic and cosmetic surgery. Rhinoplasty was often necessary in ancient India because amputation of the nose was a legally sanctioned punishment for criminals, adulterous women and prisoners of war. Sushruta used a cheek flap for nose reconstruction but the later Indian procedure involved obtaining a flap from the forehead with a pedicle (a kind of stalk containing the blood vessels that kept the flap "alive") from the region of the bridge of the nose, folding this down over the site of the nose (which had previously been prepared for the operation by cutting away the amputation scars) and stitching it in place. Without the blood supply from the supratrochlear vessels, the flap would not survive for long. This procedure is still used today.

Reports from English officers of the Indian Civil Service in the late eighteenth and early nineteenth centuries contained details of another nose reconstruction technique, based on what would nowadays be called free skin grafting. This technique was also reported by the French physician and botanist Henri Dutrochet in the *Gazette de Santé* in 1817. In this case the flap was obtained from one of the patient's buttocks, which was prepared by beating it with an old shoe until it began to swell up noticeably. A piece of skin with subcutaneous fat that was large enough for the required reconstruction was then cut out, positioned accurately on the prepared defect and held in place with adhesive plasters (Verdan, 1983).

The Dutch surgeon Johannes Esser (1878-1946) made major advances in skin grafting. In 1917 he described an improved form of split skin grafting known as "epidermal inlay grafting," while in another article the same year he proposed an axial flap that got its blood supply from the temporal artery. Vilray Blair introduced the regional flap in 1925. These were the precursors of the deltopectoral flap, popularized by Bakamjian and Littlewood in the 1960s. It was the availability of such skin grafting techniques that enabled Hayes Martin to go much further in his radical surgery than his predecessors (McGurk and Goodger, 2000).

Tumors of the extremities

Major resection of the extremities was only really possible after the introduction of general anesthesia: before that time, surgery had to be performed at breakneck speed. Nevertheless, various types of exarticulations (surgical removal of a body part at a joint) were performed during the eighteenth century and the early nineteenth century. The most important of these was the resection of the hip joint by the eminent English physician Sir Astley Cooper, surgeon at Guy's Hospital in London and surgeon to King George IV, King William IV and Queen Victoria (Hill, 1979). One of Astley Cooper's pupils was the poet John Keats, who had studied medicine at Guy's.

Oscar Creech Jr. and Edward Krementz from Tulane University in New Orleans introduced regional perfusion of the extremities with cytostatics in 1958. The idea was that if the cytostatic was only administered in the affected limb, much higher concentrations could be used without adverse systemic effects. The first case they described was that of a patient with an extensively metastasized melanoma of the lower leg (Creech et al., 1958). The range of indications was subsequently expanded to include sarcomas as well as melanomas. While this technique was initially applied at normal body temperature, it was later found to be even more effective under hyperthermic conditions – that is, when the body temperature is elevated. The roots of this approach go back more than two centuries. An article by Joachim Hartmann of the Semmelweis Institute in Germany states that a publication by the Versailles physician Dupré de Lisle in 1774 and numerous reports by his compatriot, the surgeon Stanislas Tanchou, in 1844 provided evidence that malignant diseases can be cured or improved by bacterial infection. The German physician W. Busch from Cologne gave more positive proof of this assertion in 1866 when he described the complete disappearance of histologically confirmed sarcoma of the face after the patient had twice been intentionally infected with erysipelas (a skin rash caused by streptococcal infection). Similarly, Bruns from Bonn published details in 1884 of a patient with multiple recurrent melanomas who appeared to be in a terminal phase when he became infected with erysipelas and ran a temperature of more than 40°C. All tumors disappeared, and eight years later the patient was still alive and in good health (Cavaliere et al., 1967).

These findings led a number of researchers to undertake further study of the use of fever in the treatment of cancer. In general, bacterial toxins were used to induce fever. The heyday of such therapies was the period from 1891 to 1936. The American bone surgeon William Coley (1862-1936) described in 1893 how he induced fever in cancer patients, first by infecting them with erysipelas and later by inoculation with a mixture of hemolytic streptococci and *Bacillus prodigiosus*; this mix came to be known as Coley's toxin. This led to body temperatures in the region of 40°C. Coley achieved remarkable long-term remission in a variety of inoperable, extensive malignant diseases in this way. Other doctors, both in Coley's time and later, used Coley's toxin to treat histologically proven cancers. Though some striking, verified cures of different types of cancer were reported, the toxin was not biologically standardized and its results were inconsistent. No fewer than fourteen different formulations of the toxin were in use; their efficacy was evaluated later by Dickson (1979). Coley's toxin is currently only used by alternative therapists. Nevertheless, Coley's experiments may be regarded as the first step toward immunotherapy for the treatment of cancer, as discussed further in Chapter 9.

An interesting father-and-son team deserve mention in the history of the application of hyperthermia in the treatment of cancer. Following in the footsteps of his father, Nils Westermark, a Swedish gynecologist who used diathermy (hot water) to treat cervical cancer as long ago as 1898, made an extensive study some thirty years later of the destructive effect of heat on tumors in rats (Westermark, 1927). Forty years later, Renato Cavaliere and colleagues from the department of surgery of the National Tumor Institute in Milan described how they used regional hyperthermia in human patients, with a local temperature of 43°C for 6-8 hours, to achieve remission of melanomas and sarcomas of the extremities (Cavaliere et al., 1967). At about the same time, John Stehlin from Memorial Hospital in New York perfused tumors in an extremity with blood at 40°C for two-and-a-half hours. He combined this with melphalan as a cytostatic for melanomas, and melphalan plus actinomycin D for sarcomas. In his opinion, the localized heat led to a strong reduction in the incidence of metastases, and lowered the local recurrence rate (Stehlin, 1969).

Melphalan is currently used as the cytostatic of choice in perfusions. Tumor necrosis factor (rTNF), a substance with direct cytotoxic action accompanied by effects on the tumor vasculature, has also been employed in recent years. This treatment often makes it possible to avoid amputation.

UROLOGIC TUMORS

The Italian anatomist Giovanni Battista Morgagni, mentioned above in the section on gastrointestinal tumors, may also be regarded as the founder of modern anatomic pathology of the urogenital system. He discovered prostate enlargement and classified tumors of the bladder. He also described kidney tumors (Dufour, 1981). Konig in 1826 was the first to describe renal cell carcinoma. The French biologist and histologist Charles-Philippe Robin (1821-1885) concluded in 1855 that the cancer was most probably caused by proliferation of the epithelium of the renal tubules. This was confirmed in 1867 by Heinrich von Waldeyer, professor of anatomy first at Strasbourg and later in Berlin. In 1883, after he had observed that the lipid content of cancer cells resembled that of adrenal cells, the German pathologist Paul Grawitz (1850-1932) concluded that the cancer originated in adrenal residues in the kidney. He coined the term *struma lipomatodes aberrata renis* for these clear cell tumors. They were generally referred to as Grawitz tumors for a long time thereafter. Hypernephroma, the term used for this complaint, was introduced in 1894 by another German pathologist, Felix Victor Birch-Hirschfeld (1842-1899). Since then, this conceptually incorrect term has often been used to denote all kidney cancers (Linehan et al., 2001).

Urologic cancer surgery dates from the second half of the nineteenth century. Eratus B. Walcott in Milwaukee performed the first nephrectomy (surgical removal of the kidney) on a 58-year-old man with a kidney tumor in 1861. However, the patient died fifteen days after the operation (Marston et al., 2001). Bernhard von Langenbeck (1810-1887), the founder of the journal *Langenbeck's Archives of Surgery*, performed the first successful nephrectomy for cancer in Berlin in 1875. The mortality associated with this operation was more than 50% before 1879, but fell to 17% in 1899 (Hill, 1979). At present it is less than 3%.

Philipp Bozzini (1773-1809), a physician from Frankfurt, invented the *Lichtleiter* (light guide) in 1805. This instrument made it possible to look into the bladder and the rectum with the aid of a mirror and the light from a candle and ushered in the age of endoscopy (Figdor, 2002). The French surgeon Antoine Jean Desormeaux made an improved version of the *Lichtleiter* in 1855, which served as the first functional cystoscope (instrument for inspecting the inside of the bladder). Many therefore call him the father of endoscopy' (Riskin et al., 2006). The invention of a cystoscope fitted with an electric light in 1879 by the German urologist Max Nitze (1848-1906) in Vienna greatly improved the diagnostic powers of the urologist (De Moulin, 1988). The invention of the incandescent light by Thomas Alva Edison in the United States in 1880 paved the way for a gradual improvement in the illumination with which this instrument could be equipped. Two other crucial developments were achieved by the optical physicist Harold Hopkins (1918-1994) while he was working as a research fellow and lecturer in optics at Imperial College London. He later became professor of applied optics at Reading University. In 1954, he developed a fiber-optic gastroscope at the request of Hugh Gainsborough, consultant physician at St. George's Hospital, while in 1961 he developed a rod-lens system. These two inventions formed the basis for the flexible, high-light-output endoscopes available today to help physicians in many different disciplines to get a clear picture of what is going on in many body cavities.

J. Adams, a surgeon at the London Hospital, was the first to describe a case of prostate cancer. He had confirmed the diagnosis by microscopic examination, and commented in his report that it was a very rare complaint. The modern reader will find this a remarkable statement, since prostate cancer is currently the most common form of cancer in men. There are a number of possible causes of this rise in incidence, the main one being the marked increase in life expectancy, coupled with the fact that the incidence of prostate cancer is strongly age-related.

The first radical perineal prostatectomy was performed in 1889 by Vincenz Czerny, professor of surgery at Heidelberg. Eugene Fuller (1858-1930), professor of genitourinary surgery at New York Postgraduate Medical School, removed the prostate by the suprapubic route in 1898 (Dufour, 1981). Hugh Hampton Young (1897-1941) from The Johns Hopkins Hospital in Baltimore carried out a radical perineal prostatectomy in 1904. This became the method of choice for the next forty years. The operation was initially intended as a palliative measure, but it also gradually came to be seen as a possible cure. Terence Millin (1903-1980), an Irish-born specialist in genitourinary surgery in London, introduced retropubic prostatectomy in 1945. This approach had definite advantages. The operation was easier to learn, and permitted pelvic lymph node dissection for staging purposes. However, it had the serious drawback of leading to impotence. An improved variant, nerve-sparing radical retropubic prostatectomy, was proposed by Patrick Walsh, chief urologist at Johns Hopkins, in 1983. This method made it possible to preserve erection and potency (Denmeade and Isaacs, 2002). The history of the hormonal treatment of prostate cancer is dealt with in Chapter 7.

Many different methods of treating cancer of the bladder have been tried in the course of time. The above-mentioned development of flexible endoscopes (known as cystoscopes when used for inspection of the bladder) opened the way for transurethral resection of the growth when the cancer was detected early. Nowadays this is a widely used technique with a high success rate, which leads to relatively little trauma for the patient. Before the advent of endoscopy, total resection of the bladder was the only possible treatment for bladder cancer. This operation posed serious problems to surgeons for many years, until Eugene M. Bricker (1909-2000) from the Department of Surgery at Washington University School of Medicine, St. Louis, Missouri, came up with an improved procedure in 1950 that effectively dealt with most of the outstanding issues. This involved using an isolated segment of the patient's ileum (portion of the small intestine) to make a urine reservoir that could replace the resected bladder. The existing ureters were connected between this ileal reservoir and a cutaneous stoma for drainage of the urine (Hill, 1979). One small but vital element in the success of this procedure was the development by others of a special skin adhesive to prevent the leakage of urine from the rubber collection bag attached to the stoma. Bricker himself commented that the basic concept on which his procedure was based was not new, having been described by the German surgeon L. Seiffert in 1935.

The Bricker procedure also provided a basis for total pelvic exenteration (or pelvic evisceration), in which all the contents of the pelvic cavity – the rectum and the anus, the womb and vagina in the case of female patients, the bladder and urethra – are surgically removed and a terminal colostomy and ureterostomy are performed to permit defecation and micturition (passage of urine). This procedure has allowed certain patients with a slowly growing but locally aggressive tumor in the affected organs to lead a fairly normal life after they recover from the operation, if they receive effective postoperative support (Rosenberg, 2001).

In the late 1970s, Ramon Cabanas described how examination of the "sentinel node" could improve the treatment of cancer of the penis. This provided a basis for the sentinel node biopsy technique used in the treatment of breast cancer (discussed in the section on breast cancer above) and of melanoma (Cabanas, 1977).

Gynecologic tumors

Elective surgery of the female genitalia dates from the early nineteenth century, when Ephraim McDowell, mentioned above, performed an ovariectomy (surgical removal of an ovary). General acceptance of Lister's principles for the control of sepsis about sixty years later (starting in the early 1870s) led to a sharp rise in the number of abdominal and pelvic operations. Major advances in ovariectomy were made by Thomas Spencer Wells (1818-1897), who began performing this operation before the era of antisepsis. He was appointed physician to the Samaritan Free Hospital for Women in London in 1854, but shortly after the outbreak of the Crimean War (1854-1856) he was sent to the Crimea as an army surgeon, where he gained considerable experience in dealing with sepsis. On his return, he assisted the gynecologist Isaac Baker Brown (1812-1873) in a number of ovariectomies, with generally poor results; but in 1857 he began to perform this operation on his own, with steadily increasing success. His reputation began to expand internationally, even though he initially had to overcome great resistance from leaders of opinion in the surgical world. A key factor in his success was his introduction of teamwork into the operating theatre. In 1881, he reported on his first 1000 ovariectomies to the Royal Medical and Surgical Society. The mortality rate had fallen from an initial value of about 50% to just 11% in his last 100 cases. Wells accumulated many honors toward the end of his life. He was appointed Hunterian Professor of Surgery and Pathology at the Royal College of Surgeons in 1877, and was elected president of the Royal College in 1883. He was surgeon to Queen Victoria's household from 1863 to 1896, and was knighted in 1883.

The advances in gynecologic surgery achieved by James Marion Sims (1813-1883) from Philadelphia and Howard Atwood Kelly (1858-1943) from Baltimore laid the foundation for gynecologic oncology. Between them, they designed a number of vesical and rectal specula, while Kelly invented the Kelly clamp that is so widely used in abdominal surgery. Sims is often regarded as the father of modern gynecology. There is a much-quoted anecdote about Kelly, which appears to have a basis of truth: after treating a woman whom he recognized to be the same person who, as a little girl many years before, had kindly given him a glass of milk without requesting payment when he had asked for a glass of water, he wrote off her bill for his professional services with the words "paid in full with one glass of milk." It has been commented that while Kelly often charged high fees to those who could pay, he quite frequently donated his services to those who could ill afford to pay. The story has been embellished in the retelling until it has turned into a romantic account of the rewards of unselfish good deeds.

The surgical treatment of ovarian cancer has tended to center around two key aspects. Firstly, awareness of the importance of accurate mapping of the extent of the cancer came to be recognized during the 1970s and 1980s. The FIGO (International Federation of Gynecology and Obstetrics) staging criteria were introduced, together with the staging laparotomy on which they are based. During this operation, not only the affected adnexa but also the contralateral adnexa and the uterus are removed, and omentectomy together with pelvic and para-aortic lymphadenectomy are performed for staging purposes (in other words, the omentum and the lymph glands in the pelvic area and near the aorta are removed and studied for evidence of metastases, to determine how far the disease has advanced). A number of other biopsies may also be taken for staging purposes. Secondly, C. Thomas Griffiths from Harvard Medical School pointed out the importance of a debulking operation – that is, surgical removal of as much tumor as possible, even though it is not possible to excise all of the tumor mass, to enhance the effectiveness of subsequent chemotherapy or radiotherapy (Griffiths, 1975). Although debulking is actually still prescribed in the treatment of ovarian cancer, there is currently a growing tendency to perform certain aspects of the required surgery, such as the staging laparotomy, by keyhole surgery – which precludes effective debulking.

Ernst Wertheim (1864-1920) from Vienna introduced radical hysterectomy as a treatment for cervical cancer in 1897. This operation involves removal not only of the womb but also of a large part of the parametrium and the regional lymph nodes through an abdominal incision. Wertheim based his operation on a thorough study of the pathology of the disease with the aid of postmortem examinations, and used it in a courageous attempt to remove the primary tumor together with as much of the surrounding tissue – through which the tumor normally tends to metastasize – as possible. As was the case with other surgeons before him, his chief enemy was sepsis; the mortality rate for his first series of 100 patients was 30%, but fell to 10% as greater attention was paid to details. Nevertheless, he seems to have had a slightly cavalier attitude towards the rules of antisepsis, as the following anecdote illustrates. Wertheim visited England in 1905. Cuthbert Lockyer, a renowned gynecologist who practiced in and around London, invited him to demonstrate his operation on one of his (Lockyer's) patients at St. Mary's Hospital in Plaistow (now in East London, but then in the country a few miles outside London). Lockyer drove Wertheim there in an open carriage drawn by two greys (two grey horses). The patient was a 63-year-old woman with an endocervical tumor, who was in good general condition. Lockyer assisted at the operation, and wore rubber gloves as was usual for surgeons at that time, but Wertheim did not, explaining that his hands would lose their sensitivity if he got used to wearing gloves. When the abdomen had been opened Lockyer wanted to use a retractor but Wertheim refused, saying that the wound should be held open by an assistant's hands. He saw a young man washing his hands in the corner of the operating theatre, and called him to come over and assist. Without asking any questions, Wertheim took the young man's hands and placed them in the right position for retracting the wound. The operation continued without any problems and was completed in two hours. Three days later, the patient died of fulminating peritonitis. On investigation, Lockyer discovered that the young man was a local doctor who had come to the hospital to change the dressings on a patient's septic wound, and had only come into the operating theatre to clean his hands of the blood and pus on them. A few days later, Wertheim was invited to demonstrate his operation again in St. Thomas' Hospital in London before returning to Vienna. But he refused, and is reported to have said, "Nein, nein, mein Freund, I will not. I do not want to leave a trail of blood behind me."

Friedrich Schauta (1849-1919), an Austrian surgeon and gynecologist from Vienna, modified the operation technique by removing the uterus by the vaginal route, together with the adnexa and parametric tissue. This reduced the primary mortality, but had the disadvantage of not allowing the lymph nodes to be removed. Subodh Mitra (1886-1961), an Indian gynecologic cancer surgeon from Calcutta, was a proponent of this method and defended the non-removal of the lymph nodes by saying that the patient's chances of survival were minimal anyway if the lymph nodes were affected (Stallworthy, 1979).

It is difficult to tell who had primacy in this field: Wertheim, who was an assistant to Schauta for some years, or Schauta himself. Wertheim performed the first radical hysterectomy in 1897, issued a brief report on the operation in 1900 but did not publish details about it until 1911. Schauta first performed his operation in 1901, but published details about it in 1908.

Much more recently, in 1994, a French surgeon named Daniel D'Argent introduced a new method for the treatment of limited cervical carcinoma, known as radical trachelectomy. This involves removal of the cervix together with the parametria, and has the important advantage that the patient may be able to become pregnant after the operation.

Concluding remarks

Alongside the developments in surgical oncology discussed above, new surgical techniques such as organ transplantation, vascular surgery, microsurgery and keyhole surgery (also known as laparoscopic surgery) – while not developed specifically for the purposes of cancer therapy – are also of great importance in the treatment of cancer patients.

The recognition of surgical oncology as a separate discipline and the establishment of professional organizations in this field also represented a big step forward. The birth of surgical oncology can be dated to 1912 at Memorial Hospital in New York City (the precursor of the present-day Memorial Sloan-Kettering Cancer Center), where the renowned pathologist James Ewing (1866-1943) worked. The James Ewing Society was founded in 1940 as an association of alumni of the Memorial Hospital, and its name was changed in 1975 to the Society of Surgical Oncology (O'Shea, 2004). Similar professional organizations have been set up in many other countries.

Oncology surgeons have often played a leading role in other disciplines. For example, they contributed to the introduction of certain cytostatics and biological modifiers. The introduction of the perfusion technique by Oscar Creech and Edward Krementz, Anthony Curreri's studies on 5-fluoro-uracil and those of Steven A. Rosenberg on the immune protein interleukin-2 (IL-2) are well known in this context.

The surgeon Denis Burkitt also deserves mention in this connection. His 1958 discovery of Burkitt's lymphoma, a malignant tumor of the jaw found in boys in East Africa, was described in Chapter 2. In 1965, he described the high sensitivity of this tumor to cyclophosphamide. Follow-up studies showed that a large proportion of these patients were indeed cured (Zubrod, 1979).

In summary, we may state that surgery is the oldest form of treatment for cancer. It has made, and continues to make, the greatest contribution to the cure of this scourge of mankind. Surgeons generally take the biopsies on which diagnoses are based. And where cure is not possible, surgery often offers palliative services, for example through removing gastrointestinal obstructions or the resection of tumors.

[5]

The historical development of radiotherapy

The discovery of X-rays

The discipline of radiotherapy is based on knowledge obtained in various fields of science, especially physics and chemistry. Although the ancient Greeks had been aware of the existence of electricity, it was not until the nineteenth century that this phenomenon was subjected to extensive scientific study. Many physicists at that time were interested in electric discharges in gases at low pressure and the mechanism of such discharges. One of these was Johann Hittorf (1824-1914). While studying discharge tubes in 1869, he observed energy rays emanating from the negative electrode or cathode, which produced fluorescence when they hit the glass walls of the tubes. The name "cathode rays" for these rays was coined by Eugen Goldstein in 1876. The English chemist and physicist Sir William Crookes (1832-1919) also studied these rays, and developed an improved discharge tube for the purposes of their investigation that came to be known as the Hittorf-Crookes tube or, more frequently, the Crookes tube. Further research proved that cathode rays consisted of electrons, the tiny negatively charged particles that are constituents of atoms. The electron was discovered in 1897 by the English physicist Sir Joseph J. Thomson (1856-1940). Two years earlier, in September 1895, Philipp Eduard Anton (von) Lenard (1862-1947), a Hungarian physicist who spent all his working life in Germany, reported that cathode rays caused barium cyanide crystals to fluoresce, even when he placed his hand between the vacuum tube and the crystals (Ribot, 2005). Another physicist who was interested in this effect was Wilhelm Conrad Roentgen (1845-1923) (Figure 5.1).

Roentgen was born in Lennep near Remscheid in Germany, the only child of a German father (a merchant and cloth manufacturer) and a Dutch mother. In 1845, he moved with his parents to Apeldoorn in the Netherlands and lived there until 1862. He applied to the University of Utrecht to study science in 1865, but was not admitted as he did not have the required credentials. He did however manage to secure a place at the Federal Polytechnic Institute in Zurich, and gained a degree in mechanical engineering after three years' study there. A year later, in 1869, he

CHAPTER 5

FIGURE 5.1 W.C. Roentgen (1845-1923) holding an X-ray tube in his hand. (Source: Vermey J, Van der Giessen PH, Barendsen GW, Kal HB. Honderd jaar röntgenstraling in Nederland. Meppel: Kribs repro, 1995. Reproduced with permission).

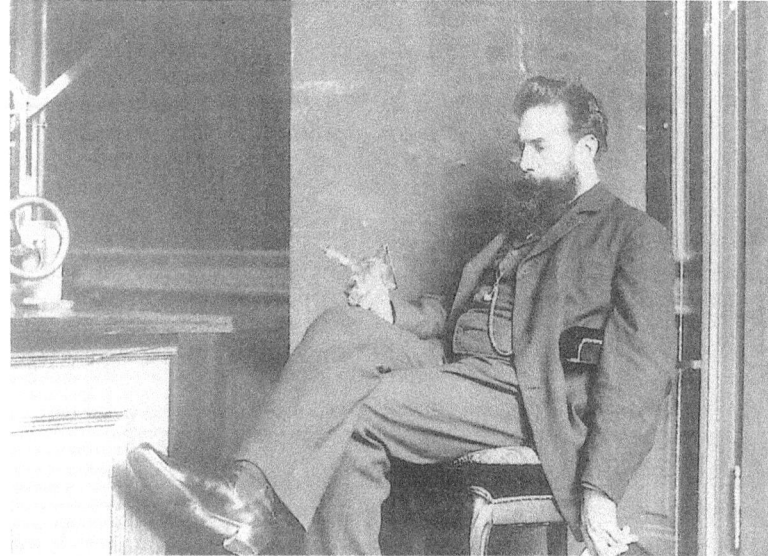

was awarded his doctorate in Zurich for a thesis entitled *Studien über Gase* (Studies on gases) (Stam, 1993). Roentgen turned down an offer to become the head of the department of physics at the University of Utrecht in 1888 but agreed to take up the same position later in the same year at the University of Würzburg, where he was made a professor.

Roentgen carried out his experiments on cathode rays with the aid of a Hittorf-Crookes tube with an aluminum window that Lenard had given him. Such a device consists of a pear-shaped glass tube from which nearly all the air has been evacuated and in which two electrodes have been mounted: the negative cathode at one end and the positive anode at the other. When these electrodes are connected to a high-voltage source, the ions remaining in the gas are given a high velocity. The cathode repels the negatively charged electrons, which then strike the opposite end of the glass tube. These fast electrons transfer their energy to the atoms of the glass, causing them to emit radiation (Bernier, 2004). On the memorable date of 8 November 1895, Roentgen observed that a barium platinocyanide screen that happened to be lying on the laboratory bench near the cathode-ray tube lit up, even though he had covered the tube with black paper so as to conceal the fluorescence of the glass at its end. Lenard had made similar observations in his experiments on the cathode-ray tube, but had dismissed them as anomalies. Roentgen realized that something important was happening, and persevered with his investigations. The cathode rays could not have been responsible for the fluorescence of the barium platinocyanide screen, so some other form of radiation of an unknown nature must have caused the effect. Roentgen called these new rays "X-rays," from the algebraic symbol x often used to represent an unknown quantity. Even today, Roentgen's term is used in the English-speaking world and in France, though in many other countries the rays are referred to as "Roentgen rays."

He carried out a series of experiments in which he held various substances in his hand between the cathode-ray tube and the fluorescent screen, to test the transparency of these substances when subjected to radiation. One day, he was astonished to see an image of the bones of his fingers on the screen. Instead of using a fluorescent screen, it also proved possible to capture the images that were observed on a photographic plate. Roentgen made his first photo in this way, of his wife's hand, at the end of December. This was the first X-ray photo in history (Figure 5.2).

Roentgen submitted his famous first paper *Ueber eine neue Art von Strahlen* (On a new kind of radiation) to the *Sitzungsberichten* (Proceedings) of the Physikalisch-Medizinischen Gesellschaft in Würzburg on 28 December 1895, and on 23 January 1896 he delivered his first lecture on his discovery to the same society. The chairman of the society was the renowned anatomist Albert Rudolf von Kölliker (1817-1905), who was so impressed by the striking new findings that Roentgen had reported that he suggested that the new rays should be called Roentgen rays instead of X-rays (Figure 5.3). Roentgen continued to use the name "X-rays," however. The

CHAPTER 5

FIGURE 5.2 The first X-ray photo ever made, taken by Roentgen at the end of 1895 and showing his wife's hand. (Source: Rosenbusch G, Oudkerk M, Amman E (Eds.), Radiologie in der medizinischen Diagnostik. Blackwell Wissenschafts-Verlag. Berlin, 1994. Reproduced with permission).

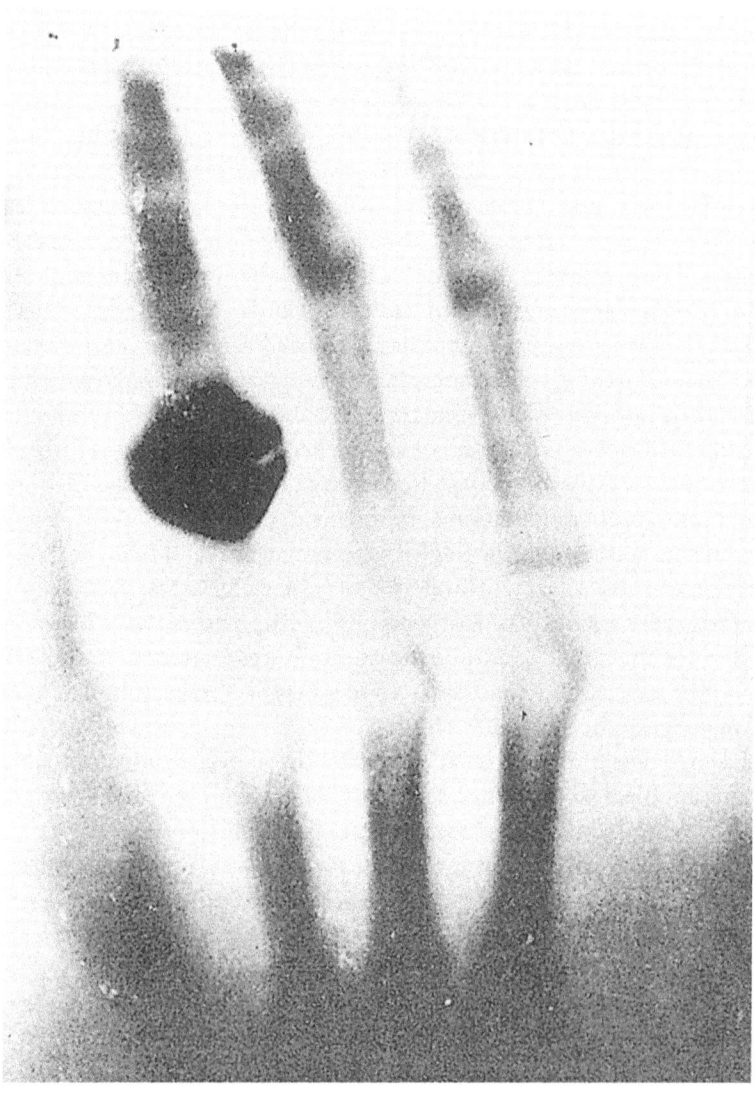

audience was so excited by the content of Roentgen's lecture that the news quickly leaked out to the popular press and was published there before it could be printed in a medical journal. The news of Roentgen's initial paper submitted to the Physical-Medical Society reached London on 6 January 1896, and was telegraphed from there around the world – in sharp contrast to the three weeks it had taken the news of anesthesia to reach London by boat from Boston nearly fifty years before, as described in Chapter 4. Physicists everywhere dropped their ongoing research and hurried to reproduce Roentgen's experiment. As Emile Bertin-Sans, professor of physics at the University of Montpellier put it, what excited people was not so much the advance that was made in the field of gas-discharge physics as the prospect of being able to photograph the skeleton, almost as if one were performing an autopsy on a living person, painlessly and in perfect safety, long before his or her death (Proux, 1983). As yet, people knew nothing of the dangers of X-rays and other forms of radiation.

Roentgen was honored in many ways for the discovery of X-rays. When the Nobel Prize for Physics was awarded for the first time ever in 1901, he was the recipient. He also received the Rumford Gold Medal of the British Royal Society and the Iron Cross – a German military order – from Field Marshal Paul von Hindenburg in recognition of the great value of X-rays in the treatment of wounded German soldiers. During the First World War Roentgen, as a good patriot, donated his Rumford medal to be melted down for the gold to support the war effort.

Roentgen was a true scientist. He refused to patent his discovery, and indignantly turned down any commercial offers. He believed that his income as a scientist gave him all the financial security he needed. However, the extreme inflation in Germany after the First World War made his savings worthless. Even the money from the Nobel Prize, which he had donated to the University of Würzburg to fund scientific research, melted away like snow in the sun (Grigg, 1965).

Philipp Lenard, mentioned above, was initially a friend of Roentgen's, but the relationship cooled when the latter won the Nobel Prize. Lenard had given Roentgen the cathode-ray tube with the aluminum window – an essential feature, since it was through this window that the X-rays left the tube (Etter, 1946). Because of this, Lenard believed that he should have received the Nobel Prize for the discovery of X-rays, and he tried to belittle Roentgen at every possible opportunity throughout the rest of his life. Lenard did win the Nobel Prize himself, in 1905, for his work on cathode rays, and he slipped some disparaging remarks about Roentgen into his acceptance speech. In fact, his attitude towards many other leading scientists in Germany and other countries was marked by suspicion and hostility. Lenard's strong sympathies for the Nazi party colored his life after the end of the First World War. He joined the Nazi party in 1924, and was regarded by the Nazis as one of Germany's leading Aryan scientists. It has been suggested that he used his privileged position at that time to claim part of the honor for the discovery of X-rays (Grigg, 1965). He compared Roentgen's contribution to the discovery of X-

FIGURE 5.3 Roentgen giving the first public lecture on X-rays, on 23 January 1896, to the Physical-Medical Society in Würzburg. This photo shows Roentgen taking an X-ray photo of the hand of the chairman of the Society, the renowned anatomist Albert von Kölliker. Von Kölliker was so impressed that he proposed naming the new radiation Roentgen radiation (Source: Rosenbusch G, Oudkerk M, Amman E (Eds.), Radiologie in der medizinischen Diagnostik. Blackwell Wissenschafts-Verlag. Berlin, 1994. Reproduced with permission).

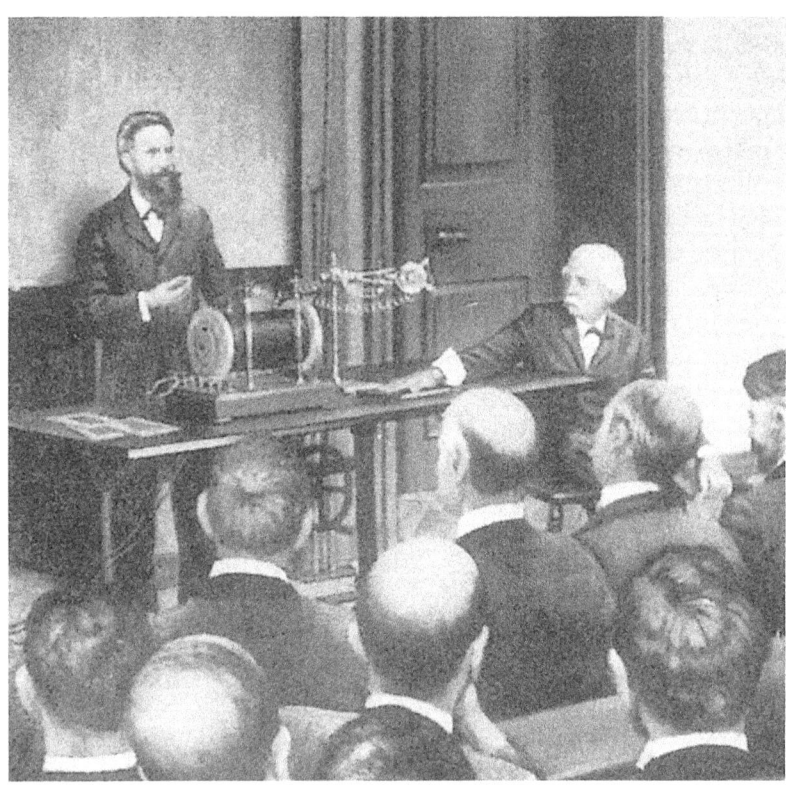

rays to that of a midwife during childbirth. It is noteworthy that a four-volume book on "German physics" published by Lenard in 1936-1937 does not mention Einstein and Roentgen at all. The foreword to the book contained an impassioned diatribe against Jewish scientists. It is therefore understandable that he did not include Einstein, but the omission of Roentgen is more puzzling. When asked whether Roentgen was Jewish, Lenard replied, "No, but he was a friend of the Jews and acted like one" (Etter, 1946).

In response to the objection that science is international, he is said to have replied, "No, it is not. Science like any other human product is racial and conditioned by blood." It has been suggested that his prejudice against Jewish scientists was not so much plain anti-Semitism as largely motivated by the difficulty he, as a skilled experimentalist, experienced in coming to terms with the increasing theorization of science, in which Einstein played a particularly dominant role. Be that as it may, the atmosphere generated by Lenard played an important role in encouraging Jewish scientists to leave Germany before the Second World War, thus largely putting an end to serious science there for a generation.

The first Dutch publication on radiotherapy dates from 1915 and was by G. F. Gaarenstroom, roentgenologist at the Antoni van Leeuwenhoek Hospital in Amsterdam. He gave the following vision of radiotherapy (Gaarenstroom 1915):

Working by trial and error, reporting our experience and comparing our results with those of others working in the same field, we are advancing slowly, step by step, but deeply convinced that there is a future for radiation therapy in the treatment of malignant tumors (Stam, 1993).

Experience since 1915 has amply confirmed the truth of his words.

The discovery of natural radioactivity

A few days after presenting his discovery of X-rays in Würzburg, Roentgen sent letters containing details of his findings to a number of scientists in other countries, including Jules Henri Poincaré (1854-1912), a French mathematician, theoretical physicist and philosopher of science attached to the Sorbonne in Paris. Poincaré is often described as a polymath. On receipt of the letter, the group around Poincaré repeated Roentgen's experiment and started a discussion of the mechanism underlying X-rays in the French *Académie des Sciences*. During the first meeting of the *Académie* after the arrival of Roentgen's letter, in January 1896, Poincaré put forward the hypothesis that the X-rays were produced by the fluorescence on the wall of the vacuum tube, and wondered whether this phenomenon also occurred in nature. This remark aroused the curiosity of his colleague Antoine-Henri Becquerel (1852-1908), a professor of physics and an expert in the field of fluorescence and phosphorescence. He began to investigate Poincaré's interesting (but in fact incorrect) hypothesis. To this end, he placed fluorescent uranium sulfate crystals on a photographic plate wrapped in black paper, with the intention of exposing

CHAPTER 5

FIGURE 5.4 The Curies, a remarkable family. Pierre (1859-1906), won the Nobel Prize for Physics; Marie (1867-1934) won two – for both Physics and Chemistry – while their daughter Irène (Joliot-Curie, 1897-1956) also won one for Chemistry, together with her husband Frédéric (Source: Shimkin, 1979, courtesy of the National Institute of Health, Bethesda, MD, USA).

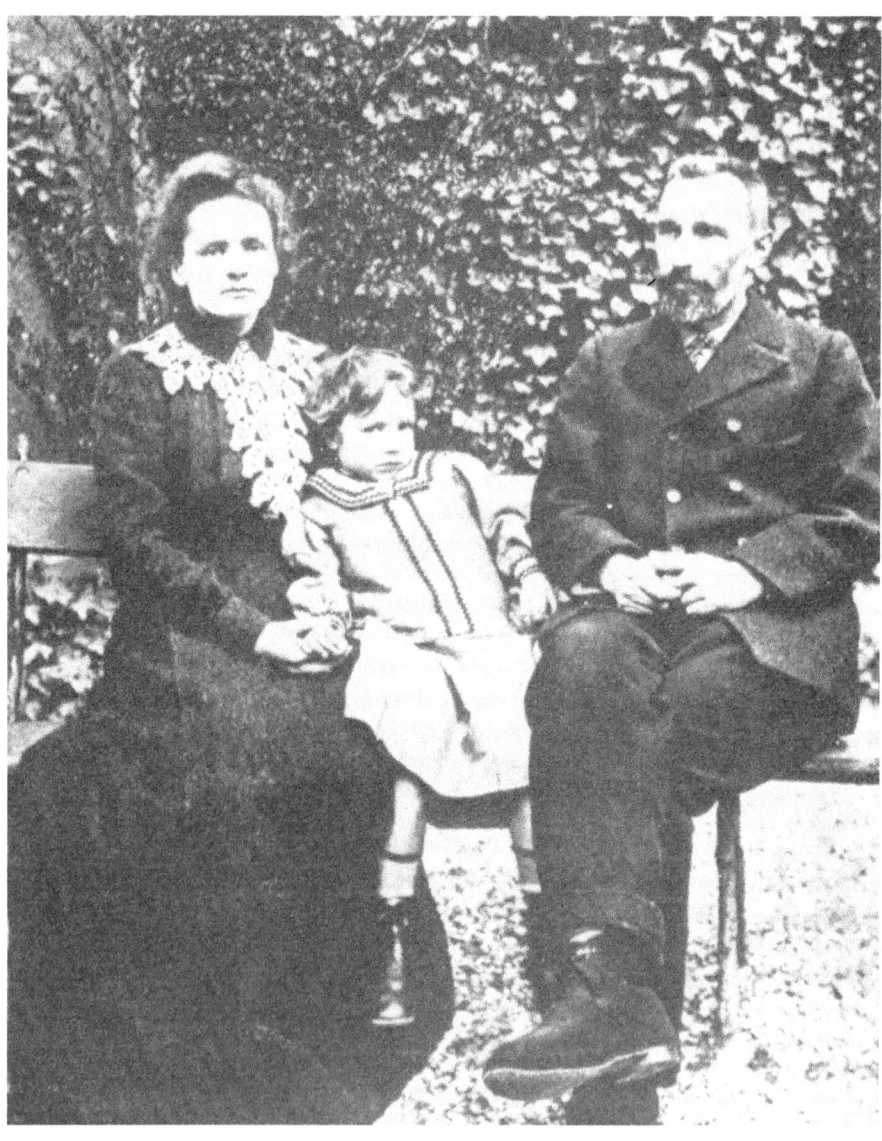

them to sunlight. According to Poincaré's theory, the light from the sun should cause the uranium sulfate crystals to emit not only visible light (as by definition they would, since the crystals were fluorescent) but also X-rays. The black paper would shield the plate from the visible light, but the X-rays would penetrate the paper and expose the plate, thus producing images of the crystals on it. Becquerel made his preparations for this experiment in the middle of the winter, and unsurprisingly the sun refused to shine for a few days so Becquerel put the assembly away safely in a dark drawer. When the sun did shine, Becquerel – as befits a good scientist – decided to use the old plate as a control while he put a new plate in the sun. To his astonishment, he found that the photographic plate that has been kept in the dark drawer with the uranium sulfate crystals was exposed! He concluded that the crystals must have been emitting radiation spontaneously, without any stimulation from heat or sunlight, and that this radiation was capable of passing through materials that were opaque to visible radiation (the black paper) and exposing a photographic plate. He had thus discovered natural radioactivity – a term coined later by Marie Curie – just a few months after the discovery of X-rays (Proux, 1983).

Marie Curie (1867-1934; Figure 5.4) was born Marya Sklodowska in Warsaw, and lived there for most of her youth. When Marie became a member of a students' revolutionary organization, however, she thought it safer to move from Warsaw, then in the part of Poland controlled by Russia, to Cracow which was under Austrian rule at that time. She longed to study at the Sorbonne in Paris, but her family could not afford to send her there. Marie therefore came to an agreement with her elder sister, Bronislava ("Bronya"): Marie would work as a governess and earn money to support Bronya while she was studying medicine at the Sorbonne. And when Bronya had completed her studies, she would help to pay the cost of Marie's studies. And this is what they did.

Marie went to Paris in 1891 to study chemistry, physics and mathematics at the Sorbonne. She met Pierre Curie (1859-1906), professor of physics, there in 1894 and married him the next year. Since Marie did not get along well with her first director of research, Professor Gabriel Lippmann (who later won the Nobel Prize for Physics in 1908 for his discovery of color photography), she did her doctoral study under the supervision of Becquerel (Ribot, 2005).

Pitchblende, the mineral that Marie Curie used as a source of uranium, proved to be four times as radioactive as pure uranium. This was a clear indication that the pitchblende must contain other radioactive components apart from uranium. Working under almost unbelievably primitive conditions, Pierre and Marie spent four years of backbreaking effort processing tons of pitchblende, obtained from slag heaps at the Joachimsthal mine in Bohemia (present-day Austria) until they had obtained tiny amounts of two new elements. This period of intense labor in their life has become legendary. They called the new elements polonium after Marie's country of origin and radium because of the latter's intense radioactivity.

FIGURE 5.5 *Report of the measurement of the amount of radium in an irradiation unit, signed by Marie Curie. This document is in the possession of the Netherlands Cancer Institute at the Antoni van Leeuwenhoek Hospital in Amsterdam (a).*

NATURE et PROVENANCE de L'APPAREIL.
Appareil à sel de Radium solide
apporté par la maison Armet de Lisle, de Nogent sur Marne.
le 23 novembre 1914   et rendu le 1 décembre 1914

CONDITIONS DE MESURES. Le rayonnement γ de l'appareil à été comparé au rayonnement γ de l'étalon du Laboratoire. L'appareil à mesurer n'avait pas atteint son rayonnement limite, et celui-ci a été déduit des mesures par le calcul (1).

Le nombre donné dans ce certificat représente la quantité de Radium contenu dans l'appareil, à la condition que la matière employée ne contienne pas d'autres substances radioactives que le Radium et ses dérivés. L'évaluation est faite en :

MILLIGRAMMES DE BROMURE DE RADIUM HYDRATÉ RaBr^2. 2 H^{2}O

L'appareil marqué n° 4695 contient 5.11 millig. RaBr^2 2H^{2}O
(Cinq virgule onze milligrammes de bromure de radium hydraté pur)

(1). La valeur ainsi calculée peut être acceptée avec confiance, mais elle ne comporte pas la même précision que la mesure directe du rayonnement limite, laquelle ne peut être faite qu'un mois après la préparation de l'appareil. Pour un appareil constitué par un tube de platine, une correction est faite afin de tenir compte de l'absorption des rayons par le platine. L'épaisseur admise est 0,5 mm. nombre donné par la maison Armet de Lisle

Le Directeur du Laboratoire.

M. Curie

a

Both elements emit radiation spontaneously. In this way the concept of radioactivity was born. After working through all those huge piles of pitchblende, the Curies ended up with 100 milligrams of pure radium. Marie Curie gained her doctorate in 1903, for her thesis entitled *Recherches sur les substances radioactives*. In the same year, the Curies' discovery was officially announced at the Royal Society in London and they were awarded the Nobel Prize for Physics, together with Henri Becquerel (Quin, 1995). Eight years later, in 1911, Marie Curie also won the Nobel Prize for Chemistry. This was a remarkable occurrence, not only because Marie Curie was a woman but because she was one of only two people who have received two Nobel Prizes in different subjects – the other being Linus Pauling, whom we met in Chapter 2; he won the Prizes for Chemistry and Peace. Although women were gradually coming to be more widely accepted as scientists, there were still large groups of scientists – and, indeed, of the general public – who did not like the idea. This is illustrated by the fact that, in the same year that she was awarded her second Nobel Prize, the proposal to make her a member of the French *Academie des Sciences* was turned down – by a single vote (Lyons and Petrucelli, 1987).

Pierre Curie died in 1906. He was crossing the road near the Pont Neuf in Paris, lost in thought, when he was run over by a heavy wagon pulled by two horses. Marie took his place as professor of general physics at the Sorbonne. Understandably, however, the tragic death of her beloved husband was quite a burden to her and she became severely depressed. She withdrew from social life, and seemed to have energy only for her scientific work.

Marie Curie died of leukemia – most probably caused by the massive doses of radiation she had been exposed to during her work (see Figure 5.5) – in 1934 at the age of 66. She was buried alongside Pierre in Sceaux on the outskirts of Paris where Pierre's family had also lived. In 1995, their remains were reinterred in the Pantheon in Paris – the highest honor that can be accorded to any French citizen. Marie Curie is the first and only woman to be buried in the Pantheon on her own merits.

The use of radiation in medical treatment

The first fully authenticated application of radiotherapy was probably that performed by A. Voigt in Germany. He reported to the Hamburg Medical Society on 3 February 1896 concerning the case of a patient with cancer of the throat whom he had irradiated in January of that year (McCarty and Million, 1995). Emil H. Grubbe (1875-1960) stated in the 1930s that he had used X-rays for therapeutic purposes in Chicago on 29 January 1896, three weeks after the report of the discovery of this new form of radiation had been telegraphed around the world; doubt has been cast on his claim of primacy, however (Mould, 1995). Grubbe was a student and a lecturer at the Hahnemann Medical College (a school of homeopathic medicine) in Chicago, and also had a small-scale business making vacuum tubes. When he

FIGURE 5.5 [CONTINUED] In 2006, the document (a) was placed on a photographic plate. The images formed before (b) and after (c) development are shown alongside. They provide visible proof that the document is still radioactive (which is hardly surprising, since radium is known to have a half-life of about 1600 years). The fingerprints on the photos show that the fingers of those who handled the document in the past must have bee contaminated with radium–a striking illustration of the lack of awareness of the health hazards of radiation in the early days of radiation research. (Reproduced by courtesy of the Audiovisual Center and the Radiation Safety Unit of the Nederlands Kanker Instituut, Antoni van Leeuwenhoek Ziekenhuis, Amsterdam).

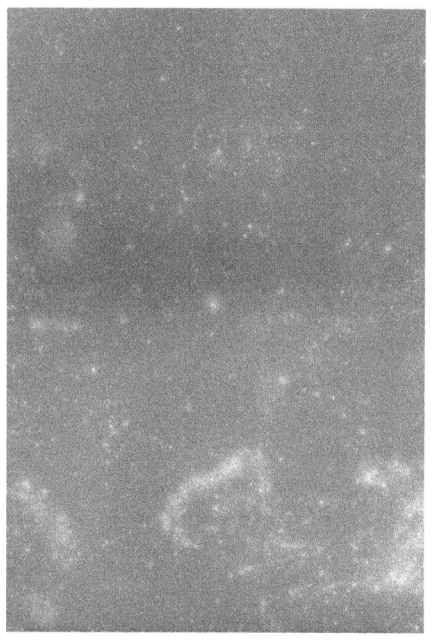

b

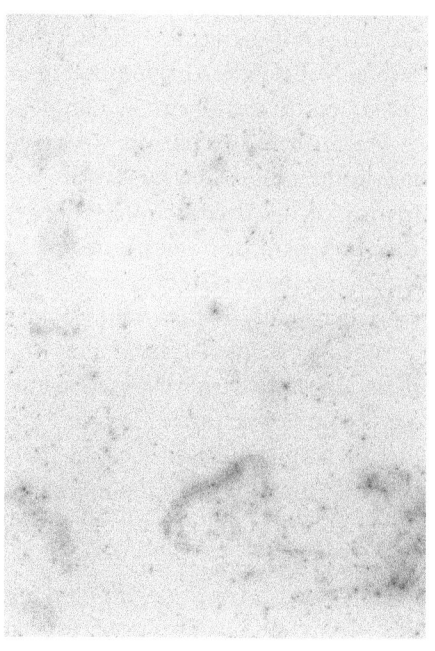

c

heard the news of the discovery of X-rays, he promptly tried them out in his workshop by irradiating his own hand. This had an adverse effect on his hand (probably some kind of burn). He mentioned this at the next Hahnemann faculty meeting, and asked for advice about suitable treatment for the lesion. A Dr J. E. Gilman, who was present at the meeting, had no therapeutic advice to offer but suggested that if X-rays cause such damage to normal tissue they might be effective in the treatment of diseases such as cancer. This idea was applauded by a number of the other doctors at the meeting, who offered to send cancer patients to Grubbe for irradiation. Mrs. Rose Lee, a patient of Dr. Ludham (another physician associated with the college), was the first. She received eighteen courses of X-ray treatment for a cancer of the left breast that had reappeared after two previous operations. The treatment relieved her pain, but she died about a month after her first visit (McCarty and Million, 1995).

Hermann Gocht (1869-1938), at that time a surgical assistant at the new General Hospital in Hamburg-Eppendorf, also tested the effect of the new radiation on two patients with breast cancer in 1896. He published his findings in the first issue of the first journal exclusively devoted to the medical application of X-rays, *Fortschritte auf dem Gebiete der Röntgenstrahlen*. One patient suffered from an ulcerating tumor, while the other, after having undergone several operations, had a recurrent cancer that affected the axillary lymph nodes. In both cases, the irradiation relieved the pain. The first patient died on the seventeenth day of treatment from cachexia and sepsis, after repeated severe bleeding from the ulcer in her breast. The second showed an increase in the size of the swellings, despite the irradiation. She died three months later. Gocht had used tubes that were no longer suitable for photography. The cathode heater voltage was quite high – at least 50 volts, according to his description. The tube was placed six or seven centimeters from the breast, and was turned on twice a day for 15 to 30 minutes a time. Lead was used to screen off the surroundings (Gocht, 1897).

An Austrian dermatologist from Vienna, Leopold Freund (1868-1943), is generally regarded as the father of both radiology and radiotherapy. In addition to studying the therapeutic effect of X-rays on patients, he also used this new form of radiation to investigate the structure of building materials. Together with a number of colleagues, Freund observed that irradiation led to hair loss. This gave him the idea of irradiating a five-year-old girl with a giant hairy nevus (birthmark) covering almost all her back. However, he was refused permission to use the X-ray equipment in the various hospitals in Vienna and was forced to turn to the Graphic School and Research Institute, the Viennese training academy for photographers, which did allow him to use its equipment. He gave the girl daily courses of radiation treatment for two weeks in November 1896 (Mould, 1995). The Swedish general practitioners Thor Stenbeck (1864-1914) and Tage Sjögren (1859-1939) were the first to cure two cases of skin cancer in 1900 – one basal cell carcinoma of the nose and one pavement cell carcinoma of the cheek – by irradiation. They used the same fractionated technique as Freund. Gösta Forsell (1866-1950), the founder of Radiumhemmet in Stockholm, followed up the first of these cases for thirty years and the second for 30 months, and found no recurrences.

Victor Despeignes (1866-1937) from Lyon was the first to perform radiotherapy in France. As early as July 1896 he gave a stomach cancer patient a course of X-ray treatment, with eighty sessions lasting 15-30 minutes twice daily, and reported a reduction in the size of the tumor and pain relief. In 1902, William Allen Pusey (1865-1940), professor of dermatology at the University of Illinois at Chicago, reported the results he had obtained by irradiating patients with lymphomas. While some patients responded so well that it was thought they were cured, later reports of recurrences and side effects from the treatment tempered the initial enthusiasm (Papac, 2001). A year later, in 1903, Nicolas Senn, professor of surgery at Rush Medical College in Chicago (a medical school with an impressive history: it was chartered in 1837, two days before the city of Chicago itself received its charter) was the first to treat a patient with pseudoleukemia (the term used to describe Hodgkin's disease in those days) by irradiation of the spleen. The response was so good that Senn assumed that he had cured the patient (Holsti, 1995).

In the first years of its use, X-rays were used to treat all kinds of diseases. J. Belot, radiologist at the Hôpital St. Louis in Paris, published a book entitled *La radiothérapie, son application aux affections cutanées* (Radiotherapy and its application to the treatment of skin complaints) in 1904. It was so well received that a second edition appeared the following year. This publication listed 56 ailments for which radiotherapy was thought to be indicated, ranging from tuberculosis, elephantiasis, syphilis, epilepsy, acne and psoriasis to breast cancer, leukemia and lymphosarcoma. This long list illustrates the enthusiasm for the new treatment and the hope felt by many that it might provide a sort of universal cure. But it soon became clear that X-rays were particularly suited to the treatment of malignant diseases and also that they could give rise to a range of unpleasant side effects, such as skin sores and inflammation, hair loss and painful irritation.

Radium was also used to treat a wide range of complaints soon after its discovery. Since radioactive materials seemed to contain a mysterious form of energy, there was initially a tendency to ascribe magical powers to them. Countless radium-containing products – such as face cream, bath salts, lipstick and even mineral water – appeared on the market around 1930. Wearing a little bag of radium in close contact with the scrotum was even recommended as a means of promoting male virility. But the death of industrialist, sportsman and man-about-town Eben Byers brought this craze to an abrupt end. Byers was the owner and managing director of the Byers Steel Company and the US Amateur Golf Champion in 1906. Between 1928 and 1930, he drank a bottle of radium-containing water a day, prescribed to him by a medical quack. He died in 1932 at the age of 51 from radium poisoning leading to severe osteolysis (disintegration) of his skeleton, in particular his jaw.

The death of this public figure was the news of the day, inspiring the *Wall Street Journal* to run the headline, "The radium water worked fine, until his jaw came off." Shortly afterwards, the use of radium in the health and cosmetics industry became subject to strict government regulation (Boerman, 2008). A similar case with far-reaching legal implications, that of the "Radium Girls" who painted luminescent watches with radium paint, was mentioned in the section on radiation-induced carcinogenesis in Chapter 2.

Radium emits three types of radiation: α (alpha) radiation, consisting of helium nuclei with a very low penetration; β (beta) radiation, high-energy electrons with a somewhat greater penetration; and γ (gamma) radiation, electromagnetic waves like X-rays but with a shorter wavelength and the highest penetration of the three. Gamma rays have the highest energy of all electromagnetic radiation, typically in the mega-electron-volt range. Only β and γ radiation are used for therapeutic purposes.

The biological effect of radium was discovered only by chance. The Curies gave Becquerel a glass vial containing a miniscule amount of radium. For fear of losing this precious sample, he kept it in his waistcoat pocket. A few days later he felt a painful itch on his skin, right next to the waistcoat pocket with the vial of radium. On closer examination, he found what looked just like a burn. He told Pierre Curie about this, and the latter repeated the experiment, this time intentionally. He too found that a rash formed near the vial, which developed into a slowly healing burn (Proux, 1983). Neither Becquerel nor Curie published this finding, but the German dentist Friedrich Otto Walkhoff (1860-1934) did. In 1900, he was the first to publish a description of the cutaneous reaction to a radium source, observed in his friend, the chemist Friedrich Giesel (1852-1927) (Mould, 2007).

Radium was first used to treat a medical condition in 1901 by the dermatologist Henri-Alexandre Danlos (1844-1912) at the Hôpital St. Louis in Paris. He irradiated a patient who had lupus (a chronic skin condition) with a small amount of radium made available by the Curies (Proux, 1983).

The first successful radium treatment of cancer was claimed in 1903 by S.W. Goldberg and Professor Efim Semenovich London (1868-1939) from Saint Petersburg, who treated two patients with a basal cell carcinoma of the face (Mould, 1995). Margaret Cleaves (1848-1917), a radiologist from New York, described the favorable effect of radium on cervical cancer in the same year (Cleaves, 1903), while Pusey and Eugene Wilson Caldwell (1870-1918) in Chicago reported on their first attempts to treat carcinoma of the uterus with glass capsules of radium placed directly in the tissue in 1904. They stated that radium offers a convenient form of radiotherapy in cases where external irradiation is very difficult or impossible (Mould, 1995). After this cautious start, the use of radium in the medical world snowballed.

CHAPTER 5

The development of external radiotherapy

External radiotherapy was initially very slow to develop. There were a number of reasons for this. To start with, of course, radiotherapy was not a recognized discipline for which training courses were available. The first medical workers to irradiate patients were dermatologists and surgeons (Kaplan, 1979). No one had any clear idea how the radiation worked. Some thought that it gave rise to electrical discharges in the tissues, while others believed that the radiation itself was responsible for the observed effect. Initially, the same type of tube, derived from the old Crookes tube, was used both for diagnosis and for irradiation. The therapists used tubes producing hard (low-wavelength and hence high-energy, high-penetration) or soft X-rays as they saw fit. The irradiation period was subject to incredible variation: some limited themselves to just a few minutes, while others irradiated for hours on end. There was moreover a constant fear of accidents, which often happened despite all conceivable precautions having been taken. The whole discipline was shrouded in mystery. The equipment was primitive, and yielded only enough energy for treatment of superficial tumors. "Empiricism rules; no one can form well-based opinions about what is going on – in short, radiotherapy is not yet a science," wrote the above-mentioned J. Belot in 1904.

Nevertheless, as early as 1899 Professor M. Levy-Dorn (1863-1929) from Berlin and the surgeon and radiologist H.E. Albers-Schönberg (1865-1921) from Hamburg took the initiative to map the field of X-ray therapy and asked all those who had any experience in this discipline to cooperate in the study. However, the credit for the first steps taken to put radiotherapy on a scientific footing must go to Robert Kienböck (1871-1953) from Vienna. He demonstrated the therapeutic efficacy of X-rays and showed that the type of radiation produced depended on the vacuum in the tube and the construction of the tube, drawing a distinction between "hard" tubes (tubes that produce high-energy, or hard, X-rays) and "soft" tubes. He also stated that the skin and internal organs could be damaged by prolonged irradiation (Proux, 1983).

One serious problem at this time was the absence of a consensus about how to measure the radiation dose. The introduction of a usable dosimeter by Guido Holzknecht (1872-1931) from Vienna in 1902 was a major step forward. His dosimeter was based on a chemical process whereby potassium sulfate fused with 0.7% sodium carbonate changed color, from ochre yellow to olive green, when irradiated. This "chromoradiometer" was not very accurate, however, in particular because the quality of the reagents used could not be kept constant. The French dermatologist Raymond Sabouraud (1864-1938) developed an improved radiometer in cooperation with Henri Noiré (1878-1937). This contained pellets of barium platinocyanide that changed color from green to ochre yellow under the influence of radiation. Holzknecht later improved this radiometer, thus providing dermatologists with an effective measuring instrument that would remain in use from 1910 until after the Second World War. Holzknecht, who specialized in the treatment of malignant diseases, died of advanced radiodermatitis caused by his exposure to radiation in the early stages of his career. Several of his fingers had to be amputated as early as 1910 and a number of other operations on his hands and arms followed. He was far from alone in his fate. The German medical journal *Strahlentherapie* (now renamed *Strahlentherapie und Onkologie*) issued a supplement in 1919 entitled *Ehrenbuch der Roentgenologen und Radiologen aller Nationen* (Roll of Honor of roentgenologists and radiologists of all nations), which listed 169 physicians who had died as the result of excessive exposure to ionizing radiation. The second edition, which appeared in 1959, added a further 190 names.

Holzknecht proposed a unit for the measurement of X-ray dosage equal to one-fifth of the dose required to produce skin erythema; however, this had the disadvantage of not being related to any established physical unit. The French chemist and physicist Paul Villard (1880-1934) had suggested as early as 1909 that the number of ionizations in air produced by radiation could be used as a measure of radiation dosage, but his proposal did not find application at the time (Ribot, 2005).

The golden age of radiotherapy began after the First World War. Improved measuring equipment finally made it possible to measure the radiation dose absorbed by the skin. From about 1920, the "ionoquantimeter" developed by the Hungarian-American physicist Leó Szilárd and the ionometer initially proposed by the German physicist Walter Friedrich and subsequently improved by Iser Solomon (a French radiologist) provided a basis for more accurate X-ray therapy. The unit of intensity of gamma radiation was named the roentgen (R) in honor of Roentgen (Proux, 1983). The *rad* was introduced in 1956 as the unit of absorbed dose of radiation (Kaplan, 1979), and after the change to the International System of Units (SI) this unit was renamed the *gray* (Gy) in memory of Louis Harold Gray (1905-1965) who had played an important role in defining the fundamental principles of radiation dosimetry.

The first major finding in the interdisciplinary field of radiobiology (study of the biological effects of radiation) was made in 1909 by the Austrian radiologist Gottwald Schwartz (1880-1959) when he observed that irradiation only has a beneficial effect when there is adequate blood flow through the tissue in question, and that the effect of irradiation is much stronger in the presence of oxygen. However, the clinical significance of this observation was not elucidated until 1953, when Gray and his colleagues showed experimentally that irradiation has much less effect on hypoxic tumor cells (Gray et al., 1953). Many researchers since then have looked for ways of making hypoxic tumor cells more susceptible to attack by radiation, for example by the administration of substances known as radiosensitizers. Such investigations have had little success so far, though studies of the effect of nicotinamide (the amide derivative of vitamin B3), which improves the microcirculation when administered in combination with carbogen (a mixture of oxygen and CO_2 gas) seem to have yielded promising results. Moreover, Overgaard et al.

(1998) in Denmark showed in a placebo-controlled phase-III trial that administration of nimorazole (a substance that reduces hypoxia) in cases of supraglottic laryngeal and hypopharyngeal carcinoma is associated with significant improvement of local tumor control and lower cancer-related mortality. An international phase-III trial is currently underway to assess the definitive value of this treatment.

Initially it was not known how often a patient needed to be irradiated. At first it was common to give a single, large dose of external irradiation, thus mirroring the attitude of the surgeon who tried to remove an entire tumor in a single sitting. Hermann Wintz (1887-1947) from Erlangen was the principal advocate of this approach, which had been proposed by the German surgeon Georg C. Perthes (1869-1927) in 1904. Ten years later, Gottwald Schwartz suggested that multiple doses might be more effective since cells are most sensitive to radiation at the moment of mitosis. The number of researchers undertaking radiobiologic studies gradually grew. In 1918, the German obstetrician Bernhardt Krönig (1863-1917) and the above-mentioned Walter Friedrich showed that the total dose needed to produce a given skin reaction in fractionated irradiation was greater than when only a single dose was given. Nevertheless, single-dose irradiation continued to find adherents in Germany, especially in Erlangen, until the 1920s.

In 1922, the French radiologist Claude Regaud (1870-1941) published a classic series of experiments in which he showed that spermatogenesis in the ram could be definitively terminated by successive daily doses of radiation, while the same result could not be achieved with a single high dose. Moreover, a single dose often led to unbearable damage to the skin of the scrotum (Holsti, 1995).

Henri Coutard (1876-1950), a French radiologist at the Radium Institute in Paris (which later became the Curie Institute), had to fractionate his X-ray treatments in order to give the X-ray tube time to cool off. They had two X-ray treatment sessions at the institute, six days a week. Coutard experimented with different fractionation schedules: he was the great pioneer in this field. He monitored his patients' condition carefully, and examined them every day. He published the results of his five years of work in the early 1930s. Coutard was regarded as a great authority in the radiotherapeutic world, both in Europe and in the United States.

Regaud, Coutard and A. Hautant, all from the Radium Institute, presented the case histories of six patients with advanced laryngeal cancer at the International Congress of Otology held in Paris in 1922. All had been given radiation therapy, and were subsequently found to be free of symptoms of the disease. This was a vitally important observation, since it was the first time that it was possible to demonstrate that radiotherapy could cure cancer without the aid of the surgeon. This moment can be seen as the birth of radiotherapy as an independent discipline.

It is appropriate at this point to mention a number of leading radiotherapists who have helped to shape the development of clinical radiotherapy. After Coutard, François Baclesse in Paris and Ralston Paterson in Manchester between 1940 and

1960 largely determined the practice in this field, followed by Gilbert H. Fletcher who was chairman of the radiotherapy department of the University of Texas M.D. Anderson Cancer Center in Houston for more than thirty years, starting in 1948.

François Baclesse (1896-1967), who was born in Luxembourg, succeeded Coutard at the Radium Institute in Paris in 1937. He developed a radiotherapy technique aimed at avoiding acute reactions of the mucous membranes and the skin. He also introduced the "shrinking field" irradiation technique, in which the area exposed to radiation was gradually reduced as the tumor shrank in response to treatment. Baclesse further increased the total treatment period to 12 or 16 weeks, and raised the dose used at the end of the irradiation period.

Ralston Paterson (1897-1981), appointed director of the Holt Radium Institute in Manchester in 1931, became the most prominent radiotherapist in England. Over the next five years, he built up his institute to become a world leader in the field of radiotherapy. He suggested in 1936 that radical irradiation was an essential element in the treatment of cancer that had been detected at an early stage, and that it was vital to give this irradiation up to the limit of the patient's tolerance. Another key contribution made by the Holt Radium Institute was the development of the standardized irradiation field concept, based on the idea that certain tumors could be treated by irradiating as uniformly as possible over a single field that covered both the primary tumor and the area in which metastases were likely. Paterson initiated radical small-field irradiation in 1935; it was an approach that remained popular for many years. His name lives on in the Paterson-Parker system of radium implant dosimetry, which he developed together with the radiation physicist Herbert Parker (1910-1984) (Holsti, 1995).

Gilbert H. Fletcher (1911-1992) was born and raised in France. His American father died young. After having gained his *baccalauréat* in Paris in 1929, he studied engineering in Louvain (Belgium), graduating in 1932, and went on to gain two further degrees in Brussels: mathematics (1935) and medicine (1941). He learned about radiotherapy during his medical studies at the Jules Bordet Institute in Brussels. The war forced him in 1942 to move to America, where he had to get used to living and working in an English-speaking environment. He joined the M.D. Anderson Cancer Center in Houston in 1948 and set up the radiotherapy department which he continued to lead until his retirement in 1981. He made a long trip to Europe to study radiotherapy practices there, where he was largely influenced by Baclesse (Ribot, 2005). He also founded a radiotherapy school in Houston, which has trained generations of American radiotherapists. He developed reproducible treatment schedules for cancers of the head and neck, breast, cervix and endometrium. His measurements of the response to the radiation dose used to control tumors of different sizes led in the 1960s to the concept of "subclinical disease," which could be effectively treated with lower radiation doses than were needed for larger tumors. Fletcher's main contribution to clinical research, however, was his systematic analysis of the failures and complications noted when

FIGURE 5.6a Orthovoltage therapy unit.(Source: Rosenbusch G, Panhuysen J, Vellenga K. and A.M. De Knecht - van Eekelen.Van Röntgenoloog naar radioloog 1901-2001 (From roentgenologist to radiologist 1901-2001). Nederlandse Vereniging voor Radiologie. Reproduced with permission).

FIGURE 5.6b Linear accelerator. (Source: Rosenbusch G, Panhuysen J, et al., 2001. Reproduced with permission).

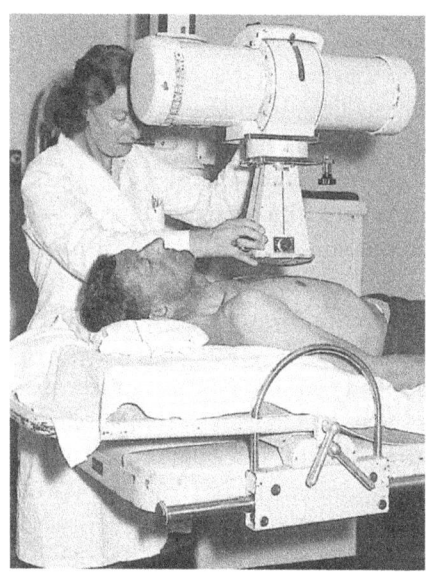

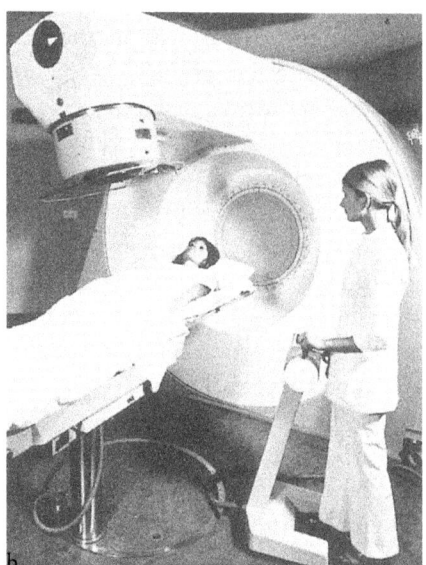

a

b

patients had undergone a standard course of treatment (Holsti, 1995). He also designed the world's first cobalt-60 clinical irradiation unit, which uses the radioactive isotope cobalt-60 as a radiation source instead of radium. This application, which made radiation treatment more effective and affordable, is discussed in greater detail in the next section.

The long-standing debate on the pros and cons of fractionated irradiation was finally settled in favor of fractionation in 1932, after thorough analysis of the data available from the literature at that time.

Another important issue was the energy of the radiation source. Early irradiation units had energies in the kilovolt range. A new generation of much more powerful irradiation units, with energies in the megavolt range, became available in the 1970s. Not everyone approved of the new equipment. Its opponents claimed that kilovolt therapy was best, so they coined the new term "orthovoltage irradiation", derived from the Greek *orthos*, meaning good or correct, for it (Figure 5.6a). Nevertheless, megavoltage irradiation gradually won the day on the basis of its many important advantages: it allows more uniform distribution of the dose and sharper focusing of the beam, causes less damage to the skin and produces lower radiation loading of bone.

The first megavoltage irradiation unit was the linear accelerator (Figure 5.6b). Like many other devices in this field, it was based on equipment originally intended (and still used) for physical research. The medical linear accelerator was developed in England, and was first used in practice at the Hammersmith Hospital in London in 1953. The Van de Graaff generator is another well-known device from the world of physics. Developed by the American physicist Robert J. van de Graaff (1901-1967) in 1929 on the basis of principles dating back to the 17th century or even earlier, it produces electrostatic voltages in the megavolt range. This is the device, familiar to many from science museums, that makes your hair stand on end. In view of the very high voltages it generates, it was thought that it might be possible to adapt the Van de Graaff generator for radiotherapeutic purposes. It was concluded, however, that the bulky nature of the equipment and the very low dose rates it produces meant that this was not a realistic option.

A much better way of obtaining very high energies is to accelerate charged atomic particles along a circular path. The basic ideas in this field, worked out by the Norwegian particle physicist Rolf Widerōe (1902-1996), famously inspired Ernest O. Lawrence (1901-1958) to develop the cyclotron – which can be used to accelerate positively charged particles such as the proton. He won the Nobel Prize for this in 1939. Cyclotrons, such as the world-famous machine built by the CERN in Geneva, have been responsible for major advances in particle physics. The same principle can be used to construct a device, known as a betatron, which accelerates electrons along a circular path to achieve energies of tens of megavolts. It seemed clear that the betatron could have important applications in radiotherapy. Widerōe worked on the betatron during the Second World War – under pressure from the Germans, who thought that the device might help their war effort. He was imprisoned in Norway for 48 days after the war as a suspected collaborator until evidence from friends and colleagues convinced the authorities of his innocence. The first successful betatron was actually made in 1940 by the American Donald Kerst (1911-1993) at the University of Illinois; he was also more interested in its possibilities as a tool for research in physics than as a therapeutic device (Bernier, 2004). The first recorded clinical application was by the German Konrad Gund (1907-1953), who is reported to have treated a patient in 1942 with a betatron he had developed himself (Ribot, 2005). Though theoretically interesting, the betatron proved to be something of a dead end in the field of radiotherapy.

James Chadwick (1891-1974) had discovered the neutron – an atomic particle with the same mass as a proton but zero electrical charge – in 1932 and was awarded the Nobel Prize for this discovery in 1935. Their absence of charge means that neutrons can penetrate much further into the body than any other ionizing radiation. This makes them potentially very suitable for radiotherapy. Some elements, such as beryllium, emit neutrons spontaneously (this is how Chadwick discovered them), but to produce the large numbers of neutrons needed for medical applications, a cyclotron is needed: it can accelerate alpha particles (helium nuclei) to very high energies, and these high-energy alpha particles can be used to bombard suitable atoms to produce neutrons in the required numbers. Patients were already being treated with neutron radiation three years after the discovery of this particle. Neutron radiotherapy is no longer used, however.

Since radium emits radiation in the megavolt range, it has also been used for the external irradiation of patients. Radium teletherapy was developed starting about 1920 by Sydney Russ, a physicist at the Middlesex Hospital in London and later professor of medical physics; Eric Lysholm in Stockholm; Sicilian-born Gioacchion Failla (1891-1961) in the United States and Lucien Mallet (1885-1981) and Robert Coliez in Paris (Proux, 1983).

The discovery of artificial radioactivity and its application

Frédéric Joliot (1900-1958) and his wife Irène Joliot-Curie (1897-1956, the daughter of Pierre and Marie) discovered artificially induced radioactivity in 1933 when they bombarded an aluminum disc with α radiation from polonium. This bombardment produced a radioactive atom, phosphorus-32, which emitted β radiation. The New Zealander Ernest Rutherford (1871-1937), professor of applied physics and Director of the Cavendish Laboratory in Cambridge, winner of the Nobel Prize for Chemistry in 1908 and later Lord Rutherford, was in fact the first to bring about the artificial transmutation of one element into another when he bombarded nitrogen gas with α radiation from radium in 1919 to produce oxygen. The Joliot-Curies, however, were the first to produce a hitherto unknown substance by a nuclear reaction – a substance, moreover, which was unstable and emitted radiation while it changed into yet another substance. This was the special significance of their discovery, for which the couple were awarded the Nobel Prize for Chemistry in 1935. Their discovery led to a massive search for new radioactive isotopes, many of which were found. This research received strong financial support from the world's largest countries in the years leading up to the Second World War, in the hope – well-founded, as it turned out – that it would lead to a powerful new weapon.

The Italian physicist Enrico Fermi (1901-1954) and his research team tackled this problem systematically in 1934, bombarding each element in turn with neutrons and noting the results. They observed that the neutron bombardment caused the nucleus of the uranium atom to split into two, a process that became known as "nuclear fission." Fermi thought that he had discovered another new element. The German phycisist and chemist Otto Hahn (1879-1968) was not so sure, and repeated the experiments. He found that bombarding a uranium atom with a neutron led to the production of two smaller nuclei, together with two new neutrons and a certain amount of energy in the form of radiation. The new neutrons can give rise to a self-sustaining chain reaction and the emission of a great deal of energy (Stam, 1993). Hahn announced his results in 1938. He won the Nobel Prize for Chemistry in 1944 for his discovery of nuclear fission, but was unable to travel to Stockholm to accept the prize until the next year because he was detained in England, together with some other prominent German scientists, by the Allies for some time after the end of the war in Europe.

The enormous amount of energy that could be released by the chain reaction involved in nuclear fission was calculated by the Danish theoretical physicist Niels Bohr (1885-1962) and Fermi, who met in the United States in 1939, where Fermi was living in exile after he was forced to leave Italy for refusing to wear the Fascist uniform when accepting his Nobel Prize in 1938. It became clear that uranium could form the basis of what came to be known as the "atomic bomb." Various European scientists felt that President Roosevelt of the United States needed to be informed of this possibility, and Albert Einstein (1879-1955) wrote him a historic letter on this subject – largely drafted by the above-mentioned Leó Szilárd – on 2 August 1939 (Proux, 1983).

This led President Roosevelt to set up the Manhattan Project to investigate the possibility of actually producing an atomic bomb. This project, under the military leadership of General Leslie R. Groves of the US Army Corps of Engineers and with J. Robert Oppenheimer (1904-1967) as scientific director, culminated in the production of the two atomic bombs, nicknamed "Little Boy" and "Fat Man," that were dropped on Hiroshima and Nagasaki in August 1945 and led to the beginning of the end of the war.

An important spin-off of this military project for the medical world was the availability of radioactive isotopes that could be put to both diagnostic and thera-

CHAPTER 5

peutic use. The main benefit of these new substances in the field of diagnosis was that many of them were gamma-emitters with a much shorter half-life than natural radiation sources, making them much safer for patients. Such radioactive isotopes are currently used in bone scintigraphy and PET (positron emission tomography) scans. Radioactive isotopes that emit gamma rays also proved very useful for therapeutic purposes, in particular because many of them accumulate preferentially in certain organs thus permitting specific irradiation of tumors present in those organs. A good example of this is the use of radioactive iodine to treat thyroid cancer.

One gamma-emitter made available by the atomic energy industry that proved to be of particular benefit for medical applications was radioactive cobalt (cobalt-60), first produced in a cyclotron in 1941. By 1945 the physical properties of this isotope had been largely determined. It was found to have a half-life of only 5.3 years, compared with approximately 1600 years for radium (Proux, 1983). This has the important advantage of ensuring that any traces of the radioactive isotopes left in the body will decay reasonably quickly.

Although the idea of using cobalt-60 as a teleradiotherapy source came from the eminent English radiotherapist Joseph Stanley Mitchell (1909-1987), later Regius Professor of Physic[1] at Cambridge University from 1957 to 1975, it was the American physician Leonard G. Grimmett together with the engineer Bailey Moore at the M. D. Anderson Cancer Center in Houston who, at the urging of the above-mentioned Gilbert H. Fletcher, realized the first working cobalt-60 unit in 1948. This unit had a source intensity of 10 curie. Two years later, Grimmett drew up plans for a 1000 curie unit (corresponding to a kilogram of radium). However, the American team fell apart due to Grimmet's early death and General Electric – the company that would have built the unit – did not see promise in the concept. The first unit of this size was actually built in Canada, at the Chalk River nuclear reactor facility in Ontario (Proux, 1983) for delivery to the team headed by Harold Elford Johns (1915-1998) – one of the founders of medical physics – at the University of Saskatchewan in Saskatoon. The first patients were treated with it – successfully – in 1951 at the Victoria Hospital in London, Ontario, by Dr. Ivan Smith and Roy Errington, the designer of the machine (Litt 2002). These cobalt bombs, as they were called, became so popular that thousands of them were built.

Eventually, however, cobalt bombs were superseded by the above-mentioned linear accelerator, which has a number of advantages compared with the cobalt bomb: there is no need to replace the radiation source, and it delivers more energy with higher penetration and less scattering of the radiation (Bernier, 2004).

---

1 "Physic" is an old-fashioned word for 'medicine' that is no longer used in everyday language. It only survives in the noun 'physician' (a synonym for 'doctor') and in this academic title at Cambridge.

The 1930s saw a major shift in radiotherapy, from a mainly palliative approach to a realization that this technique offered real opportunities for curing certain cancers.

Major breakthroughs were achieved after the Second World War, for example in the treatment of Hodgkin's disease. Thanks to improved staging and the development of total lymph node irradiation, the five-year survival rate in this previously incurable disease could be improved to better than 80 percent if treatment was given early enough. The American radiologist Henry S. Kaplan (1918-1983) at Stanford University was the great pioneer in this field. High cure rates could also be achieved in the radiotherapy of various youth cancers and seminoma (a type of testicular cancer). Irradiation can furthermore often cure laryngeal cancer and other cancers of the head and neck, endometrial, bladder and prostate cancer, thyroid and cervical cancer if these conditions are detected early enough, and can improve the survival rate in rectal cancer and breast cancer.

Developments in the field of internal irradiation

Internal isotope treatment is known as brachytherapy, from the Greek work *brachy*, meaning short or nearby. This term refers to the treatment of tumor tissue with the aid of a small radioactive source implanted in or very close to the tissue in question. It was coined by Gösta Forsell, mentioned above in the section on the use of radiation in medical treatment. There are two main types of brachytherapy: *afterloading*, with the use of source holders connected to tubes that are implanted in the tumor or body cavity, and direct implantation of radioisotope "seeds" in the tumor. Brachytherapy can be given as a separate treatment or in combination with external irradiation.

Internal irradiation has been used in the treatment of cancer since the start of the twentieth century. The report by Margaret Cleaves in 1903 of the favorable effect of radium in the treatment of cervical cancer was already mentioned above. H. Strebel, a physician from Munich, also used a form of afterloading in 1903 – not so much in the interests of radiation safety, as is the case nowadays, but for the sake of convenience. He used trepanation needles to make a hole in the tissue, thus facilitating the insertion of the radium sources (Mould, 1995).

The American physicist William Duane (1872-1935) developed the use of glass "seeds" filled with radon gas, a decay product of radium with a half-life of no more than 3.82 days (Ribot, 2005). William Duane was a descendant of Benjamin Franklin, the famous American scientist, politician and diplomat. He worked for some time in Marie Curie's laboratory in Paris. It is reported that when Madame Curie visited America some years later and was asked what she particularly wanted to see in the United States, she replied, "Niagara Falls, the Grand Canyon and William Duane."

The gynecologist James Heyman (1882-1956) from Radiumhemmet in Stockholm (the first cancer treatment clinic in Sweden) was the great advocate of gynecologic brachytherapy. This approach was strongly opposed by gynecologic surgeons, especially in Germany, as the following anecdote illustrates. Carl Gauss, a pupil of the above-mentioned Bernhardt Krönig in Freiburg in Germany, was invited to read a paper on the radiotherapy of gynecologic tumors to the Berlin Society of Gynecology and Obstetrics, in view of the excellent results they had been getting with this form of treatment at the Freiburg clinic. However, the lecture ended in turmoil when many members of the audience loudly expressed their disbelief of the results presented. The Berlin gynecologists left the lecture theatre en masse, leaving Gauss alone on the field of battle (Mould, 1995).

Modern afterloading techniques – known as remote afterloading brachytherapy – were introduced in 1953 by Ulrich Henschke and colleagues at Ohio State University, and further developed at the Memorial Hospital in New York City (Henschke et al., 1963). Since then, interest in this method has taken a rollercoaster ride, with a succession of peaks and troughs. The availability of new isotopes such as cesium-137 and iridium-192 about 1960 led to a surge of interest in brachytherapy performed with the aid of source holders. Iridium-192 can be placed in the tumor via removable tubes, which is very convenient for afterloading applications. This technique was pioneered by the Frenchman Bernard Pierquin (Bernier, 2004). Interest in brachytherapy then declined again until the early 1970s when Willet Whitmore (1917-1995) from Memorial Hospital described an open implantation technique for the use of radioactive iodine in the treatment of prostate cancer. The isotope was sealed in tiny titanium capsules that could be placed in the prostate: without any imaging system that could provide a precise check on their position, however. This method was initially very popular, but the irregular dose distribution (with excessive doses at some points and inadequate doses at others) led to unpredictable results and side-effects and a consequent loss of interest.

The sharp improvement in brachytherapy facilities during the past couple of decades has led to yet another rise in interest. High-dose brachytherapy units were introduced about 1980. These units make it possible to implant radium in body cavities or interstitially and to remove it again in-between treatment sessions, thus giving short irradiations that can be administered on an outpatient basis. It is no longer necessary to place the radioactive sources in the source holders by hand: a simple push on a button is currently sufficient (Bernier, 2004). Details of a device known as the "Royal Marsden gun" (after the renowned cancer hospital in London where it was developed) that could be used for the implantation of radioactive gold-198 seeds were published by Hodt et al. (1952); while H. Holm, a urologist from Copenhagen, described a technique for guiding the implantation of radioactive seed-bearing needles by ultrasonography in 1983 (Denmeade and Isaacs, 2002).

Recent developments

Digital technology brought about major changes in radiotherapy at the end of the twentieth century. Much of the progress can be ascribed to the availability of smaller, faster computers that permit improved planning of the irradiation schedule. Radiotherapy-planning CT (computed tomography) permits a more accurate determination of the target field and its immediate vicinity. It may be noted that the first CT unit was built in 1971 by the English electrical engineer Godfrey Hounsfield (1919-2004) and his team on a theoretical basis elaborated by the South Africa-born American physicist Allan McLeod Cormack (1924-1998). Cormack began work on his ideas in this field in the Groote Schuur Hospital in Cape Town, famous as the site of the world's first successful heart transplant operation, performed by the surgeon Christiaan Barnard in late 1967. Hounsfield and Cormack won the Nobel Prize for Medicine in 1979 for their development of computed tomography. It seems possible that *magnetic resonance imaging* (MRI) may replace CT in coming years. PET-CT and functional MRI will probably ensure further improvement in the near future, because they allow functional information to be combined with anatomic data. The above considerations apply to both external and internal irradiation. Recent developments like IMRT (*intensity-modulated radiation therapy*) and tomotherapy also increase the scope for further improvement of the quality of external irradiation. IMRT allows the intensity of the radiation beam to be adjusted in any field and at any desired moment. Tomotherapy can be regarded as a further refinement of IMRT, in which the radiation beam is rotated around the tumor in the course of treatment, while the intensity of the beam can be regulated from moment to moment. These new techniques also allow the form of the radiation beam to be better adapted to the sometimes irregular contours of the tumor, thus helping to give a higher dose within the target field while sparing surrounding normal tissue.

The latest development is 4D irradiation, which allows the irradiation schedule to take not only the three spatial dimensions but also the fourth dimension of time into account. A CT scanner with a conical beam, rather than the conventional fan-shaped beam, mounted on the linear accelerator performs a 4D scan of the target area during irradiation. This allows the radiotherapist to adjust the irradiation unit to take into account the movement of the tumor due to the patient's respiration and heartbeat.

The combination of radiotherapy with hyperthermia (high body temperature) is another trend that deserves mention. The application of hyperthermia in the treatment of cancer was discussed in Chapter 4, in the section on tumors of the extremities. Hyperthermia increases sensitivity to irradiation by enhancing the circulation of the blood, thus improving the oxygenation of the tissues. The main reason for the intensification of the effects of irradiation, however, is that hyperthermia interferes with the repair of DNA in tumor cells damaged by irradiation.

In particular, radiotherapy combined with local heating of the tumor seems likely to have a bright future.

Radiotherapy has also been increasingly combined with surgery and chemotherapy. This has led to a substantial improvement in the prognosis for many types of cancer. The present-day cure rate for cancer is about 50%. About 14% of patients are currently cured by radiotherapy alone, another 13% by combined therapy (which almost always includes radiotherapy) and the rest by surgery and chemotherapy.

The combination of radiotherapy with other forms of treatment also has the important advantage of leaving the patient less severely mutilated in many cases. While in the past the treatment for breast cancer usually involved surgical removal of the entire breast, it is currently generally possible to spare the breast by surgical removal of the tumor alone followed by radiation treatment to deal with local metastases. This is a great beneit to the psychosocial well-being of the patient. Another field in which combined treatment has made an enormous difference is that of advanced laryngeal and hypopharyngeal cancer. In the past, these diseases often required total excision of the larynx and the consequent loss of the ability to speak. Even with the means available to alleviate this condition, the patient never recovered a normal voice. A combination of chemotherapy and irradiation treatment means that it is currently generally possible to avoid removing the larynx, with the immeasurable benefit of allowing the patient to retain his or her voice.

The recognition of radiotherapy as a separate specialism, independent from radiology, had important implications for the status of the discipline and the effectiveness of its practitioners. For example, it allowed radiotherapists to devote themselves exclusively to the therapeutic use of radiation, thus improving the quality of the treatment given. This development took place at different times and in different ways in different countries. Radiology societies were founded in many countries throughout the world in the couple of decades after Roentgen's discovery of X-rays. However, it gradually came to be realized that having one professional body that covered both those who used X-rays and other forms of radiation for diagnosis and those who used such radiation for therapy was not effective. In Britain, for example, the Roentgen Society – the first medical X-ray society in the world – was founded in 1897, and the British Association of Radiologists in 1934. One year later, the Society of Radiotherapists of Great Britain and Ireland was set up to represent the interests of those using X-rays and radium in the treatment of cancer. In 1939, these two bodies merged again to form the Faculty of Radiologists, which was renamed the Royal College of Radiologists in 1979. This body has two different types of members: clinical radiologists, who specialize in diagnostic imaging systems, and clinical oncologists, who specialize in radiotherapy. A similar development may be seen in the United States. The Western Roentgen Society was founded in late 1915. This organization changed its name in 1919 to the Radiological Society of North America (RSNA), which still exists today. A separate body for radiotherapists, the American Society for Therapeutic Radiology and Oncology (ASTRO), was set up in 1958.

The Dutch professional body for radiotherapists, the Nederlandse Vereniging voor Radiotherapie en Oncologie (nvro), was set up in 1978 – 77 years after the foundation of the Nederlandse Vereniging voor Radiologie (NVvR) – and the European Society for Therapeutic Radiology and Oncology (estro) was founded in Milan in 1980.

[6]

The development of chemotherapy

The introduction of cancer chemotherapy – that is, the treatment of cancer with appropriate chemical substances – in the 1950s and 1960s resulted in the development of curative and palliative treatments for almost all solid tumors and malignant blood diseases. While it emerged that chemotherapy alone can lead to a cure, the combination of chemotherapy with surgery and radiotherapy gave a significantly higher chance of recovery.

The main problem associated with treating cancer with cytostatics (substances that are capable of killing cells) is that they attack normal tissue as well as cancer cells and can thus often lead to unpleasant and sometimes serious side effects. The discovery, discussed in Chapter 2, that the cause of cancer lies in the DNA of the nucleus opened up new ways of combating the disease by attacking the problem at its root. This approach, described in greater detail in Chapter 8, is known as targeted therapy. It offers the prospect of concentrating therapeutic action on the tumor alone while sparing healthy tissue. But targeted therapy is still in its infancy, so conventional chemotherapy will doubtless continue to be needed in the immediate future though it is expected to eventually become obsolete. Since this form of therapy is currently still very much in demand, however, a detailed overview of how it came about will be given in the present chapter.

Chemotherapy in the distant past

Remedies for cancer and other diseases, in the form of ointments, pastes, plasters, powders, aromatic liquids, wines, medicinal herb mixtures and the like have been known since the dawn of history. Details of these ancient formulations, dating back to about 2000 BC, have been discovered in Sumerian, Chinese, Indian, Persian and Egyptian records. Even in those days, of which we have such an imperfect understanding, each civilization had a long list of folk cures for all sorts of complaints. While most medicines were made from herbs, minerals such as iron, copper, sulfur, arsenic and mercury and animal products such as leather, bones and urine were also used in their preparation (Wolff, 1907).

An important source of information about ancient remedies, including some for cancer, is the 37-volume Natural History by Pliny the Elder (AD 23-79), a Roman lawyer, scholar and encyclopedist who found time amidst his busy public life to write at least 75 books and 160 unpublished notebooks, of which Natural History is the only one to have been preserved. The last 18 volumes of this work describe remedies from plant and animal sources, and stones and minerals and their use in medicine and architecture. Pliny's keen interest in natural history actually led to his death: as commander of the Roman fleet in the Bay of Naples, he took his boats too close to Mount Vesuvius during the famous eruption of AD 79 in order to investigate the cause of the eruption and to calm the populace, and probably perished in the fumes from the volcano. This event was described by his nephew and adopted son, Pliny the Younger (AD 62-113). Pliny is known for the saying, "true glory consists in doing what deserves to be written; in writing what deserves to be read; and in so living as to make the world happier for our living in it." In his Natural History, he tended to replace the simple remedies recommended by earlier herbalists, such as cabbage juice for the treatment of cancer, with more complicated formulations. For example, he recommended a boiled mixture of the ash of sea crab, egg whites, honey, stinging nettles with salt and a powder made from the dried feces of falcons for the treatment of internal cancers. The Natural History remained an authority for many centuries and was one of the first scientific texts to be printed in Venice – probably the world center for the early printing of scientific and medical works – after the printing industry became established there in 1469.

The Roman author Celsus thought that cancer could be cured by means of a special diet, medicines and surgery. His ideas were, however, rejected by Galen, who adhered strictly to the dogmas of the humoral theory. He believed that cancer was caused by a build-up of black bile. It followed that in order to cure cancer, the patient's entire body had to be purged of this excess of black bile. Galen prescribed simple remedies and herb mixtures to this end.

Galen's ideas persisted for many centuries: the monks in the monasteries of medieval Europe prepared their medicines in accordance with his writings. It was generally accepted at that time that cancer first had to be thinned out in the body using sugar water, after which it could be cleared up with the aid of laxatives and the like.

One non-herbal remedy much used at the time was Blatta bizantina, an oil-based preparation of dried cockroaches used to treat warts, ulcers, skin cancers and other cancers.

Painkillers were also prescribed alongside anti-cancer agents. One of the most popular analgesics used in the treatment of internal diseases (including non-superficial cancers) was a mixture of arsenic, camphor, licorice root, honey, alcohol and boiled viper meat. Dried frog could be added as an optional extra.

Medieval European medicine took over a number of features from the flourishing Arabic medical tradition, including some occult therapeutic methods derived from alchemy. But there were also some more rational practices, such as the writing of prescriptions and the establishment of pharmacies. The *quid pro quo rule*, in the currently unusual sense that when one medicine is not available it can be replaced with another, was also introduced at this time.

There was a gradually perceived need for a move away from a more or less haphazard approach to the preparation of medicines and towards a more orderly, standardized procedure. An important step in this direction was the posthumous publication of the Nuremberg *Dispensatorium* (book of prescriptions) by Valerius Cordus in 1546. The introduction by Paracelsus (mentioned in Chapter 2) of the iatrochemical hypothesis of disease and treatments based on this also made an important contribution to the standardization of medicine. Paracelsus was a Swiss physician who studied metallurgy, alchemy and chemistry at the University of Basel, while he learned medicine from his father and from barber-surgeons. He was a skilled doctor and an original thinker. He did not accept arguments simply because they were supported by tradition, and in particular he rejected the centuries-old humoral theory that lay at the heart of much of Galen's teachings. He travelled widely throughout Europe and made many enemies because of his controversial ideas. He was ultimately forced to flee Basel and settle in Salzburg, and he died shortly afterwards from injuries he sustained in a café brawl.

Iatrochemistry is the name given to the hypothesis that health depends on a balance of the chemical substances in the body. Paracelsus believed that any disease – cancer included – was caused by the precipitation of chemicals in the body, and could only be cured by chemical means. According to him, cancer could be successfully treated with chemical elements or compounds administered in gradually increasing doses. He introduced the medical use of many chemicals, including mercury, lead, sulfur, iron, copper, arsenic, iodine and potassium, and wrote several monographs on medicines.

In the period immediately following Paracelsus' death, mercury was used as a caustic agent for treating external cancers, while a solution of mercury salts was recommended for internal tumors (in particular sarcomas) such as cancer of the tongue. Arsenic to be taken by mouth was prescribed as a remedy for the hemorrhaging of tumors (Hadju, 2005).

Antonius Nück (1660-1692), professor of medicine at Leiden, and the well-known surgeon and anatomist Govert Bidloo (1649-1713) from The Hague, however, saw no advantage in treating cancer with the aid of medicines (De Moulin, 1988).

The London *Pharmacopoeia*, printed in many editions between 1621 and 1851, was the main guide to the prescription of drugs in England until the introduction of the British *Pharmacopoeia* in 1864. The 1721 edition, produced under the auspices of Sir Hans Soane, omitted many of the more ridiculous remedies, while the 1746 edition introduced a much greater degree of standardization. One of the more popular prescriptions from the earlier editions, intended to combat an accumulation of malignant acids, was *tinctura vitriolata* in a dosage of two drops a day and an alkaline solution of camphor, chalk, gold, silver and lead salts. Another formulation that was supposedly very effective in treating the same complaint was composed of crab's eye (20 grains), red coral (20 grains), salt of tartar (15 grains), oil of cloves (12 droplets), oil of cumin (12 droplets) and 5 grains of opium. The mixture was fermented to a powder and divided into seven portions, one of which was given each day (Hadju, 2005).

In 1767, the English physician John Burrows summarized the development of the treatment of metastasized cancer as follows in his publication, "A new practical essay on cancers":

_____ *Everything that has ever been produced to cure cancer is simply a palliative remedy. From the time of Hippocrates until now no real medicine has ever been discovered against this fatal affliction, although doctors from all countries have carried out countless experiments using all manner of things that can be found in nature, from the most harmless substances to the most venomous poisons originating from minerals and from the plant kingdom. Nevertheless the illness is still mightier than the power of medicine.*

Francis Arthur Bainbridge (1874-1921), professor of physiology at Durham University from 1911 to 1915 and then at St. Bartholomew's Hospital for the rest of his life, wrote in a similar vein in 1914:

_____ *Throughout the centuries, the sufferers of this disease have been the subject of almost every conceivable form of experimentation. The fields and forests, the apothecary shop and temple have been ransacked for some successful means of relief from the intractable malady. Hardly any animal had escaped making its contribution of hide or hair, tooth or toenail, thymus or thyroid, liver or spleen, in the vain search for a means of relief* (Papac, 2001).

Modern chemotherapy

The roots of present-day cancer chemotherapy lie in chemotherapy for infectious diseases. The story begins with Jesuit missionaries in Peru around 1630, who learned from the natives that tea made from the bark of a certain tree could be used to cure malaria. The natives called it *quiniquina* ("the bark of barks"), from which name the modern word *quinine* is derived. It was imported into Europe under the name of Jesuit's bark or Jesuit's powder and was highly prized as a remedy for fevers.

The next major step in the development of chemotherapy came about 200 years later, in 1865, when Heinrich Lissauer of Breslau demonstrated that potassium arsenite is effective in the treatment of chronic lymphatic leukemia (Burchenal, 1975). He stated that administration of this substance led to an improvement in the condition of his patients, but he did not carry out any blood cell counts. The beneficial effects on the peripheral blood cell level were not described until about 13 years later (Papac, 2001). Billroth stated that potassium arsenite was also effective in the treatment of malignant lymphomas. Potassium arsenite had been well known under the name of "Fowler's solution" as a tonic and remedy for various diseases, including leukemia, since its introduction by a Dr. Fowler of Stafford in England in 1786. It was still being prescribed in the United States for the treatment of malaria, chorea and syphilis until the late 1950s.

Then, around the turn of the century the great Paul Ehrlich (1854-1915), pupil of Robert Koch, demonstrated that an azo dye was effective in curing mice that had been infected with *Trypanosoma equinum*, the causative agent of trypanosomal encephalitis, or sleeping sickness, in horses. The dye was renamed "trypan red" in honor of this discovery. Ehrlich had been interested in the aniline dyes discovered by the English chemist Sir William Henry Perkin (1838-1907) since 1878, but for many years he had concentrated on their application in staining tissues as an aid to their microscopic examination. This gave him the idea that certain molecules bind specifically to given cell receptors, like a key in a lock. Taking this one step further, Ehrlich developed the side-chain theory of antibody formation – a key concept in the understanding of immunity for which he shared the Nobel Prize in Physiology or Medicine with Ilya Mechnikov in 1908. Before that, Ehrlich had another brilliant idea: perhaps these azo dyes or similar compounds could act as "magic bullets," targeting the active site responsible for specific diseases. He set up a major research program, screening hundreds of compounds for possible therapeutic activity. It was during this screening program that the curative action of trypan red was established in 1904. The discovery that a synthetic organic substance derived from known chemical materials could be used to cure a disease was a huge step forward. An even more important discovery was made in 1909, when the Japanese bacteriologist Sahachiro Hata, who was working in Ehrlich's laboratory, found that the 606th substance to be screened – which combined both azo groups and the arsenic whose therapeutic action has been noted above – was active against *Spirochaeta pallida* (now generally known as *Treponema pallidum*) the infective agent causing syphilis, at that time a widely prevalent and debilitating sexually transmitted disease (Burchenal, 1975). This drug came to be known as 606 or Salvarsan.

It was Ehrlich who coined the term *chemotherapy*, by which he meant the use of chemical substances to treat infections. His use of an *in vivo* rodent model to test means of chemotherapy in the treatment of infectious diseases inspired George Clowes (1877-1958) of the Roswell Park Institute in Buffalo, New York, to develop inbred rodent breeds with transplanted tumors for the screening of potential anticancer drugs during the first years of the 20th century. This *in vivo* system became the basis for the mass screening of new cytostatics (Chu and DeVita, 2001).

There were no noteworthy developments in the field of antibacterial treatment during the next thirty years. The medical world was slow to take up the above-mentioned new therapeutic agents. In hindsight, it is clear that the positive results obtained with quinine, trypan red and salvarsan demonstrated that medicines acting at a systemic level could cure a variety of diseases. Bacteriologists were on the whole not impressed, however, since they argued that while these agents might be able to cure protozoan diseases such as malaria and sleeping sickness they were not suitable for treating bacterial diseases. (It may be noted that *Spirochaeta pallida*, the infectious agent causing syphilis, was thought to be a parasite at that time, though it is now classified as a bacterium.) Thus, all the highest authorities in the first decade of the 20th century kept echoing the message that there was no point in trying to combat bacterial infections using chemotherapy.

Although the description in 1919 by the American pathologists E.B. and H.D. Krumbhaar of autopsy findings on soldiers who had been exposed to mustard gas in the trenches of Verdun came from an entirely different field, it was still significant for the later development of cancer chemotherapy. They found atrophy of lymphatic and testicular tissue and damage to the bone marrow. This prefigures the later important research on nitrogen mustard as a cytostatic, described below under the heading alkylating cytostatics. The description by Alexander Fleming (1881-1955) in 1929 of the antibacterial effect of penicillin cultures on *Staphylococcus aureus* was also of crucial importance. But neither the observations of Krumbhaar and Krumbhaar nor those of Fleming received the attention they deserved for many years. The time was not yet ripe for them (Burchenal, 1975).

The German pathologist and bacteriologist Gerhard Domagk (1895-1964) discovered an important new antibacterial agent in 1932, while he was working at the research institute for pathological anatomy and bacteriology that had been set up a few years before by the chemical giant IG Farben. IG Farben's interest in this topic is understandable. The company's name stands for "syndicate of dyestuff industries." At this time, Germany was the world leader in the production of synthetic dyes, after they had been discovered in England. When Ehrlich discovered the therapeutic properties of trypan red as described above, it was IG Farben that took the initiative to set up a large-scale screening program for new drugs derived from dyestuffs, since if such substances could be found it would open up a new and hugely profitable market for the company. Then in 1932, Domagk discovered that the red dye prontosil (a derivative of sulfanilamide, discussed in greater detail below) protected mice and rabbits against lethal doses of staphylococci and streptococci. The first medicinal use of this compound took place later the same year – and the patient was none other than Domagk's own daughter, who had a serious streptococcal infection. Domagk gave her the prontosil in desperation, and she made a complete recovery. Domagk did not publish news of his discovery until 1935, after the compound had been subjected to more extensive clinical trials. In 1939 he was awarded a Nobel Prize for his work. However, the Nazi authorities then in power in Germany forced him to turn down this prestigious award: the Nazis considered the Nobel Prize to be "anti-German," since Carl von Ossietzky, a vehement critic of their repressive regime, had won the Nobel Peace Prize in 1935. Domagk was able to go to Stockholm to accept his Nobel Prize medal in 1947, after the war – but he did not get the substantial sum of money that normally goes with it, since according to the rules of the Nobel Committee, the monetary prize reverts to the Nobel Fund if it is not used within a year (Chast, 2003).

Jacques Tréfouël (1897-1977) together with his wife Thérèse and their team at the Pasteur Institute in Paris showed in 1936 that prontosil is broken down in the body to produce the colorless sulfanilamide, so that in fact prontosil should be regarded as the precursor of sulfanilamide, which is the real chemotherapeutic agent.

Sulfanilamide was actually synthesized as early as 1908 by the young chemist Paul Gelmo (1879-1961) in Vienna, as part of his doctoral research. This relatively simple compound formed the basis for a large number of synthetic dyes. IG Farben was initially interested mainly in the excellent bonding of these dyes with wool and silk, and their colorfastness. It has been suggested that IG Farben was already aware that sulfanilamide had an antibacterial effect before it introduced prontosil to the market as a drug, but since the patent on sulfanilamide had lapsed they could not make big profits from its manufacture. Consequently, they were looking for related compounds based on sulfanilamide but sufficiently different that they could patent, and this led to the discovery of prontosil (Comroe, 1976). When the excellent antibacterial effect of sulfanilamide became widely known, more than five hundred "sulfa drugs" were prepared during the late 1930s and early 1940s. One of these was sulfapyridine, which is reputed to have saved Winston Churchill's life when he came down with pneumonia just before the Casablanca Conference in 1943 (Chast, 2003).

The discovery of the bacteriostatic properties of sulfanilamide (that is, its ability to halt the growth of bacteria) inspired medical researchers Sir Howard Walter Florey (1898-1968) and Ernst Boris Chain (1906-1979), both from Oxford, to continue the investigations started by Fleming. Chain succeeded in purifying penicillin and found it to be a stable compound. An article by Florey and Chain in *The Lancet* in 1940 brought Fleming's work to a much wider audience. Penicillin's moment had arrived. The world was already embroiled in World War II, and an effective antibacterial drug was of inestimable importance to the war effort. Industry threw itself into the task of producing as much penicillin as possible: the age of antibacterial therapy had dawned (Burchenal, 1975).

Just like the development of chemotherapy for infectious diseases, the development of cancer chemotherapy was very largely a matter of trial and error. Nevertheless, a valuable store of knowledge about useful cytostatics was gradually built up and transferred to clinical practice. Cytostatics are classified according to their mechanism of action, and the following overview of the history of this type of chemotherapy is structured on the same basis.

Alkylating cytostatics

The physiologist Isaac Berenblum – mentioned in Chapter 2 in connection with his important theory of the way cancers are formed – was studying carcinogenesis (the factors leading to the formation of cancers) at the newly created department of Experimental Pathology and Cancer Research at Leeds University in England at the end of the 1920s. His basic approach was to apply tar to the skin of experimental animals under various conditions, and examine what effect this had on tumor formation. It occurred to him that the known irritant sulfur mustard (the active component of mustard gas, which had been used as a chemical weapon in the First World War because of its vesicant properties – its ability to raise blisters on the skin) might enhance the carcinogenic effect of tar. He therefore applied a solution of the sulfur mustard to the skin of the experimental animals in the expectation that the local irritation it produced would lead to hyperemia (increased blood flow through the tissues near the point of application) and hence enhanced growth of the tumors. To his surprise, the mustard had precisely the opposite effect, actually slowing tumor growth. Further research suggested that this was due more to the action of the mustard gas on the experimental animal than to interaction with the carcinogen. Berenblum continued his study by investigating whether sulfur mustard also slowed the growth of tumors induced by other carcinogens such as dibenzanthracene. This did indeed prove to be the case (Berenblum, 1929; 1935).

A further development was initiated by Dr. James Ewing (1866-1943), a pathologist working at Memorial Hospital in New York. During the First World War, while working in the United States Military Museum at West Point, Ewing was struck by the highly specific nature of the burns caused by nitrogen mustard gas. In 1931 he suggested to Frank Adair and Halsey Bagg, researchers at Memorial Hospital's Douglas Laboratory, that it might be fruitful to study the effect of mustard gas on experimental tumors. They followed Ewing's suggestion and applied a solution of this gas to a tumor in a mouse induced by a carcinogen. The skin tumor disappeared, but an autopsy revealed a metastasis in the animal's lung. The response of the skin tumor encouraged them to subject the skin of a rabbit to various doses of mustard gas, to determine the optimum dose for use on the skin. On the basis of this information, they applied mustard gas locally to skin lesions in twelve patients and also used it to treat a tumor in another patient by injecting a solution of mustard gas into the tumor. The skin cancers responded very well to the topical treatment, while the tumor that had received the mustard-gas injection disappeared almost completely. In histological terms, the skin lesions treated consisted of a melanoma, an epithelial cell carcinoma, a neurofibrosis, a neurosarcoma and two metastases of penis cancer. The reduction in size caused by the mustard gas persisted for months in all cases, and the authors concluded that mustard gas was an effective means of treating local skin cancers (Adair and Bagg, 1931). In spite of the positive results of this rarely cited work, it still took more than two decades for this treatment to be introduced into general clinical use. The topical application of nitrogen mustard did not become common until 1956, when it was found to be of use in the treatment of *mycosis fungoides*.

Renewed interest in nitrogen mustard gas arose at the start of World War II. At that time a contract was signed between Yale University and the Federal Office of Scientific Research and Development to research chemical weapons. Louis S. Goodman and Albert Gilman (1908-1984) were given the task of carrying out the research into nitrogen mustard gas, with support from Frederick S. Philips and Roberta P. Allen. It may be noted that Albert Gilman was the father of Alfred G. Gilman (born 1941) – also a pharmacologist – who shared the Nobel Prize in 1994 with Martin Rodbell for their discoveries concerning G-proteins. An excellent review of the work by Goodman and Gilman is given by Gilman (1963). One of their main findings was that lymphatic tissue is very sensitive to nitrogen mustard gas. They then contacted Thomas Dougherty from the department of anatomy at Yale, who made more detailed studies of the sensitivity of lymphomas in mice to nitrogen mustard. It was found that this treatment caused the lymphomas to disappear completely. The effect of nitrogen mustard on leukemia in mice was also tested. In this case, some of the animals responded while in others there was no response at all. In the course of his review Gilman wrote:

> *I have often thought that if we had coincidentally taken one of these leukemias where absolutely no effect had been seen, we might have stopped with the project altogether.*

CHAPTER 6

He also reported that, contrary to what is often suggested, a great deal of preclinical research was carried out before nitrogen mustard was used to treat patients.

When the results of these successful animal experiments were shown in December 1942 to Gustav E. Lindskog, who was Assistant Professor of Surgery at the Yale Cancer Center at the time, this encouraged him to use nitrogen mustard to treat a 48-year-old patient who was in the final stages of a radiation-resistant non-Hodgkin lymphoma. Lindskog observed a dramatic reduction in the size of the lymphomas but also a sharp drop in the white blood cell and thrombocyte counts (Figure 6.1 and 6.2). After the bone marrow had recovered, new tumor growth was observed. The patient then received a second course of treatment with a somewhat lower dose of nitrogen mustard. When a third course of treatment led to no further tumor response, the treatment was stopped. After this finding, patients with other forms of cancer were also treated with nitrogen mustard and intensive research was carried out into the mechanism of action, pharmacology and toxicology of this substance, and into the synthesis of chemicals related to mustard gas (Gilman, 1963). The activity of nitrogen mustard has been found to be due to its alkylating effect.[1] This can lead to breaks in single- or double-strand DNA, or to cross-link formation between DNA strands, causing cell division to stop.

Many authors have suggested that the history of chemotherapy began with a German bomb attack on the Italian port of Bari towards the end of the Second World War. The Allies using the harbor for provisioning when, on the night of 3 December 1943, the German *Luftwaffe* mounted a massive bombing raid. Sixteen ships were sunk, including the USS *Liberty*. This ship had an ultra high secret store of a hundred barrels of mustard gas on board, intended for use during the war. The barrels sprung leaks. The American cancer researcher Cornelius Packard Rhoads was serving in the US Army Medical Corps at the time, as chief of the medical division of the Chemical Warfare Service, and he was called on to treat many of the more than six hundred survivors who had been on the *Liberty*. He observed that

---

1 A substance is said to have an alkylating effect if it can add an alkyl group on to another molecule–DNA in the present case. In fact, when we call nitrogen mustard an alkylating agent, the situation is somewhat more complicated. Readers who are interested in the chemical background can read the following explanation; it can however be skipped without seriously affecting the main lines of the message here. There are different types of nitrogen mustards. The chemical name of the type discussed here is bis(2-chloroethyl)methylamine, corresponding to the chemical formula $Cl-CH_2-CH_2-N(CH_3)-CH_2-CH_2Cl$. Chemists call this type of compound a substituted hydrocarbon. The corresponding hydrocarbon would be $CH_3-CH_2-CH_2(CH_3)-CH_2-CH_3$. If we leave off an atom at the beginning of this hydrocarbon, we get the alkyl group $-CH_2-CH_2-CH_2(CH_3)-CH_2-CH_3$. And if we leave off an atom at the end of the nitrogen mustard molecule, we get the substituted alkyl group $-CH_2-CH_2-N(CH_3)-CH_2-CH_2Cl$. The reason why nitrogen mustard is called an alkylating agent is that it can add this last-mentioned substituted alkyl group to a molecule such as DNA. It seems almost self-evident that the addition of large numbers of such a relatively large molecule will seriously interfere with the function of the DNA.

FIGURE 6.1 *The first patient ever to receive systemic chemotherapy. The photo shows clearly that the patient, who is suffering from non-Hodgkin lymphoma, has enlarged lymph nodes in the armpits and the neck, and a puffy face.*

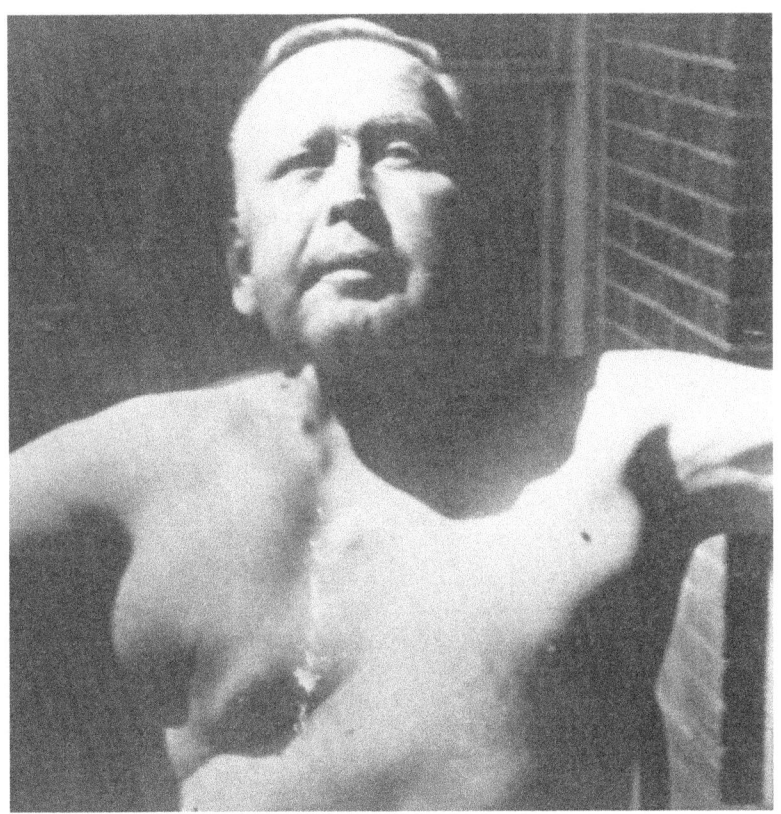

FIGURE 6.2 *The same patient after treatment with nitrogen mustard. Note the reduction in the size of the lymph nodes and in the facial edema (Source: Shimkin, 1979, courtesy of the National Institutes of Health, Bethesda, MD).*

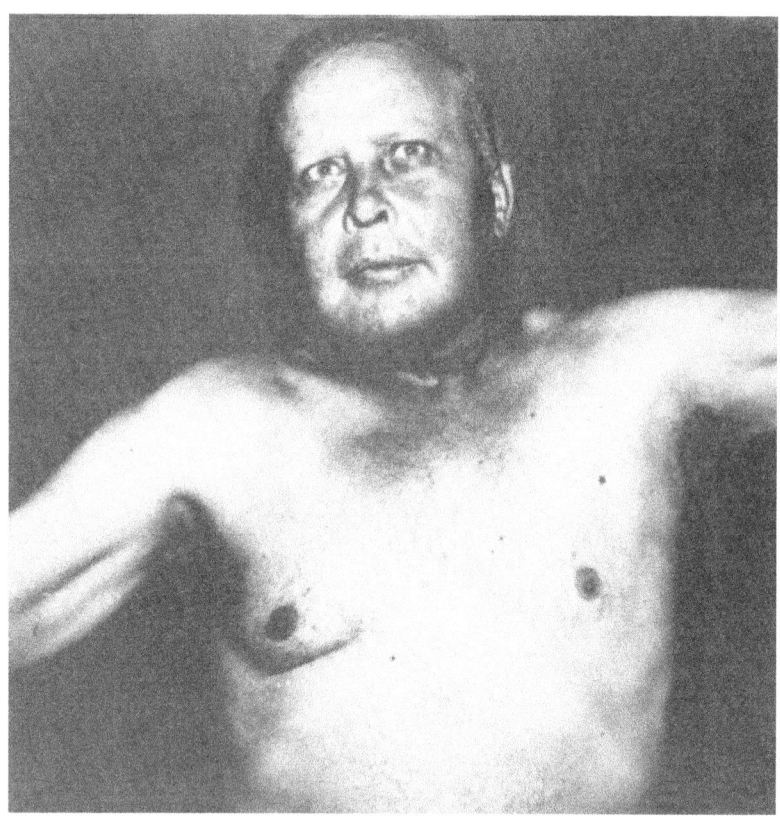

their blood cell counts were dramatically lowered, while the rest of their tissues appeared to be normal. It occurred to Rhoads that this characteristic of mustard gas might be useful in the treatment of cancers associated with an excess of white blood cells, such as cancer of the lymph glands and leukemia. Clearly, however, the above-mentioned research by Gilman and colleagues at Yale predated this event (Zubrod, 1979; Papac, 2001).

Goodman and Philips did not publish the results of the Yale research until 1946, after the embargo on the details of investigations related to the war effort had been lifted. Even the doyen of American cancer research, William H. Woglom, had not been aware of this study. He said in 1945 that devising a systemic therapy for cancer would be as difficult as finding a substance that dissolved the left ear while leaving the right one intact (Burchenal, 1975; Woglom, 1947).

It should be mentioned that John F. Wilkinson, Director of the Department of Haematology at Manchester Royal Infirmary in England, had been working with F. Fletcher on nitrogen mustards since 1942, but they had also been unable to publish their results until 1947 because of the need for secrecy during the war. They gave no reason for their decision to embark on this research, but commented that in general, nitrogen mustards affect the blood system in much the same way as radiation. They treated eighteen patients: eight with chronic myeloid leukemia, three with chronic lymphatic leukemia, four with Hodgkin's disease and three with *polycythemia vera* – an abnormal increase in the number of blood cells (in particular red blood cells). The patients with chronic myeloid leukemia responded best, though those with Hodgkin's disease also clearly benefited (Papac, 2001).

After the initial discovery that an effective alkylating cytostatic could be derived from mustard gas, a search for similar substances began. The Chester Beatty group in London made use of the finding that the action of a substance on blood cells was an indication of its utility in the treatment of hematological malignancies to develop busulfan for chronic myeloid leukemia, chlorambucil for chronic lymphatic leukemia and melfalan for multiple myeloma. All three substances were found to be effective in preventing the conditions in question, though they did not cure them once they were established.

Another alkylating agent with an interesting history is cyclophosphamide. The assumptions on the basis of which it was concluded that this compound would make an effective drug later turned out to be incorrect, but it still worked. It was synthesized in 1958 at Asta Werke in Germany by Herbert Arnold, Friedrich Bourseaux and Norbert Brock, who thought that phosphates and phosphoramides occurring in tumors could convert cyclophosphamide into an active metabolite. It was later shown that this conversion did not take place in the tumor but was carried out by microsomes in the liver. No matter where the conversion occurs, this means that cyclophosphamide – like the above-mentioned prontosil – is a "prodrug," a chemically and pharmacologically inactive derivative of the active agent that is metabolized *in vivo* to produce the active form. The clinical activity of this substance was first demonstrated by Rudolf Gross and Klaus Lambers from the University of Marburg in Germany (Gross and Lambers, 1958). Despite the initially false assumptions about its mechanism of action, cyclophosphamide has proved to be a very effective drug, which offers a cure for Burkitt's lymphoma, non-Hodgkin lymphoma and various juvenile cancers. The screening of more than eight hundred chemicals related to cyclophosphamide led to the discovery of iphosphamide, which is an even stronger anti-tumor agent than cyclophosphamide itself (Brock et al., 1988).

Alkylating nitrosourea derivates such as lomustine were synthesized and investigated by John A. Montgomery at the Southern Research Institute in Birmingham, Alabama (Montgomery, 1976). They are active against tumors localized in the central nervous system and against malignant lymphomas. Alkylating cytostatics are still in clinical use today.

Antimetabolites

In 1940, Donald O. Woods of Oxford University and Sir Paul Gordon Fildes carried out some very important studies on sulfanilamide, the antibacterial effect of which had been discovered by Domagk and Tréfouël as described above. Sir Paul Fildes (1882-1971) was the head of the biology department at Britain's top secret Porton Down research establishment during the Second World War, where he supervised the country's first attempts to develop biological weapons. The son of Luke Fildes, a famous painter who had illustrated books by Charles Dickens, he had studied medicine but later turned to bacteriology. He was knighted in 1919. Woods and Fildes used sulfanilamide in their elucidation of the mechanism of action of antimetabolite drugs – a very important piece of theoretical work. They grew cultures of bacteria that require folic acid (a form of water-soluble vitamin B9) for their metabolism. Normally, bacteria can synthesize the folic acid it needs by a process in which para-aminobenzoic acid (often known by its abbreviation, PABA) acts as an intermediate. As Figure 6.3 shows, the chemical structure of sulfanilamide is closely related to that of PABA. This allows sulfanilamide to act as a competitive inhibitor of PABA, supplanting it in the metabolism of the bacteria so that no folic acid is formed and the bacteria stop multiplying. (The phenomenon of competitive inhibition had first been studied, and named, by Judah Quastel at Cambridge in 1931.) A number of important cytostatics have been developed on the basis of this principle, that certain substances can take the place of essential metabolites in an organism's metabolic pathways, thus disrupting the function of that organism.

FIGURE 6.3 Schematic representation of the mode of operation of antimetabolites, based on the studies of Donald Woods and Sir Paul Fildes (PABA=para-aminobenzoic acid).

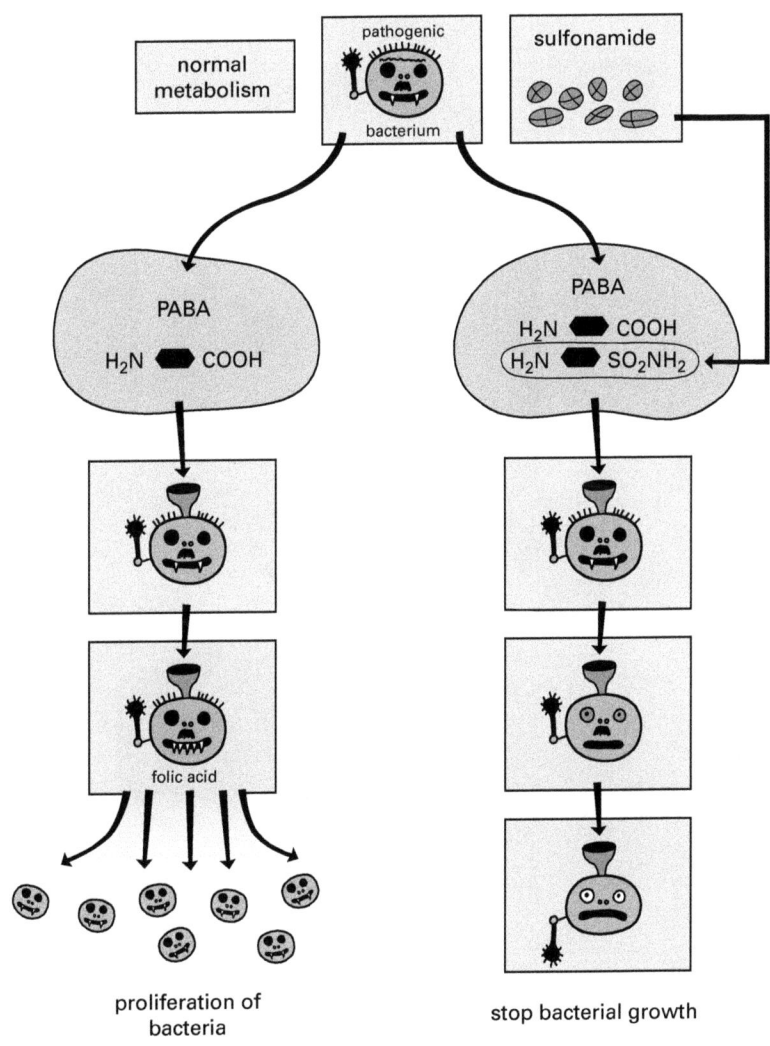

FIGURE 6.4 Dr. Yellapragada SubbaRow (Source: Shimkin, 1979 courtesy of the National Institutes of Health, Bethesda, MD, USA).

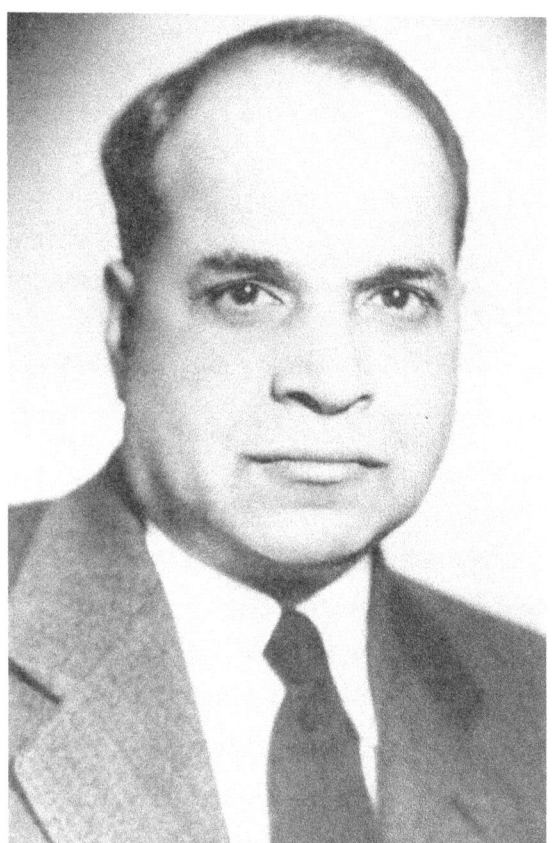

The fact that the first chemotherapeutic agent to be tested was an antagonist of folic acid was due to an intelligent observation by Sidney Farber, head of pathology at Children's Hospital Boston, and his team. He had found that the recently discovered folic acid stimulated the growth of red blood cells in his patients. He therefore gave it to a number of leukemia patients in the hope that it would improve their condition; but in fact, they got worse (Chu and De Vita, 2001). Farber then reasoned that if folic acid speeded up the progress of leukemia, a substance that countered the action of folic acid might slow down the disease. Confirmatory evidence was provided in 1944 and 1945 by Rudolf and Cecilie Leuchtenberger and colleagues at Mount Sinai Hospital in New York, who succeeded in halting the growth of sarcomas and spontaneously arising breast cancers in mice using L. *casei* factor, which they called folic acid but which later proved to be a weak antimetabolite of folic acid (Kardinal, 1985).

On the basis of these findings, together with the theoretical framework provided by the metabolite/antimetabolite theory, Farber (who is often called the father of cancer chemotherapy) asked the chemists at Lederle Laboratories (at that time the pharmaceutical division of the chemical giant American Cyanamid but currently owned by Wyeth – one of the largest pharmaceutical companies in the world, originally founded in Philadelphia in 1860) to make a substance that would block the action of folic acid. A team led by the biochemist Yellapragada SubbaRow (Figure 6.4) undertook this task. Using information that had recently become available about the structure of folic acid, the workers at Lederle managed to make inactive analogs of folic acid that could halt the growth of tumor cells in the laboratory. This research project was the first logically reasoned approach to the problem of making chemotherapeutic agents with a desired set of properties (Patlak, 2002).

The first substance to be clinically tested was pteroylaspartic acid, a nonfunctional analog of folic acid. It was given to a patient who was dying of progressive myeloid leukemia. In fact, the treatment only led to a severely hypocellular bone marrow without any obvious clinical advantages. Nevertheless, the researchers were sufficiently encouraged by the effect on the bone marrow to continue testing similar compounds. They gave a stronger folic acid antagonist, aminopterine, to children in the advanced stages of leukemia (Chu and De Vita, 2001). The first patient was treated on 3 December 1947 by Sydney Farber (Figure 6.5) and his team. They managed to bring one young patient with acute leukemia into remission through the aminopterine treatment – the first time this had been achieved with any drug. Moreover, ten of the first sixteen patients that they treated showed temporary hematologic and clinical improvement (Farber et al., 1948). It is striking that the considerable contribution to this investigation made by SubbaRow and his team was not mentioned in the publication describing this form of therapy and its results, nor in any of the subsequent publications (Pearson, 2002).

CHAPTER 6

FIGURE 6.5 Sidney Farber. (Source: Shimkin, 1979, courtesy of the National Institute of Health, Bethesda, MD, USA).

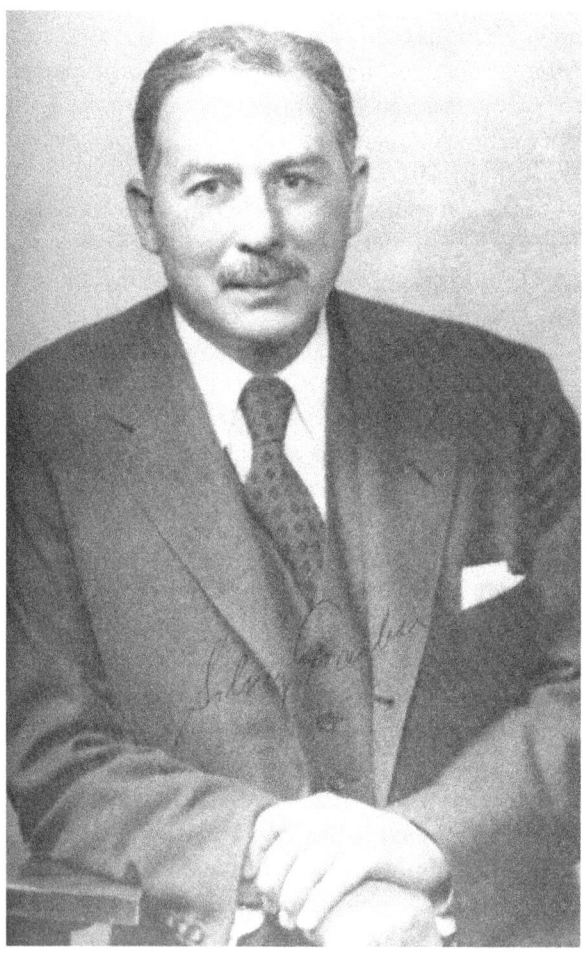

Methotrexate (formerly known as amethopterin) was developed in 1949. It soon replaced aminopterin for the treatment of leukemia because it had a better therapeutic index when used in an experimental L1210 leukemia model in mice. Methotrexate is an anti-metabolite that inhibits the reduction of dihydrofolic acid to tetrahydrofolic acid, an essential step in the synthesis of nucleic acids during cell division. It took some time for methotrexate to be used for cancers other than leukemia. In 1956, Chinese-born Min Chu Li successfully treated a disseminated choriocarcinoma patient with methotrexate (Figure 6.6). Choriocarcinomas are malignant tumors that can grow from trophoblast cells – cells that feed the embryo and develop into a large part of the placenta. They are generally formed in the uterus, but often metastasize to other parts of the body. The patient Li treated had lung metastases. A chance observation held the key to this discovery. Li had recently come to work at the endocrinology department, headed by Dr. Roy Hertz, at the National Cancer Institute (NCI) in Bethesda, MD. In his previous position at the Memorial-Sloan Kettering Institute in New York, Li had treated a melanoma patient who had unusually high gonadotrophin levels and observed that these levels fell after treatment with methotrexate. Li therefore decided to try methotrexate therapy on his choriocarcinoma patient with lung metastases, who was known also to have elevated gonadotrophin levels. D.B. Spencer used a quantitative biological method to measure the secretion of gonadotrophin as a check on the efficacy of the treatment. Li consulted Abraham Goldin, a leader in the development of experimental models of human malignancy, and pharmacologist Paul Condit – both also of the NCI – about the best distribution of the methotrexate dosage to use. Condit suggested use of a single high dose since the patient urgently needed treatment, but Li eventually decided to spread the methotrexate over a four- or five-day period for safety reasons (Li, 1973). The patient's gonadotrophin levels were found to drop steadily, and several weeks later the lung metastases disappeared (Li et al., 1958). This was the first recorded case in which a treatment schedule had been devised that was able to cure metastasized solid cancers. Further studies on a large number of patients showed that that quantitative determination of the tumor boundaries allowed the recession of the tumor to be predicted and assessed.

Isaac Djerassi, born in 1925 in Sofia, Bulgaria, introduced the therapeutic approach known as leucovorin rescue (which involves administering the drug leucovorin to counter the toxicity of methotrexate) while working at the Children's Hospital of Philadelphia in 1960. It then became possible to give patients high doses of methotrexate without adverse toxic effects. It was then found that methotrexate was also active against lymphosarcomas and carcinomas (Zubrod, 1979). Another very important development, in particular with regard to the treatment of acute leukemia, was J.A. Whiteside's 1958 demonstration, first in dogs and later in humans, that methotrexate could be given intrathecally (that is, by injection into the spinal

FIGURE 6.6 Reaction of a patient with disseminated choriocarcinoma to intermittent treatment with methotrexate. The vertical arrows represent the times of administration of methotrexate, and the graph the variation of the measured gonadotropin levels in the patient's urine. The X-ray photo on the left, taken in September, shows widespread light patches in the lungs that reveal the presence of metastases. The lungs in the X-ray photo on the right, taken a month later, are uniformly dark, indicating healthy lung tissue. (Source: Shimkin, 1979 courtesy of the National Institutes of Health, Bethesda, MD).

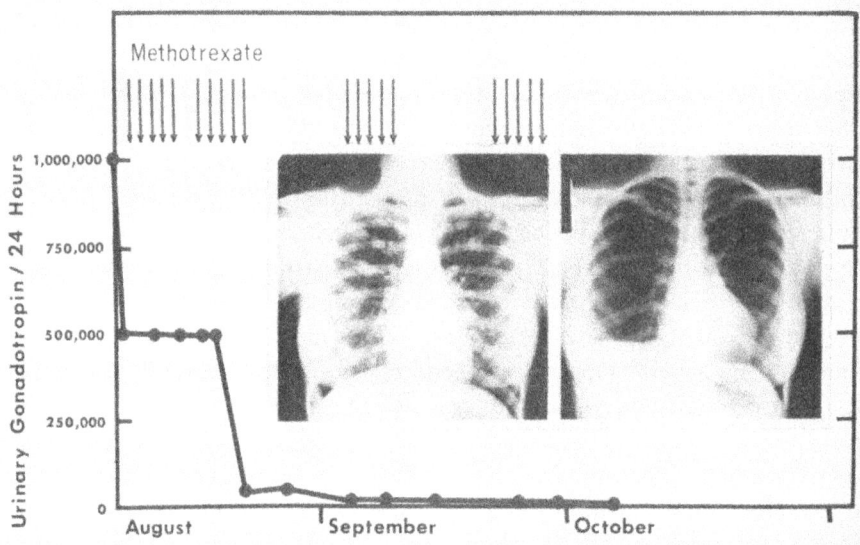

cavity – thus bypassing the blood-brain barrier which stops oral and intravenous drugs from getting into the brain). This made it finally possible to eradicate the leukemia cells on the meninges (the membranes that cover the brain and the spinal cord), which are particularly known for hiding these cells.

Metabolite/antimetabolite theory also stimulated George Herbert Hitchings (1905-1998) and Gertrude Bell Elion (1918-1999) and their team at the Burroughs Wellcome Laboratory at Tuckahoe NY to carry out systematic screening of antimetabolites of the naturally occurring purines and pyrimidines. They shared the Nobel Prize in 1988 with Sir James Whyte Black (born 1924), of King's College Medical School in London (who had been working on beta-receptor antagonists, more commonly known as "beta blockers"), for their discoveries of "important principles for drug treatment." The research by Hitchings and Elion led to the synthesis of tioguanine in 1948 and 6-mercaptopurine in 1951. The clinical use of these molecules in the treatment of leukemia was pioneered by David A. Karnofsky (1914-1969), R.R. Ellison, Irwin Krakoff and M.L. Murphy. The work by Hitchings and Elion also led to the synthesis and use of the xanthine oxidase inhibitor allopurinol (which is of great use in the prevention and treatment of high uric acid levels in the blood – an abnormality which is sometimes seen when cytostatics cause a very sudden breakdown of tumor cells, and of course also in gout) and of the immunosuppressant azathioprine.

The original observation in 1954 by Robert J. Rutman, Abraham Cantarow and Karl E. Paschkis from Jefferson Medical College in Philadelphia of an elevated level of labeled uracil in the nucleic acids of transplanted tumors led Charles Heidelberger (1920-1983) and his team at the McArdle Memorial Laboratory of the University of Wisconsin to synthesize the antimetabolite 5-fluorouracil (FU) and its derivatives in 1958 (Burchenal, 1975). This cytostatic proved to be important in the treatment of many different types of intestinal tumors and breast cancers. In view of its limited absorption when given orally, 5-FU was most effective when administered intravenously. The pharmaceutical industry launched an intensive, logically structured search for possible ways of improving the absorption through the use of pro-drugs (substances that are converted into active drugs in the tumor), and by slowing down the breakdown of the drugs. This led to the discovery of capecitabine, which was developed by a group of researchers from the Japanese division of Roche. The design process of this compound was described by Miwa et al. in 1998. This patient-friendly oral cytostatic has largely replaced the intravenous use of 5-FU (Budman et al., 1998).

Another antimetabolite, cytosine arabinoside – better known as ara-C – was isolated from the sponge *Cryptotethya crypta* by E.R. Walwick and colleagues in 1959. John Evans and his team at an Upjohn research laboratory demonstrated its effectiveness on leukemias in mice. It was initially found to be of limited efficacy in humans due to its short half-life, but a change in the treatment regime has made it one of the most important drugs for the treatment of acute myeloid leukemia.

Antibiotic cytostatics

The American biochemist and microbiologist Selman Abraham Waksman (1888-1973), often called the "father of antibiotics," discovered actinomycin D in 1940 during his search with H. Boyd Woodruff for anti-tuberculosis drugs – even before he found the antibiotic streptomycin, for which he received the Nobel Prize in 1952. Actinomycin D was forgotten for a decade, because it was too toxic to be used as an anti-bacterial drug. In 1952, when the idea that the treatment of cancer by chemotherapy was not an impossible dream became widespread, the German C. Hackmann and the above-mentioned Sydney Farber showed that this substance was active against mouse tumors. Farber and his colleagues reported in 1956 that actinomycin D was effective in the treatment of Wilms' tumor, a kidney cancer in children. Stimulated by the research of M.L. Murphy and David Karnofsky, who had shown in the laboratory that various drugs had a strong effect on embryonic tissue, the above-mentioned Min Chu Li determined in 1960 that actinomycin-D was effective in combination with methotrexate and chlorambucil against the very malignant embryonic cell carcinoma of the testicle. G. Schulte was the first to use the drug in the treatment of Hodgkin's disease (Burchenal, 1975), while its activity against Ewing's sarcoma was discovered in 1968 by H.O. Hustu.

The favorable results obtained with actinomycin D encouraged much wider investigation of the activity of other antibiotics in slowing tumor growth. This led to the discovery of a large number of antibiotics that were effective against cancer, such as the anthracyclines. These antibiotics were isolated from *Streptomyces peucetius* and were discovered independently by the Italians Grein, Spalla, Canevazzi and DiMarco, and by the Frenchman Dubost and his colleagues. The structure of the anthracycline daunorubicin was determined by Federico Arcamone at Farmitalia in Milan (now a division of the pharmaceutical giant Pfizer). Its clinical effectiveness against leukemia in children was demonstrated in 1965 by Charlotte Tan at the Memorial Sloan-Kettering Cancer Center in New York and a year later in the clinic of the hematologist Jean Bernard (1907-2006) in Paris. Because daunorubicin had a limited field of application and sometimes led to death from heart failure, the anthracyclines were not rated highly as therapeutic agents until Arcamone discovered the anthracycline doxorubicin, better known as adriamycin, in 1967. This cytostatic was isolated from the mold *Streptomyces peucetius* which was found on the ruins of a tower overlooking the Adriatic sea, hence the name. Like daunorubicin, adriamycin blocks the synthesis of DNA and RNA. Aurelio DiMarco reported that this drug showed strong activity in experimental tumor models. Professor Gianni

Bonadonna, Director of the Oncology division of the National Tumor Institute in Milan, quickly showed its clinical activity in a broad spectrum of solid tumors and also determined its dose-dependent cardiotoxicity (Zubrod, 1979).

Professor Bonadonna related how he came to administer adriamycin.

_____ *At the start of 1968, a young lab assistant came into my office with thirty tubes of adriamycin, a short description of its chemical properties and the preclinical results. "A present from Dr. DiMarco to test on your patients," she said.*

Bonadonna asked for some extra details, discussed the matter with his colleagues and decided to start a phase-I trial. The first patient was a 22-year-old man with lung metastases from a fibrosarcoma. Three weeks into the trial, the patient refused further therapy because it was making him too ill. He did, however, agree to have a chest X-ray. This showed that all the metastases were considerably smaller. Encouraged by this success, the research team concluded the phase-I trial and found that a remarkably high number of test subjects had shown a positive response. A phase-II trial was therefore started, again with excellent results. On this basis, adriamycin was cleared for general clinical application (Bonadonna, 1984). While looking for alternatives to adriamycin with lower cardiotoxicity and higher efficacy, Arcamone discovered the anthracycline epirubicin in 1975.

Another important cytostatic antibiotic was discovered in Japan by Hamao Umezawa (1914-1986). This brilliant researcher had been working on antibiotics since 1955, and in 1966 he found bleomycin after investigating various strains of *Streptomyces verticillus*. This cytostatic is not a single compound but a mixture of a number of substances. Since it has no toxic effect on bone marrow, it is often used in combination with other cytostatics. In view of the fact that bleomycin accumulates in the skin, Tukuji Ichikawa and colleagues tried it out on squamous cell carcinomas and found it to be very effective. The main field of indication has in the course of time come to be nonseminomatous testicular cancer (Zubrod, 1979).

Yet another drug from this group is mitomycin C, which can be obtained from *Streptomyces caespitosus*. T. Hata and his team from the Kitasato Institute in Japan isolated two mitomycins in 1956, which they called A and B. Both were found to be highly toxic in mice. S. Wakaki later isolated mitomycin C from the same mold. This had a stronger anti-tumor activity and was less toxic (Remers, 1979). It was found to be effective against chronic myeloid leukemia and carcinomas of the stomach and pancreas.

The most important mechanism of action of most antibiotic cytostatics is based on DNA intercalation – that is, the insertion of a flat ring molecule between the two neighboring base pairs in the DNA which distorts the double helix, thus blocking DNA synthesis and stopping cell growth.

Antraquinones

During the search for drugs with greater effectiveness and lower toxicity than the anthracyclines, two groups independently discovered a new class of cytostatics, the anthraquinones, in 1979. These are derivatives of anthracene, a substance that has been widely used as the basis for synthetic dyestuffs – for example, in the textile industry – since the beginning of the twentieth century. The first group was working at Lederle Laboratories under the leadership of K.C. Murdock, while the second was under the supervision of Randall K. Johnson at Stanford University. The research gave rise to the cytostatic mitoxantrone, which is structurally related to doxorubicin and has strong anti-tumor activity. It is effective against breast cancer, non-Hodgkin lymphoma and various other solid tumors (White and Durr, 1985).

L-asparaginase

While L-asparaginase had already been discovered in 1904 by S. Lang, and A. Clementi had demonstrated its presence in guinea-pig blood in 1922, it was not until 1953 that evidence was provided that it could be used as a cytostatic. In that year, John Kidd found that serum from guinea-pigs led to a decrease in tumor growth in mice and rats, while J.D. Broome suggested in 1961 that the efficacy of the guinea pig serum was due to L-asparaginase. In 1964, L.T. Mashburn of the Research Institute for Skeletomuscular Diseases of the Hospital for Joint Diseases in New York and J.C. Wriston Jr. from the department of chemistry at the University of Delaware found that L-asparaginase derived from E. coli was also effective against mouse tumors. Serum from the agouti, a South American relative of the guinea pig, gave T. DeBarros and colleagues the opportunity to try out L-asparaginase on a cancer patient in 1965. William C. Dolowy, at the Medical Research Laboratory of the University of Illinois at Chicago, tested guinea pig L-asparaginase on a child with leukemia in 1966. The efficacy of E. coli L-asparaginase in humans was first shown by J.M. Hill and H. Oettgen and their respective teams in 1967. The drug, derived from E. coli, is today primarily used to treat acute leukemia in children (Zubrod, 1979).

Cisplatin

One of the most effective cytostatics is cisplatin. It was discovered by Barnett Rosenberg in 1965, largely by chance. Rosenberg was working as a biophysicist at the University of Michigan and was particularly interested in the effect of electrical current on bacterial growth. He placed a platinum rod on either side of a colony of intestinal bacteria (E. coli) and applied an AC voltage between the two rods. To his amazement, he observed a drop in the density of the bacteria in the vicinity of the electrodes. Microscopic investigation showed that the coccal (spherically shaped) bacteria had turned into long filaments. Rosenberg eventually came to the conclusion that the change in the shape of the bacteria was caused by a substance originating from the platinum electrodes. After two years of experimentation he succeeded in identifying this substance as a complex compound of platinum, cis-diamminedichloroplatinum, which today is well known globally (under the shorter name of cisplatin) for its strong anti-tumor activity (Rosenberg, 1985). Its mechanism of action resembles that of the alkylating cytostatics. This compound forms platinum cross-links between the DNA chains of the cells it acts upon. The drug was introduced by Lawrence Einhorn for the treatment of testicular cancer.

During his training at the M.D. Anderson Hospital in Houston, Einhorn came into contact with M.L. Samuels from the hospital's department of medical oncology, who had introduced the use of vinblastine combined with bleomycin for the treatment of testicular cancer. This combined therapy led to the largest number of complete recoveries in patients at that time, but the recovery was only short-lived. Einhorn himself carried out a phase-I trial of cisplatin. Initially, it seemed that the drug would not prolong patients' lives by many years due to its serious kidney toxicity, but Hayes, Cvitkovic and colleagues showed that this problem could be avoided by aggressive prehydration (Hayes et al., 1977). When Einhorn was subsequently appointed professor of medicine at Indiana University, he added cisplatin to the vinblastine/bleomycin mix. This combined therapy proved very successful, making it possible to cure about 70% of patients with extensively metastasized testicular cancer. Previously they would have died within nine months. The use of cisplatin thus represents an enormous step forward in the cytostatic treatment of tumors.

The success of cisplatin encouraged researchers to synthesize and test many other platinum compounds. This led to the discovery of carboplatin, which had the same efficacy as cisplatin but lower toxicity. Another new compound was oxaliplatin, a cytostatic from the diamminecyclohexane-platinum family. Further development of this drug was stopped in the United States after a phase-I trial of tetraplatin – another drug from the same family – yielded very poor results. It was Georges Mathé of Paris who had the vision to introduce oxaliplatin into clinical practice. He set up a somewhat unorthodox phase-I trial of this compound, which showed no kidney or liver toxicity, and no loss of hearing due to its administration. Despite a general lack of interest in this drug, researchers at the Hôpital Paul Brousse in Villejuif, a suburb of Paris, kept working on it and found it to be effective against carcinomas of the colon (Cvitkovic, 1998). It has become an important addition to the therapeutic arsenal available to treat this form of cancer.

CHAPTER 6

Topoisomerase inhibitors

Topoisomerases are enzymes that cause controlled breaks in DNA, needed to permit the separation of the closely interwined DNA strands during cell division. This is necessary for DNA replication and gene expression. The cytostatics that disrupt the function of these enzymes are called topoisomerase inhibitors. They are divided into topoisomerase I and II inhibitors: the former lead to single-strand breaks in the DNA, and the latter to double-strand breaks.

The history of topoisomerase inhibitors dates back to 1971, when James Chuo Wang (born 1936) from the department of chemistry of the University of California, Berkeley, discovered topoisomerase I in E. coli bacteria. Since then, many researchers have isolated other topoisomerases. M.E. Wall, director of the Eastern Regional Research Laboratory in Philadelphia, and his team were looking for sources of cortisone in plant extracts when they discovered the first topoisomerase I inhibitor. This was camptothecin, which they isolated from *Camptotheca accuminata*, a tree originating in China, in 1965. An extract of this tree was used in traditional Chinese medicine for the treatment of many ailments, including tumors (Potmesil, 1994). Camptothecin was found to be highly effective against cancer, but had too many adverse side effects to be useful in clinical practice. A systematic screening program for camptothecin analogs was therefore set up. The first ten analogs isolated were also found to be too toxic, but in 1984 Yokura and colleagues succeeded in isolating irinotecan (also known as CPT-11, since this was the eleventh camptothecin analog to be screened). The demonstration by Hsiang et al. (1985) that camptothecin worked by inhibiting topoisomerase I led to great interest in this drug. Irinotecan was found to be effective in the treatment of tumors of the colon and rectum. Topotecan, a camptothecin analog that was also developed at the Eastern Regional Research Laboratory, is another topoisomerase I inhibitor. It is effective against ovarian cancer (Chen and Liu, 1994). CPT-11 has been successfully developed in Japan and France, and topotecan in the US.

Etoposide, a semi-synthetic derivative of a toxin isolated from the plant *Podophyllum peltatum* (the American mayapple), is a topoisomerase II inhibitor. Although extracts of this plant had long been used as folk medicine in the Himalayas and in North America as laxatives and anti-worm drugs, the curative effect against genital warts (condylomata acuminata) was not demonstrated until 1942, by I.W. Kaplan. The molecular structure was determined by Hartwell and Schrecker in 1951. Since then, several other analogs of this compound have been isolated and synthesized and their anti-tumor activity tested. Etoposide underwent clinical trials in 1973, and its efficacy against small-cell lung carcinomas and lymphomas was well known within a year (Stähelin and Von Wartburg, 1991).

It was later established that adriamycin, mentioned above in the section on Antibiotic cytostatics, also acts as a topoisomerase II inhibitor.

Spindle poisons

All the cytostatics described so far act by influencing the DNA in the cell nucleus in some way. A completely different class of cytostatics comprises substances that influence the structure and function of the microtubules of the mitotic spindle that ensures proper migration of chromosomes leading up to cell division. In view of their mechanism of action, these substances are known as mitotic inhibitors or "spindle poisons." Two groups may be distinguished here: the vinca alkaloids, which inhibit the production of the microtubules; and the taxanes, which block microtubule depolymerization.

Vinca alkaloids

The vinca alkaloids are natural or semisynthetic substances derived from the periwinkle (*Vinca rosea Linn*, now called *Catharanthus roseus G. Don*). It was long known that extracts of this plant could give rise to hypoglycemia, as a result of which they have been used in many countries as a traditional cure for diabetes.

Two groups were interested in this plant: a small academic team led by Robert Noble, Professor of Medical Research in the laboratory headed by James Bertram Collip, FRS (1892-1965) at the University of Western Ontario (UWO) in Canada and the research laboratory of the pharmaceutical giant Eli Lilly in Indianapolis. In 1955, Collip's team observed that injection of periwinkle extracts in rats led to leukopenia and severe depression of bone marrow. Charles Beer, an English-born chemist working in the laboratory, isolated, purified and crystallized the active agent responsible. At the same time, and independently, Irving Johnson and his team at Eli Lilly discovered, as part of a massive screening program for pharmaceutically interesting compounds, that extracts of *Vinca rosea* caused remissions in P-1534 leukemia (an acute lymphocytic leukemia) in mice. The two research groups now joined forces, and Norbert Neuss and his team at Eli Lilly isolated and characterized a number of alkaloids, the most important of which were vinblastine and vincristine.

Dr. M.E. Hodes from the University of Indianapolis School of Medicine and Harold Warwick, Dean of Medicine at UWO, showed in 1960 that vinblastine was effective against Hodgkin's disease, while Roy Hertz, M.B. Lipsett and R.H. Moy found it to be active against choriocarcinoma. M.R. Karon reported in 1962 that vincristine was much more active against acute lymphoblastic leukemia than vinblastine, and the year after P.P. Carbone demonstrated its activity against Hodgkin's disease (Zubrod, 1979). Chemical modification of vinblastine led to the development of vindesine, which shows cytostatic activity against lung cancer (Pierce and Miller, 2005).

Taxanes

The taxoids or taxanes are a group of natural or semisynthetic substances that occur in various trees of the yew family and that prevent breakdown of the mitotic spindle. The first cytostatic to be identified in this family of compounds was taxol. This discovery was the result of a massive search for natural anti-cancer products headed by Dr. Jonathan Hartwell of the National Cancer Institute (NCI). The NCI had signed an agreement with the United States Department of Agriculture for USDA botanists to collect plant samples from various parts of the United States. Arthur Barclay from the USDA brought back samples of the Pacific yew (*Taxus brevifolia*) from Gifford Pinchot National Forest in the southwest of Washington State (which includes Mount St. Helens, the site of a huge volcanic eruption in 1980 – the biggest in the US excluding Alaska and Hawaii since 1915) in August 1962, and taxol was isolated from the bark of this tree. It was shown in 1964 that this substance was active against many different types of tumors in mice (Suffness and Wall, 1995), and the next year Dr. Monroe Wall (1916-2002) succeeded in fractionating large amounts of taxol from the parent material (McGuire and Rowinsky, 1995). Mansukh Wani and colleagues determined its structural formula (Wani et al., 1971).

In 1979, Peter Schiff and Dr. Susan Horwitz elucidated taxol's unique mechanism of action. It stabilizes the microtubules that form the mitotic spindle, thus "freezing" them in their new position and stopping cell division (Wall and Wani, 1995).

Two problems had to be solved before taxol could be used on a large scale for cancer therapy. Firstly, it is insoluble in water. No matter how effective a substance may be in fighting cancer, if it cannot be dissolved in water it cannot be administered to patients. The NCI's drug formulation team finally came up with an answer after a year's experimentation: the non-ionic surfactant Cremophor EL could be used to prepare a stable emulsion of taxol in water, thus opening the way for its use in humans.

The second problem was that the raw materials from which taxol was prepared were very scarce. It initially took six Pacific yews to get enough taxol to treat one patient – and the yew is one of the slowest-growing trees in the world. To make matters more complicated, a very rare white owl nested in the Pacific pine, and conservationists protested because they were afraid that cutting down too many trees would lead to the extinction of the bird. Bristol-Myers Squibb, the company that marketed taxol, had to promise to plant a new tree for every one that was cut down.

All the efforts devoted to bringing this drug on the market finally paid off. Taxol was found to show strong activity against ovarian cancer, and later against a range of other tumors. It was given the generic name paclitaxel in 1993, but retained the brand name Taxol (Cortes and Pazdur, 1995).

The high activity and unusual action mechanism of this drug and the difficulty experienced in producing it in sufficient quantities sparked the search for semisynthetic alternatives. The French pharmacist and natural-products chemist Pierre Potier succeeded in producing the related substance docetaxel in 1986 at the Institut de Chimie des Substances Naturelles (ICSN) in Gif-sur-Yvette, southwest of Paris, in cooperation with the Centre National de la Recherche Scientifique (CNRS) and the French chemical and pharmaceutical company Rhône-Poulenc (at the time of writing, part of Sanofi-Aventis, the third largest pharmaceutical company in the world). The raw materials for this substance are extracted from the needles of *Taxus baccata* (the European yew) and subjected to a series of chemical reactions to arrive at the desired chemical structure (Chast, 2003; Cortes and Pazdur, 1995). Docetaxel is also known for its great anti-cancer activity.

Combined chemotherapy

Animal experiments by Daniel S. Martin, Howard E. Skipper (1915-2006) and Frank M. Schabel (1918-1983) at the Southern Research Institute in Birmingham, AL, and Abraham Goldin (1912-1988) at the National Cancer Institute showed that using cytostatics in combination enhanced their efficacy. In addition, pharmacologic studies demonstrated that different classes of cytostatics have different action mechanisms and different toxicity spectra. This led to the idea of combined cytostatic therapy in humans. The basic principle was that each of the substances to be combined should attack the cell at a different point, should have a different pattern of side effects and should have proven efficacy as a monotherapy.

Jean Bernard in Paris was the first to use combined cancer chemotherapy, for the treatment of acute lymphoblastic leukemia in children in 1951. He gave his patients a mix of cortisone and methotrexate. His decision to try out this approach was partly motivated by the good effects observed in the combined therapy of syphilis and the effectiveness of combined antibiotic treatment of sepsis and tuberculosis. Bernard's combined therapy of leukemia produced markedly better results than treatment with methotrexate alone. He also introduced the principle of short induction chemotherapy of leukemia with vincristine and prednisone – that is, giving the patients high doses of the drugs for a short period at the start of their treatment (Burchenal, 1975); O.S. Selawry and Emil Frei III reported in 1964 that this combination led rapidly to complete remission in a high proportion of acute lymphoblastic leukemia patients (Zubrod, 1979).

Once the cortisone-methotrexate and vincristine-prednisone combinations had proved their effectiveness, the time was ripe to go a step further. VAMP therapy, involving the combined use of vincristine, amethopterin (methotrexate),

6-mercaptopurine and prednisone for the treatment of acute leukemia, was introduced in 1964 by Jay Freireich, Emile Frei III and Myron Karon at the NCI. It is noteworthy that these authors only published their results in the form of an abstract, as they were so excited about the success of the new treatment that they were keen to hurry on and look for even better combinations.

The encouraging results obtained with VAMP therapy inspired Vincent DeVita and his team, also at the NCI (DeVita is currently director of the Yale Cancer Center), to design the MOPP regimen (mitoxine, oncovin (vincristine), procarbazine and prednisone) in 1967. This combination of cytostatics proved highly successful in the treatment of Hodgkin's disease, curing many patients in whom the disease had progressed so far that they would have died in the short term without it. About 75% of the patients who were given this treatment showed a complete remission, and half were cured.

MOPP therapy was particularly important because the impressive results obtained with its aid indicated that it might be possible to achieve similar success in the chemotherapy of solid tumors. It would be more than a decade before this hope became reality – at least to a certain extent – when the combination of cisplatin, vinblastine and bleomycin was found to be effective against metastasized testicular cancer, as mentioned above in the section on cisplatin.

In order to improve the prospects for patients who did not respond to MOPP therapy, Bonadonna and his colleagues in Milan developed a combination of four cytostatics not included in the MOPP regimen for the treatment of Hodgkin's disease. This ABVD therapy, consisting of adriamycin, bleomycin, vinblastine and DTIC (dacarbazine), was introduced in 1977. It showed much the same activity as the MOPP combination, and also proved effective for second-line therapy (DeVita et al., 1978). (Second-line therapy is used when patients do not respond, or no longer respond, to the initial (first-line) therapy.) In addition, it had the important advantage of reducing the induction of secondary malignancies. A combination of the last-mentioned two regimens, known as the MOPP/ABV hybrid therapy, was subsequently used for a while as the treatment of choice, until a recent American study showed that this hybrid regimen is no better than ABVD on its own. Consequently, ABVD is currently the gold standard for first-line treatment of advanced forms of Hodgkin's disease.

Multidisciplinary treatment and adjuvant chemotherapy

The introduction of multidisciplinary treatment and adjuvant chemotherapy represented a major milestone in the treatment of cancer. It was Sidney Farber and his team, already mentioned in the section on antimetabolites, who suggested that patients who still had a poor prognosis despite treatment with surgery, radiotherapy or a combination of both should also receive chemotherapy. While both surgery and radiotherapy can be used to remove large tumors, they are not effective in dealing with micrometastases. Conversely, the above-mentioned Skipper, Martin and Schabel had demonstrated convincingly in experimental tumor models that chemotherapy can clear up micrometastases but is generally unable to destroy large tumors. By combining the different forms of treatment, it should be possible to use each therapy to cancel out the shortcomings of the other. It was time to test this idea in clinical practice. The multidisciplinary approach was first applied to Wilms' tumor, a kidney tumor occurring in children. In the period from 1940 to 1958 only 17 to 23% of patients with this condition were cured, while Farber achieved an impressive 80% cure rate with the aid of surgery, radiotherapy and chemotherapy using actinomycin D, thus emphatically validating the concept under trial. It was subsequently found that radiotherapy was no longer necessary in this combination. The multidisciplinary approach also proved to be effective against a number of other childhood cancers such as non-Hodgkin lymphoma, embryonic cell carcinoma, Ewing's sarcoma and osteosarcoma (Burchenal, 1975).

Multidisciplinary treatment could often benefit adults too. For example, it often made it possible to use a breast-sparing form of therapy in the treatment of breast cancer and to avoid surgical removal of the larynx when treating head and neck tumors, such as advanced laryngeal and hypopharyngeal carcinomas; this latter option had the enormous benefit of allowing the patient to retain his or her natural voice.

Adjuvant chemotherapy treatment is in fact a form of multidisciplinary treatment, where the macroscopic cancer has already been cleared up by surgery combined if necessary with radiotherapy before chemotherapy (and possibly hormonal therapy) is used to deal with any micrometastases that may remain.

It was Michael Shimkin of the NIH and George Moore, chief of surgery and director of the Roswell Park Memorial Institute, who took the initiative to set up the first clinical trial of this approach in 1957. At that time, surgeons were concerned about the fact that cancer cells were found in patients' blood after surgical operations. Shimkin and Moore thought that the administration of cytostatics for three days before, during and after the operation might destroy the cells in circulation. They therefore proposed that patients who were being operated on for breast, colorectal and lung cancer should also be given the cytostatic thiotepa. The results of this trial were disappointing. A ten-year follow-up study revealed that only premenopausal breast cancer patients showed a small but significant increase in the survival rate.

However, laboratory studies gradually provided more support for this approach. For example, Linda Simpson-Herren and her team from the Southern Research Institute showed in 1974 that there was an excellent kinetic basis for adjuvant chemotherapy. They found that small metastases are more sensitive than the primary tumor, because they contain a larger number of proliferative cells. Soon after, Frank Schabel from the same institute found that adjuvant chemotherapy produced strikingly high cure rates in mouse models.

The increase, albeit slight, in breast cancer survival rates found by Shimkin and Moore continued to intrigue surgeons, and further trials were carried out to clarify the situation. In 1971, the Norwegian breast cancer researcher Roar Nissen-Meyer reported the results of an investigation by the Scandinavian Adjuvant Study Group, where patients were given six courses of cyclophosphamide after radical mastectomy. The patients treated with cyclophosphamide showed a lower recurrence rate. A number of other large randomized trials performed since then have shown that adjuvant chemotherapy, with or without hormonal therapy, yielded significant benefits in both pre- and postmenopausal women (Zubrod, 1979). As a result, this has become a standard treatment for breast cancer patients where the prognosis is unfavorable.

Many multi-institutional trials have also been set up to assess the utility of adjuvant chemotherapy in the treatment of colon cancer, especially in more advanced stages such as Dukes' B2 (corresponding to TNM stage II), where the tumor has penetrated through the bowel wall and the five-year survival rate is 75%, and Dukes' C (corresponding to TNM stage III), where the tumor has led to involvement of the lymph nodes and the five-year survival rate is 45%.

Initially, little or no benefit was seen. The big step forward came through a study set up by the NCCTG (North Central Cancer Treatment Group) and the Mayo Clinic (with locations in Arizona, Florida and Minnesota) (Laurie et al., 1989). These groups investigated the value of postoperative administration of levamisole, a substance with immunomodulating properties, alone or in combination with 5-fluorouracil in patients with resected colorectal cancer in Dukes' stages B2 and C. The favorable results of this study were confirmed by a multi-center trial carried out by the NCCTG, ECOG (Eastern Cooperative Oncology Group) and SWOG (Southwest Oncology Group). The five-year survival rate for patients in Dukes' stage C was found to be significantly improved. This led to many large-scale trials of adjuvant therapy in colon cancer, and the introduction of adjuvant chemotherapy as standard treatment for this condition (Skibber et al., 2001).

Bone marrow transplants

Any discussion of the history of chemotherapy would be incomplete without mention of bone marrow transplantation, which permits chemotherapy in some cases where the high dose of cytostatics needed for cure would otherwise be precluded by the toxic effect these cytostatics would have on the bone marrow.

The story of bone marrow transplantation goes back to the studies of Leon O. Jacobson (1911-1992) at the department of medicine of the University of Chicago in 1949, which showed that screening the spleen of a mouse would allow it to survive an otherwise lethal dose of radiation (Jacobson et al., 1949). Egon Lorenz at the Argonne National Laboratory in Lemont, Illinois, reported that irradiated mice could also be protected by an infusion of spleen or bone marrow cells after irradiation (Lorenz et al., 1951).

It was initially thought that this protection against radiation effects was due to humoral factors. It gradually became clear, however, that it was the infused cells that were providing the protection. C.E. Ford from the Radiobiological Research Unit of the Atomic Energy Research Establishment at Harwell in the UK finally demonstrated this in 1956 by showing that the bone marrow of mice that had survived a lethal radiation dose due to bone marrow infusion had the cytogenetic characteristics of the donor (Ford et al., 1956).

Dick van Bekkum and Jan de Vries from the Radiobiological Institute of the TNO (Netherlands Organization for Applied Scientific Research) in Rijswijk showed in the 1950s that successful allogeneic bone marrow transplants in mice induced an immune reaction against the host, currently known as graft-versus-host disease (GVHD). It was later found that methotrexate could prevent this condition.

In 1954, Peter Miescher and Marthe Fauconnet from the New York University School of Medicine discovered antibodies induced by blood transfusions and pregnancies that reacted with antigens on white blood cells. Jean Dausset from the Institute of Research into Blood Diseases at the University of Paris VII and Jon van Rood from Leiden University used these antibodies to describe human leukocyte antigen (HLA) groups. This approach was used to improve the characterization of these antigens in the years that followed. It is now known that these antigens induce immune reactions whenever tissues are transplanted from one person to another, and that the genetic control of these antigens resides on chromosome 6 in a "supergene" region known as the *major histocompatibility complex* (MHC). Dausset shared the Nobel Prize in 1980 with Baruj Benacerraf and George Snell for their work on the MHC.

It was shown in the 1960s that dogs from which bone marrow cells had been removed and that were then given two to four times the level of a lethal dose of body irradiation could still survive if their bone marrow cells were replaced after the irradiation. Dogs given allogeneic bone marrow cells could also survive if they received chemotherapy with cyclophosphamide or busulfan. The antigenic composition of the blood cells also proved to be of importance in this connection: the graft generally took if the donor leukocyte antigens matched those of the host (Thomas, 1999).

In 1956, David W.H. Barnes (1923-1998) of the Radiobiological Research Unit of the Atomic Energy Research Establishment at Harwell in the UK described the treatment of leukemic mice after a supralethal dose of irradiation followed by infusion of normal bone marrow. E. Donnall Thomas, the great pioneer in the field of bone marrow transplantation, described the application of this technique in humans at practically the same time. He shared the Nobel Prize in 1990 with Joseph E. Murray for this groundbreaking work. Initially, transplantations were only successful between identical twins. Georges Mathé from Paris was the first to get an allogeneic bone marrow graft to take in a leukemia patient, but the patient died shortly after, probably as the result of graft-versus-host disease.

Thomas and his group went on with their work undaunted. By the end of the 1960s blood platelet infusions became available alongside better antibiotics and cytostatics, all important developments for successful bone marrow transplantation. Our knowledge of the human histocompatibility system continued to grow, and it became routine practice to test each donor and recipient for tissue compatibility.

Evaluation of the results of bone marrow transplantation in the 1970s was hindered by the fact that practically all patients received a bone marrow transplant at a time when their disease had recurred in greater intensity after failure of the initial conservative treatment. The medical team gradually learned how to better select candidates for transplantation. By the end of the 1970s, leukemia patients were only given a bone marrow transplant during their first remission or when the initial signs of a recurrence had just been observed. This group of patients had a much better survival rate. Bone marrow transplantation gradually became a standard treatment for acute leukemia, and the indication expanded to include other blood cancers.

Autologous bone marrow (that is, bone marrow taken from the patient's own body) was also used for a while, but it was not found to yield any clear benefit because it proved impossible to destroy all the leukemia cells before the bone marrow was returned to the patient.

Another important development was described in 1986 by Shimon Slavin of the Hadassah University Hospital in Jerusalem. He had given a patient who had suffered a recurrence of acute lymphoblastic leukemia a bone marrow transplant followed by a transfusion of donor lymphocytes, and was able to report that the patient had remained in remission for eight years after this treatment. Further reports of successful treatment with donor lymphocytes followed. This type of treatment can in fact be regarded as a kind of immune therapy in which the lymphocytes react with antigens of the MHC or the recipient's minor antigens in case of a mismatch.

The way in which bone marrow cells are collected has also changed in the course of time. Initially, the bone marrow was taken from the bones of the pelvis using a needle and syringe, under general anesthetic. It later proved possible to harvest the stem cells from the donor's bloodstream with the aid of an apharesis machine as an outpatient procedure. (The stem cells are essentially filtered out of the donor's blood by the machine, which then returns the blood minus the stem cells to the donor.) The yield of stem cells can be increased by chemotherapy and the administration of hematopoietic growth factors.

Dr. Elaine Gluckman and colleagues from the Hôpital St. Louis in Paris found another important source of stem cells in 1989, when they succeeded in isolating these cells from cord blood (the blood in the umbilical cord) (Thomas, 1999).

All in all, bone marrow transplantation has become an indispensable new addition to the arsenal of methods available for the treatment of blood cancers.

Conclusion

Chemotherapy has not been with us for very long, but it has already become an important weapon in the battle against cancer. It was initially developed at a time when the cause of cancer was not understood. The early researchers were looking for substances that could stop cell division. As a result, the agents they found attacked healthy cells as well as cancer cells. They could thus be highly toxic, especially for cells that undergo rapid division – and there are plenty of those in the body. For example, every second we make three million new red blood cells, 1.5 million new white blood cells and lots of hair cells, mucosal cells, sperm cells and the like. Each DNA molecule would be about 4 cm long if we could pull it out straight, and we have 46 of them in each cell. It follows that if we laid all the DNA molecules we produce in a day end-to-end, they would be about 500 million kilometers long. When I told that to my students, one said: "Now I understand why I am so tired in the evening". We need these new cells to replace the old ones that die off from natural causes. And when we use chemotherapy, we interfere with this delicate mechanism of cell division. It may be regarded as a miracle that this does not lead to disaster. The fact that the benefits of some of the substances we have discovered outweigh their drawbacks is the foundation on which this form of cancer therapy rests.

The number of cytostatics is still increasing steadily. The search for new active agents in this field is continuing, as is the search for possible ways of getting around the side effects of the existing remedies. We have succeeded in making chemotherapy somewhat patient-friendlier with the aid of antiemetics, growth factors, antibiotics etc., but cancer treatment still represents a heavy burden for the patient. This makes it important for physicians that use chemotherapy in the fight against cancer to have specialized training in this field, in order to optimize patient safety and to be able to select the optimum treatment modality on the basis of the clinical data. Medical associations have long been aware of this. For example, the American College of Physicians set up a committee in 1957 to determine the role of the internist in the treatment of cancer patients. The recommendations of this committee led in 1972 to the recognition of medical oncology as subspecialism of internal medicine in the United States. The Dutch Association of Internists made the same move twenty years later.

The establishment of professional organizations of medical oncologists was also necessary, in the interests of developing higher standards of treatment and representing the joint interests of members. Seven American doctors got together in Chicago in 1964 to found the American Society of Clinical Oncology (ASCO), thus breaking away from the American Association of Cancer Research (AARC) that had been set up in 1907 (Krueger, 2004). The European Society for Medical Oncology (ESMO) was founded in 1975.

[7]

The history of the hormonal treatment of cancer

Hormone therapy of tumors has two advantages compared with the surgical, radiotherapeutic and cytostatic approaches discussed in previous chapters. Firstly, it does not cause severe damage to the patient's tissues. And secondly, it can contribute to the long-term palliative care of patients with extensively metastasized tumors that are sensitive to hormones without causing serious side effects. In other words, it can in general be characterized as a mild treatment. It has the disadvantage that it can only help to cure the patient when used as an adjuvant to other forms of treatment, and it can no longer serve this purpose if the cancer has metastasized.

Breast cancer, endometrial cancer and prostate cancer respond best to steroid hormones (hormones that are related to cholesterol), but thyroid cancer, malignant lymphomas and some other tumors may also be hormone-sensitive. Hormones other than sex hormones can also be used in the treatment of cancer.

This chapter is largely devoted to a summary of key moments in the history of the hormone therapy of breast cancer; it then goes on to discuss prostate cancer. There is so little to be said about endometrial cancer, thyroid and malignant lymphomas in this connection that they have been omitted from the present review.

Breast cancer and hormones

The Italian physician Bernardino Ramazzini (1633-1714) was the first to observe that certain groups of women were more susceptible to breast cancer than others. Ramazzini is considered to have been the founder of occupational medicine, and published a book entitled *De Morbis Artificum Diatriba* (On the Diseases of Workers) in Modena in 1700 where he described how people's work in some 50 different professions affected their health. His initial objective in studying the conditions in convents was to investigate how the work the nuns performed impinged on their health. His most striking conclusion, stated in 1713, was that nuns were more likely to get breast cancer than other women (Petrakis, 1979). "You seldom find a convent," he wrote, "where this accursed canker is not encountered within the walls" (Patterson, 1987). He was at a loss to explain this fact, but thought that it might be related to the celibacy and consequent childlessness of the nuns. This supposition has been echoed by many authors after him.

The German anatomist, surgeon and botanist Lorenz Heister (1683-1758), professor of anatomy and surgery at the University of Altdorf and later, from 1720 until his death, at Helmstadt, stated in 1714 that breast cancer was frequently found in unmarried and infertile women, while the German physician and chemist Friedrich Hoffmann (1660-1742), professor of medicine in Halle, Prussia, published the same conclusion in 1739. In 1842, the Italian physician Domenico Rigoni-Stern issued a statistical analysis of death rates for various types of cancers by "sex, age, organ and certain social conditions." He concluded that the frequency of breast cancer increased with age, and he confirmed the finding that the disease occurred more often in nuns than in other women. T.H.C. Stevenson, from the General Register Office in London, who was mentioned in Chapter 2, reported in 1913 that the mortality rate from breast cancer for unmarried women over the age of 45 was much higher than that for married women in the same age range. Dr. Jane Lane-Claypon from the Ministry of Health in London extended Stevenson's study by collecting data on a large number of breast cancer patients and control subjects. She stated in 1926 that statistical analysis of her data showed that breast cancer patients generally married later, underwent fewer pregnancies and had a lower frequency of breastfeeding. Abraham M. Lilienfeld, of The Johns Hopkins School of Hygiene and Public Health, reported in 1956 that artificial menopause was associated with a reduction in the frequency of breast cancer, while J. Staszewski from the Institute of Oncology in Gliwice, Poland, stated in an article published in 1971 that the incidence of breast cancer is related to the age of menarche (the age at which a girl has her first period). Brian MacMahon (1923-2007) and his team at the Harvard School of Public Health demonstrated that the age at which a woman had her first child was more important in determining the risk of breast cancer than the total number of children she had (Petrakis, 1993). More recently, Valerie Beral and her team at the Cancer Epidemiology Unit at Oxford University, which was later responsible for coordinating the Million Women Study of women's health in the United Kingdom, reported in 1993 that the number of pregnancies increased the risk of breast cancer in younger women but actually reduced it in women over 45 years of age (Beral and Reeves, 1993). All these data indicated the existence of a relationship between the occurrence of breast cancer and the duration of the fertility period (that is, the time between menarche and menopause), the age of the first pregnancy and the number of pregnancies.

The relationship between hormones and cancer has also been studied extensively in animal models. Abbie Lathrop (1868-1918), a commercial mouse breeder from Granby, Massachusetts, was concerned about the high incidence of tumors among the mice she was breeding for experimental purposes, and published a series of papers on this topic together with Leo Loeb (1869-1959) from the University of Pennsylvania. They showed in 1916 that sterilizing newborn female mice from a strain that was very susceptible to breast cancer led to practically complete eradication of this complaint. They also noted the importance of the timing of sterilization. When ovariectomy was performed between the fifth and the seventh month, breast cancer occurred less often and at a higher average age than in controls, while carrying out the operation after the eighth month had hardly any effect on the occurrence of breast cancer. This time dependence is reminiscent of the clinical observation of the occurrence of cancer of the penis in relation to the timing of circumcision. This form of cancer is not found in Jewish men, who are circumcised on the eighth day after birth, but does occur when circumcision is performed later, in particular between the ages of three and fifteen (Raven, 1990).

Antoine Lacassagne (1884-1971) at the Radium Institute in Paris (which he headed from 1937 to 1954) and Harold Burrows from the Royal Cancer Hospital in London took an entirely different approach to the investigation of the relationship between breast cancer and hormones, in studies published in 1932 and 1935, respectively. Instead of stopping hormone production, they actually gave their experimental animals additional amounts of hormones. They found that both male and female mice developed breast cancer in response to the continuous administration of estrogens (Bett, 1954). It became clear that the early sterilization of female mice can reduce the occurrence of breast cancer while the administration of estrogens can induce this condition.

Animal experiments also indicated that hereditary conditions can play a role in this connection. In a study published in 1919, after Abbie Lathrop's death, Lathrop and Loeb had shown that when mice from a strain where the incidence of cancer is typically high are crossed with mice from a strain with low cancer incidence, the chance of developing breast cancer is mainly determined by the genetic makeup of the mother. The father has a much less important, but still measurable, influence.

The mechanism of the influence of hormones on the development of breast cancer has been subjected to extensive study. This led to the key discovery of estrogen receptors in the uterus and in vaginal tissue in 1967 by Elwood V. Jensen (born 1920) and his team at the University of Chicago's Laboratory for Cancer Research, which proved to be of particular clinical significance. These receptors were later also found in the breast and other tissues (Raven, 1990). Jensen received the prestigious Albert Lasker Award for Basic Medical Research in 2004 for these investigations.

Estrogen receptors are proteins present in certain body cells that are able to bind estrogens and transport them to the cell nucleus where they activate specific genes. Research has shown that if estrogen receptors cannot be detected in tumor tissue, the chance for the successful hormonal treatment of the tumor is less than 10%, while if the estrogen receptors can be detected then the chance of successful hormonal treatment is about 60% (which means, of course, that the treatment is still likely to fail in 40% of the cases). Kathryn Horwitz, a professor of endocrinology and molecular biology at the University of Colorado Health Sciences Center in Denver, postulated that this failure of estrogen-receptor-positive tumors to respond to treatment was due to a defect in the route followed by the estrogen within the cell after binding with the estrogen, leading to autonomous growth. This led to a search for an examination technique that would give a better indication of the link between the presence of estrogen and its effect.

Based on the observation that estrogens induce progesterone receptors both in reproductive tissue and in human breast cancer cells, it was hypothesized that the progesterone receptor might be a better indicator of treatment prognosis than the estrogen receptor. Kathryn Horwitz and William McGuire of the University of Texas at San Antonio succeeded in detecting this receptor in human breast cancer tissue in 1975 (Horwitz and McGuire, 1977). However, determination of the progesterone receptor alone proved to be no more predictive of the therapeutic response than that of the estrogen receptor alone. Combined determination of both receptors was found to give the best prediction of the therapeutic response.

Both receptors are currently routinely determined in breast cancer patients. We now know that when both receptors are found to be positive in primary breast cancer, the patient has a better than 70% chance of responding to hormone treatment. The search for hormone receptors has continued, and has led to the discovery of receptors for androgens and corticosteroids in addition to the above; however, these are of less clinical importance (Raven, 1990).

Ablative hormone therapy of breast cancer

The original idea that the prognosis for young women with breast cancer could be improved by ovariectomy dates from 1889, and was put forward by the German surgeon Albert Schinzinger (1827-1911) from Freiburg im Breisgau. He had observed that young women have a poorer prognosis than older ones, and thought that prematurely aging patients by removing their ovaries might improve their prognosis. He went no further than this theoretical suggestion, however.

The first major step forward in this field was the historic paper entitled "On the treatment of inoperable cases of carcinoma of the mamma: suggestions for a new treatment with illustrative cases" read to the Edinburgh Medico-Chirurgical Society on May 20, 1896, by Sir George Thomas Beatson (1848-1933, Figure 7.1), consulting surgeon to the Glasgow Cancer Hospital, and published the same year in The Lancet. In this article, Beatson described three patients, one with a local recurrence of breast cancer and two with extensive primary mammary carcinoma. He had treated all three with bilateral ovariectomy, and all had shown marked remission of the disease (Beatson, 1896). Beatson went into detail in the about the line of reasoning that had led him to this new therapeutic approach. Shortly after graduating from the University of Edinburgh in 1874, he had lived on a large estate in

FIGURE 7.1 *Sir George Thomas Beatson.*

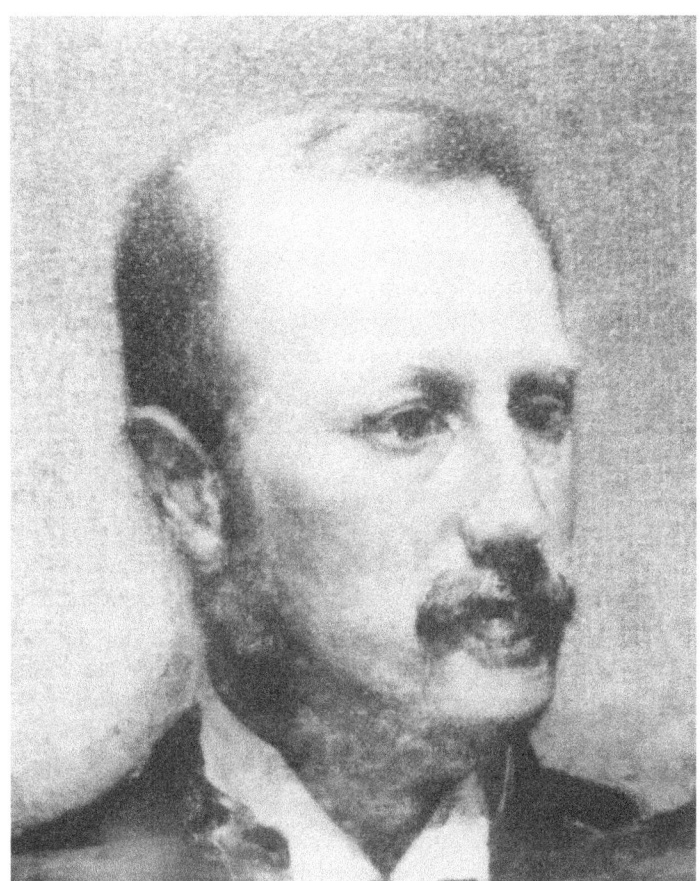

CHAPTER 7

the west of Scotland while providing medical care for the Scottish laird who owned it. There was a large sheep farm adjoining the estate, and Beatson was so enthralled by the weaning of the lambs there that he initially intended to take lactation as the topic for his MD thesis. Though he later changed this topic to investigation of the cerebral cortex, he retained his interest in lactation and the factors that determined it. He noticed that the histological changes taking place in the lactating breast after pregnancy were similar to those observed in cancer. He also learned that farmers were well aware that cows could give milk indefinitely if their ovaries were removed after calving, and that it was common farming practice to have cows served by the bull again when their milk production fell off after calving, since it was known from experience that milk production was maintained while the cows were in calf. Farmers also knew that cows started menstruating every three weeks shortly after they had calved but that they did not menstruate while they were in calf, indicating that the ovaries were no longer functional during this period. Beatson concluded from these observations that the breast was controlled by the ovaries. This led him to write:

_____ That we must look in the female to the ovaries as the seat of the exciting cause of carcinoma, certainly of the mamma, in all probability of the female generative organs generally, and possibly of the rest of the body. I have felt for some time that the parasitic theory of cancer is an unsatisfactory one in many ways, and that in directing all our energies to working it out we are losing time and searching for what will never be found simply because it does not exist.

He went on to state that he did not think that it was time to replace the current treatment for breast cancer, surgical removal of the breast in question, by this still unproved method; he was however convinced that the cancer was caused by some kind of effect proceeding from the ovaries, and that removal of the ovaries could improve the patient's condition.

Beatson provided extensive details about the patients he treated. The first was 33 years old and had an extensive local tumor, which was judged to be inoperable. He discussed his ideas with the woman and her husband and she gave him permission to remove her ovaries, which he did. The patient's condition gradually improved after the operation, to the extent that eight months later all signs of breast cancer had disappeared and the patient appeared to be completely healthy. Encouraged by this result, Beatson performed the same operation on two other patients, who also showed marked postoperative improvement.

At a meeting of the Royal Medical and Chirurgical Society in London in 1905, Sir Hugh Lett, surgeon at the London Hospital, reported that he had performed an ovariectomy on 99 patients with inoperable breast cancer after becoming acquainted with Beatson's results. Lett had observed marked improvement in 23.2% of the cases and clear but less extensive improvement in 13.1%. Thus, a total of 36.3% of Lett's patients benefited from the operation, and one was even alive and in good condition five years postoperatively. The best results were obtained in women between 45 and 50 years old, while hardly any benefit was found in women over 50. During the discussion after Lett's lecture, James Stanley Boyd of the Charing Cross Hospital commented that he had seen the best effects from this operation in chronic cases of breast cancer. Boyd also mentioned that in two cases he had removed the patient's breast as well as the ovaries, and claimed that the results of this treatment surpassed anything he had been able to achieve by removal of the breast alone (Raven, 1990). This was the first example of adjuvant treatment, which later came to be routine practice for certain patient categories.

In connection with the relatively high mortality associated with ovariectomy in those days, the German radiologist Ludwig Halberstädter (1876-1949) introduced the use of radiation for ablation of the ovaries as early as 1905 (Stoll, 1950).

The encouraging results of removal of the ovaries in cases of extensive and metastasized breast cancer suggested that ovariectomy might play a role in preventing local recurrences and metastases after mastectomy. The first published study on this topic was by George Smith and O. Watkins Smith from the Fearing Research Laboratory of the Free Hospital for Women, Brookline, Massachusetts, in 1953. This and subsequent investigations showed that benefit could be derived from both prophylactic ovariectomy and radiation-induced ovarian ablation. Roar Nissen-Meyer compared the results obtained with surgery and postoperative irradiation alone with those of the same treatment combined with prophylactic castration (Nissen-Meyer, 1965; 1967). He found that the survival curves for the first four years were better after ovariectomy, but that after five years there was little difference between the two treatments. He therefore concluded that there were no grounds for expecting that castration could prevent recurrences, but it could delay them and thus possibly increase the survival time of patients who could not be cured by the primary surgery with irradiation. Meta-analyses carried out since that time have shown however that prophylactic ovarian ablation used as an adjuvant therapy in women with hormone-sensitive tumors can contribute to a drop in the risk of recurrence.

Bilateral adrenalectomy (surgical removal of both adrenal glands) was introduced as a treatment for metastasized breast cancer in cases where ovariectomy did not yield the desired improvement because of a low residual level of estrogen production. We now know that this residual estrogen production is derived from androgens secreted by the adrenal glands, since androgens can be transformed into estrogens. This new approach was first described in 1952 by Charles Huggins (1901-1997) and Delbert M. Bergenstal from the Ben May Laboratory for Cancer Research and the Department of Medicine at the University of Chicago. They were able to perform this operation after cortisone acetate had become available as substitution therapy for adrenal insufficiency (see Figure 7.2). (Readers may find it useful to consult this schematic overview of the relationship between the various hormones that play a role in breast cancer, the hormonal therapies that have been used in the past and those that are used in the present. We will refer to it from time to time where appropriate in this chapter.) In their first group of six patients with extensive breast cancer, two enjoyed definite improvement, one showed a slight benefit and three showed no improvement (Raven, 1990). This form of treatment was used quite widely for a while but became obsolete after aromatase inhibitors (discussed in the next section) were introduced in 1970.

Hypophysectomy (surgical removal of the pituitary gland) was also used for a while as a treatment for extensive or metastasized breast cancer (Figure 7.2). Since the adrenal glands are controlled by the pituitary, it was hoped that removing the latter would stop estrogen production by the former. This view was supported by evidence gained from animal experiments. For example, Remmert Korteweg and Frédéric Thomas from the Dutch Cancer Institute in Amsterdam had shown that breast cancer in mice grew more slowly after hypophysectomy (Korteweg and Thomas, 1939). This operation was first described in humans by the endocrinologist Rolf Luft (1914-2007) and the neurosurgeon Herbert Olivecrona (1891-1980; often described as the father of modern neurosurgery in Sweden) from Stockholm University in 1951. The pituitary is notoriously difficult to get to, being situated at the base of the brain and protected by the *sella turcica* bone; Luft and Olivecrona chose to approach it by the transcranial route. The results were comparable with those achieved by adrenalectomy. The transcranial route was later replaced by the transnasal-transsphenoid route, which while technically more demanding is less hazardous for the patient (Raven, 1990). Hypophysectomy was also used for a while for pain relief in patients who were suffering severe pain. Fortunately, this operation is no longer used for these indications, since drugs are now available that can achieve the same ends without invasive surgery.

Use of drugs in the hormone therapy of breast cancer

ESTROGENS

Edward Charles Dodds (1899-1973) from the Courtauld Institute of Biochemistry at Middlesex Hospital in central London discovered stilboestrol, a substance with a biological activity comparable with that of the estrogens, in 1938 (De Moulin, 1983). (Founded in 1745 as the Middlesex Infirmary, the Middlesex merged with University College London Hospital in 1994, and ceased to exist in 2005.) Interest in the treatment of extensive breast cancer with estrogen analogs was stimulated by the discovery that these substances could slow tumor growth under certain circumstances. In 1943, Dr. W.M. Biden, an Edinburgh graduate practicing in Pitlochry (a small town and popular tourist resort in the Scottish Highlands) wrote a letter to the *British Medical Journal* in which he described how a 78-year-old patient of his with an extensive breast tumor showed marked improvement when treated with stilboestrol. He wrote, "The great interest in this case was the clearly visible tumour, which could be seen during its retrogression. It is unfortunate that microscopical sections could not be obtained, but one felt much indebted to the patient's horror of an operation for an instructive experience" (Biden, 1943). The next year, Alexander Haddow (1907-1976; later Sir Alexander Haddow FRS) and his team at the Chester Beatty Cancer Research Institute (now called the Institute of Cancer Research) in London published the results obtained from the treatment of 73 patients suffering from different forms of cancer with three estrogen analogs. Of the 22 breast cancer patients treated with the nonsteroid estrogen triphenylchloroethylene, ten showed a significant but temporary retardation of tumor growth, while one actually showed prolonged regression of the cancer. Five of the 14 breast cancer patients treated with stilboestrol also showed a temporary slowing of tumor growth (Raven, 1990).

In 1955, Olof H. Pearson and colleagues at the Sloan-Kettering Institute reviewed the combined results obtained by several clinics that had been treating breast cancer with estrogens (see Figure 7.2). Objective remission was observed in 44% of the patients. The average duration of the remission was eight months, and the median duration 4.5 months. The authors pointed out, however, that about 50% of breast cancer patients have estrogen-dependent tumors, so the administration of estrogens to patients in this group is potentially hazardous (Pearson et al., 1955).

Androgens

While the testes are the main source of androgens, experimental studies showed that both the ovaries and the adrenal glands can produce these male sex hormones. The Viennese physiologist and endocrinology pioneer Eugen Steinach (1861-1944) and colleagues demonstrated as early as 1936 that estrogens are in fact metabolic products of androgens. They gave androsterone to rats and observed increased excretion of estrogens in the urine of both normal and castrated animals, which proved that the conversion did not take place in the testes.

The main male sex hormone, testosterone, was isolated the same year in the pharmacology laboratory of Professor Ernst Laqueur (1880-1947) in Amsterdam. It did not take long for other groups to learn to make this hormone by a semisynthetic process (DeMoulin, 1983).

The use of androgens in the treatment of breast cancer has attracted a great deal of interest for many decades. A.A. Loeser, consultant gynecologist to St. Saviour's Hospital in London, and P. Uhlrich independently reported in 1939 on two cases each where androgen therapy appeared to have benefited patients with advanced breast cancer. Similarly, F. E. Adair in 1947 and Basil Stoll in 1950 published reports of favorable results of androgen treatment in patients with metastasized breast cancer.

Michael Shimkin from the National Institutes of Health (mentioned in Chapter 6 in the section on multidisciplinary treatment) published the results of his treatment of 450 patients with testosterone propionate in 1957. He concluded that androgens are indicated for both pre- and postmenopausal patients with advanced breast cancer who can no longer be considered for radiotherapy (see Figure 7.2). He stated that more than 50% of the patients reported subjective improvements, but that objective effects were found in no more than 10-15% of the cases involving bone metastases and 10-25% of the cases with soft-tissue metastases. The duration of the improvement varied from a few weeks to more than two years. Virilization was a common side effect of this treatment.

The great interest in androgen treatment half a century ago was reflected in the introduction of several new drugs, the most important of which was 19-norandrostenolone phenylpropionate (marketed under the name of Durabolin); 19-norandrostenolone is currently known as norandrolone, and is a powerful anabolic steroid in addition to possessing a limited androgenic potency (Raven, 1990). It is very popular among bodybuilders as a means of building muscle mass, and its use is forbidden in competitive athletics; several athletes have been banned from competing after they tested positive for this substance. Today, androgens are rarely used in the treatment of breast cancer, as other substances with higher therapeutic activity and fewer side effects have been discovered.

Antiestrogens

Antiestrogens were discovered in the late 1950s, and were initially regarded as possible contraceptive agents. Tamoxifen was developed in 1962 and introduced as an anti-cancer drug by Arthur L. Walpole, head of the fertility control program in the pharmaceutical division of Imperial Chemical Industries (ICI) – now known as Astra-Zeneca Pharmaceuticals – in Macclesfield in the north of England. Tamoxifen, a derivative of the above-mentioned nonsteroidal estrogen triphenylchlorthylene, was found to be an effective postcoïtal contraceptive in rats, and it was hoped that it might form the basis of a morning-after pill for use in humans. But further investigation showed that the physiology of ovulation and implantation in rats differed from that in humans. When it was tested on women, it was found to induce ovulation rather than suppressing fertility. It is still marketed in some countries as a means of stimulating ovulation in women with fertility problems.

Walpole, who had previously been engaged in the development of cytostatics, now focused his attention on the fact that tamoxifen bonded with estrogen receptors and might thus be used to prevent estrogen from stimulating breast cancer growth (see Figure 7.2). This made tamoxifen the first of the selective estrogen receptor modulators (SERMs), and it is currently the most widely used oral anti-breast-cancer drug in the world. It would probably never have achieved this status, however, without Walpole's personal enthusiasm for this project. He encouraged specialists at the Christie Hospital and the Holt Radium Institute in nearby Manchester to test tamoxifen as a means of breast cancer therapy, thus spearheading the introduction of this substance as a breast cancer drug (Jordan, 1988). M.P. Cole and his colleagues at the Christie Hospital in 1971 were the first to describe the favorable effect of tamoxifen in breast cancer (Cole et al., 1971). It was found to combine good efficacy with relatively few side effects. Tamoxifen was initially only used for the provision of palliative care in the treatment of breast cancer, but was later also used as a form of adjuvant therapy. The first positive results of two big randomized trials, the Christie Hospital Adjuvant Trial (Ribeiro and Swindell, 1985) and the NATO (Nolvadex Adjuvant Treatment Organisation) trial, were published in 1985 (Baum et al., 1985). As in a subsequent investigation performed within the framework of the National Surgical Adjuvant Breast Project (NSABP), adjuvant treatment with tamoxifen was found to lead to a significant reduction in the risk of recurrence in women with estrogen-receptor-positive (ER+) tumors (Fisher et al., 1996).

The NSABP, under the energetic chairmanship of Bernard Fisher from the University of Pittsburgh, also introduced tamoxifen as a preventive measure in persons with an elevated risk of breast cancer. In a large-scale study with nearly 14,000 participants, the results of which were published in 2005, it was found that tamoxifen reduced the likelihood of actually developing breast cancer in high-risk women by 45% (Fisher et al., 2005).

Tamoxifen proved, however, to have certain drawbacks, such as the increased proliferation of endometrial cells and hence a slight risk of endometrial cancer and other estrogenic effects such as an increased tendency to blood clotting. In recent years the study of antiestrogens has therefore focused on a search for improved SERMs with a strong antagonist effect against tumor cells but an agonist effect on the beneficial action of estrogens on the skeleton, lipid metabolism and the processes that lead to hot flashes and mucosal damage in cases of estrogen depletion.

Robert Bucourt, head of chemistry at Roussel-Uclaf, a French company active in healthcare, agrochemicals, animal health and related fields, and his team showed that side chains could be attached to the estradiol core without reducing the bonding to the estrogen receptor. Systematic studies at the ICI on the basis of this insight led to the synthesis of a series of pure steroid antiestrogens (Carlson et al., 2004). The first of these to be used clinically was fulvestrant, synthesized in 1987 by Alan E. Wakeling and J. Bowler (Wakeling and Bowler, 1987). Like tamoxifen, it bonds with the estrogen receptor, but it differs from tamoxifen in that this bonding leads to reduced transport of the estrogen receptor to the cell nucleus and to accelerated degradation and loss of the receptor. It also switches off the two activating functions on the estrogen receptor (Carlson, 2005).

Another of these second-generation SERMs is raloxifene, which has higher estrogenic activity on bone and is therefore prescribed for osteoporosis. The NSABP carried out a phase-III randomized trial of the efficacy of tamoxifen and raloxifene for the prevention of breast cancer in post-menopausal women. They found no significant difference between the two drugs, but raloxifene was associated with fewer thromboembolic complications and a lower incidence of cataracts (Vogel et al., 2006).

Aromatase inhibitors

As mentioned above, estrogens are formed from androgens in the body. The conversion is catalyzed by the enzyme system cytochrome P450, usually known as aromatase, since the transformation process in question involves aromatization (a selective increase in the proportion of aromatic – benzene-like – rings in the molecule). This reaction is the final step in the conversion of cholesterol and androgens into estrogens, and occurs in the adrenal cortex as well as the liver, muscle and adipose tissue. Y. J. Abul-Hajj and colleagues from the University of Minnesota reported that this reaction also occurs in tumor tissue in breast cancer (Abul-Hajj et al., 1979), and this finding was confirmed by Daniel Rabe and colleagues from the University of Oklahoma Health Sciences Center in 1983. Inhibition of this enzyme blocks estrogen synthesis. The first aromatase inhibitor to be used in clinical practice was aminoglutethimide. It was originally intended for use as an anticonvulsant, but was found to have serious and sometimes fatal side effects of adrenocortical insufficiency. This led researchers to look for other possible uses for this substance. Ralph Cash, a pediatrician at the Sinai Hospital in Detroit, reported that its properties included the inhibition of aromatase activity (Cash et al., 1967). As mentioned in the section on ablative hormone treatment, since surgical adrenalectomy had sometimes proved effective in the treatment of metastasized breast cancer but was associated with appreciable morbidity and sometimes mortality, it was replaced by the administration of aminoglutethimide combined with good glucocorticoid replacement (see Figure 7.2). Richard J. Santen and colleagues from Pennsylvania State University provided the scientific basis for this therapy. They compared the administration of aminoglutethimide and hydrocortisone with surgical removal of the adrenal glands, and found no significant difference between the two forms of treatment (Santen et al., 1981).

Another selective aromatase inhibitor, anastrozol, soon came on the market. It was synthesized by Michael Dukes and F. Thomas Boyle from AstraZeneca. This substance bonds reversibly with aromatase. Unlike aminoglutethimide, it has no effect on the synthesis of steroid hormones in the adrenal cortex and hence has far fewer side effects. Its clinical activity as a palliative treatment for breast cancer was first described by B.J. Nathan Griffiths from Cardiff University in 1973. Its suitability for adjuvant treatment – which means that it can contribute to the cure of cases of breast cancer – was reported in 1996.

The third-generation aromatase inhibitor letrozole has also been found to be highly effective in the treatment of breast cancer (Iveson et al., 1993; Dombernowsky et al., 1998). Exemestane, developed by Enrico di Salle at the laboratories of Pharmacia & Upjohn in Nerviano, Italy (this establishment, later taken over by Pfizer and recently renamed Nerviano Medical Sciences, is the biggest pharmaceutical R&D facility in Italy) is a steroidal aromatase inhibitor that owes its very high activity to the fact that it binds irreversibly to the enzyme, thus permanently preventing it from converting androgens into estrogens. It was launched on the market in 1992 (Evans et al., 1992).

LHRH ANALOGS

Andrew Schally, born in Poland in 1926, later emigrated to the United States and is now an American citizen. He determined the structure of a hormone produced in the hypothalamus, known as luteinizing hormone-releasing hormone (LHRH) or gonadotropin-releasing hormone, in 1971 while he was a professor of medicine at Tulane University in New Orleans. This hormone triggers the production of follicle-stimulating hormone (FSH) and luteinizing hormone (LH) in the pituitary, which in turn regulate various maturation and development processes in both male and female gonads (see Figure 7.2). Schally also determined how this substance could be synthesized, and made peptide agonists of it (Denmeade and Isaacs, 2002). He shared the Nobel Prize in Physiology or Medicine in 1977 with Roger Guillemin and Rosalyn Yalow for their "discoveries concerning the peptide hormone production of the brain."

Chronic administration of an LHRH agonist results in an initial rise in gonadotropin, rapidly followed by a drop in the secretion of this substance and then by a drop in circulating estrogen to a postmenopausal level in women and a drop in testosterone production in men. The ultimate effect is thus drug-induced castration.

Professor Jan Klijn, a medical oncologist from Erasmus Medical Center in Rotterdam, was the first to publish a description of the clinical effect of an LHRH agonist (Klijn and de Jong, 1982). The substance he selected was goserelin, an LHRH agonist that is preferably given in the form of a time-release preparation. C.W. Taylor and colleagues at the University of Arizona Cancer Center in Tucson showed in a multicenter randomized trial that patients who were treated with this substance had rates of freedom from recurrences and total survival times that were comparable with those for surgical ovariectomy in premenopausal patients with metastasized breast cancer, without the drawbacks associated with surgery (Taylor et al., 1998). Other randomized trials published since then confirm the value of LHRH agonists in the adjuvant treatment of premenopausal patients with estrogen-positive tumors. Because LHRH agonists allow the ovaries to resume their function after treatment is stopped, this approach is theoretically best for young women. Their definitive place in the therapeutic arsenal still remains to be determined, however (Sharma et al., 2005).

FIGURE 7.2 Schematic overview of the hormonal system in women and the various possible ways of manipulating it so as to inhibit tumor growth. The main events represented in the central part of this figure may be recapitulated as follows: the hypothalamus makes luteinizing hormone-releasing hormone (LHRH), which stimulates the pituitary (also known as the hypophysis) to produce luteinizing hormone (LH) and follicle-stimulating hormone (FSH). These last-mentioned hormones cause the ovaries to produce estrogens, progesterone and androgens (andronstenedione and testosterone). The pituitary also secretes adrenocorticotropic hormone (ACTH), which stimulates the adrenal cortex to produce androgens, among other substances, and these androgens can be converted into estrogens by a chemical process known as aromatization (a selective increase in the proportion of aromatic (benzene-like) rings in the molecule) which is catalyzed by an enzyme known as aromatase. Androgens are also aromatized to estrogens in tumor cells. The treatments for various types of breast cancer are shown on the outside of the figure; those which are rarely or no longer used are given between brackets. (Source: CJH van de Velde, JHJM van Krieken, PHM De Mulder and JB Vermorken (eds.), Oncologie. Bohn, Stafleu van Loghum, Houten, 2005).

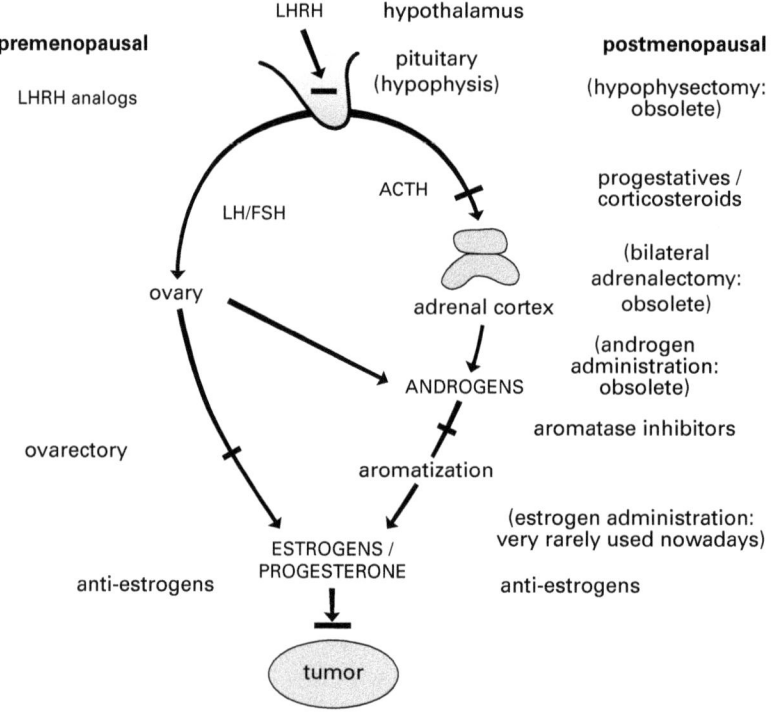

Progestins

Progesterone is one of the hormones that promote growth of the breast. Since the mid-twentieth century considerable interest has been shown in various synthetic analogs of progesterone, known as progestins. For example, Taylor and Morris in 1951 and Gordon and colleagues in 1952 described a number of patients with advanced breast cancer who responded favorably to the administration of pharmacologic doses of progestins (Stoll, 1969) (see Figure 7.2). Two representatives of this group, medroxyprogesterone acetate and megestrol acetate, were regarded as especially promising at the end of the 1960s: when given in sufficiently high doses, they were found to be effective in the treatment of postmenopausal patients with metastasized breast cancer. Italian researchers, in particular F. Panutti and colleagues and Mario De Lena and colleagues from the Cancer Hospital in Bari reported favorable objective and subjective results when very high doses of medroxyprogesterone acetate were used to treat women with metastasized breast cancer (Panutti et al., 1979; De Lena et al., 1979). Treatment with high doses of megestrol acetate produced similar results (Muss et al., 1990). These therapies gave rise to a great number of side effects, however, and in recent years have come to be regarded as a treatment of last resort for breast cancer. Their anabolic and glucocorticoid properties are however currently put to good use in another field, since high doses of progestins have proved to be effective in the treatment of cachexia.

A Brief Summary of Hormone Therapy for Breast Cancer

The interest in hormone treatment for breast cancer has shown marked ups and downs over the years. After its introduction, around 1900, ovariectomy soon fell into disrepute when it was found to be ineffective in curing breast cancer. Interest was revived in the period between 1940 and 1960 as a whole series of ablative measures such as ovariectomy, adrenalectomy and hypophysectomy became available, together with many different hormone-based drugs such as estrogens, androgens and progestins. The arguments advanced in favor of using hormones that basically promoted tumor growth in order to limit the growth of malignant tumors were not very scientific. It is probably due more to good luck than to good judgment that the relatively high doses (in the milligram range) of these substances used at the time actually brought about tumor regressions in many cases.

The introduction of chemotherapy between 1960 and 1970 led to a renewed loss of interest in hormonal therapies, which produced unpredictable results and yielded objective improvement in only 20-30% of cases – and that after a delay of six to eight weeks – while chemotherapy could produce a 60-70% response rate with much less delay. The scope for endocrine therapy increased again around 1980 when methods to determine the content of estrogen and progesterone receptors in tumor tissue became available, thus allowing the response to hormone treatment to be predicted in advance. In addition, new, less toxic hormone drugs came onto the market, such as tamoxifen and SERMs, aromatase inhibitors and LHRH analogs, which presented a useful alternative to surgical measures. This made the use of estrogens, progestins and androgens the treatment of last resort for breast cancer (Kardinal, 1992).

Hormone therapy of prostate cancer

The Scottish surgeon John Hunter (1728-1793), who was regarded as one of the most outstanding medical men and scientists of his time, and in honor of whom the Hunterian Society of London was named, was the first to provide evidence suggesting that the prostate depended on the testes for its development and probably for its very existence. In a paper published in 1786, entitled "Observations on the glands situated between the rectum and bladder, called vesiculae seminales," he stated that the prostate atrophied after castration and that the vesiculae seminales in eunuchs were much smaller than in men who had not undergone this operation. Removal of a single testicle did not lead to atrophy of the vesiculae seminales, however. Hunter added a range of corroborative evidence, taken from both the human and animal kingdom. He noted, for example, that there is little difference between boys and girls before puberty, and that after menopause women lose some of their female characteristics and show a trend towards virilization. He also observed that birds and mammals with a marked, limited breeding season showed striking differences in the size and external appearance of the gonads and accessory genital organs at different times of year. He further noted that the rudimentary spur of the hen developed into a good-sized male spur when transplanted to the foot of a rooster, while the small spur of a young male bird failed to develop properly when transplanted to the foot of a hen. All these original experiments performed by Hunter demonstrated the hormonal function of the testes. The mechanism underlying these effects was however not well understood at that time.

A.A. Berthold, professor of physiology at the University of Göttingen in Germany, threw new light on these phenomena in 1849. He postulated that the testes influenced the operation of various parts of the body by producing a certain substance that is then carried around the body in the bloodstream, allowing it to act on the various organs it reaches. Such substances were given the name "hormone" (from the Greek *ormi*, meaning "impetus") by the Cambridge physiologist Sir William Bate Hardy (1864-1934). This classical idea that the growth of certain normal tissue was regulated by hormones led to the supposition that the growth of tumors might also be subject to hormonal control (Raven, 1990).

In 1893, W. White, a surgeon from Philadelphia, observed a reduction in the weight of the prostate in dogs after castration. He therefore recommended castration as a treatment for obstruction of the bladder (Denmeade and Isaacs, 2002).

Clyde Deming, a urologist at Yale Medical School, and his team reported in 1935 that castration in primates led to a reduction in the size of the normal prostate, but that the operation did not help men with benign hypertrophy of the prostate. A few years later, Robert Moore and Allister McLellan found that estrogen injections led to atrophic changes in prostate epithelium, but once more had no effect on prostate hypertrophy.

An important step forward in our knowledge of hormones was made in 1929 and in subsequent years, when several researchers succeeded in isolating a number of these substances. For example, in 1929 the American biochemist Edward Doisy (1893-1986) and the German Adolf Butenandt (1903-1995) independently isolated estrone (the first estrogen to be prepared in this way) in pure crystalline form (Huggins, 1966). Butenandt later isolated pure crystalline androsterone in 1931 and progesterone in 1934, and synthesized testosterone from androsterone in 1939. He won the Nobel Prize in 1939 for his work on sex hormones, while Doisy went on to share the 1943 Nobel Prize with Henrik Dam from Denmark for their work on vitamin K.

In the late 1930s, Alexander Gutman and his wife, Ethel Benedict Gutman, of the department of medicine at Columbia University, New York, discovered that the acid phosphatase level in the blood was elevated in metastasized prostate cancer; this discovery provided an important basis for monitoring the treatment of prostate cancer. Charles B. Huggins, urologist and professor of surgery at the University of Chicago, also introduced methods for measuring the effect of various hormonal manipulations on prostate function at about the same time. He found that castration or the administration of estrogen led to atrophy of the prostate, which could be reversed by the administration of androgens. He also showed that acid phosphatase production fell after androgen ablation in dogs (Kardinal, 1985).

The measurement of the acid phosphatase level was gradually displaced by the determination of prostate-specific antigen (PSA), which has now become the method of choice for detecting pathologic changes in prostate tissue. PSA was discovered by Professor Richard Ablin and his team at the University of Arizona Health Center, who published their groundbreaking work in 1970 – nine years before T.J. Wang from the research and development department at Hybritech, a subsidiary of Beckman Instruments in San Diego, California, who is often cited as the discoverer of PSA. Wang did, however, purify and characterize PSA (Zaviačić, 1997). It may be noted that, after having discovered PSA, Richard Ablin has devoted much energy over several decades to warning against the dangers of indiscriminate reliance on the PSA test as an unambiguous sign of prostate cancer and an indication for prostate surgery.

The introduction of the PCA3 urine test, with its higher specificity and sensitivity, represented a major improvement on the PSA test. PCA3 stands for prostate cancer gene 3, which was first described in 1999 by Marion Bussemakers, a member of the team led by Jack Schalken, a professor of experimental urology at Radboud

University Nijmegen, in the Netherlands, and Bill Isaacs from The Johns Hopkins University. The test is performed on a urine sample after digital rectal examination (Bussemakers et al., 1999; De Kok et al., 2002).

The favorable effects of androgen ablation in metastasized prostate cancer were first observed in 1941 by Charles Huggins and Clarence Hodges (who was still a medical student at the time) at the University of Chicago. They had treated prostate cancer patients with orchiectomy (surgical removal of the testicles) or the administration of oral estrogens in the form of stilboestrol. This was the first example of a systemic approach to the treatment of prostate cancer. Orchiectomy led to an increase in weight, appetite and hematocrit – and more importantly, to a reduction in pain. Huggins won the 1966 Nobel Prize for his discoveries concerning the hormonal treatment of prostate cancer, sharing it with Francis Peyton Rous, who was recognized for the discovery in 1910 that viruses can cause cancer – which was discussed in Chapter 2 (Denmeade and Isaacs, 2002).

The demonstration of the favorable effects of androgen ablation triggered many large-scale clinical trials. One of the most important of these was the randomized trial begun in 1960 by the Veterans' Administration Cooperative Urologic Research Group (VACURG) in the US, which led to the conclusion in 1967 that treatment with diethylstilboestrol is just as effective as orchiectomy. It was also found, however, that systemic hormonal therapy had two drawbacks: the increased risk of cardiovascular complaints (including thromboembolic complications), and the fact that neither orchiectomy nor the administration of estrogens offers a cure for prostate cancer.

In an attempt to avoid thromboembolic complications, diethylstilboestrol was converted into a prodrug by adding two phosphate groups to create phosphestrol, an inactive transport form of the drug. The idea was that this would be converted back into the active form in prostate tissue with its high acid phosphatase activity (Brock et al., 1988). Unfortunately, however, most of the phosphestrol was hydrolyzed during its passage through the wall of the intestine, thus doing away with most of the intended reduction in toxicity and increase in activity.

It was again Charles Huggins, working with another of his students, W.W. Scott, who observed the temporary benefit brought about by bilateral adrenalectomy on the recurrence of tumor growth after orchiectomy. Others found that hypophysectomy has a similarly good effect.

New avenues of investigation explored from the 1960s to the 1980s concern the blocking of androgen production in the adrenal glands and the inhibition of the interaction of androgen with target tissue. Andrew Schally, mentioned in the section on the hormonal treatment of breast cancer for his determination of the structure of LHRH in 1971 and his preparation of LHRH agonists, was also involved in the clinical investigation of the use of this substance in the treatment of prostate cancer. He and other researchers found that the administration of LHRH initially led to a temporary rise in the testosterone level, coupled with pain and urinary obstruction. If however the treatment was continued with LHRH agonists, the LHRH receptors in the pituitary were down-regulated and the LH and FSH levels fell. This eventually caused a drop in testosterone levels similar to that found after orchiectomy. Schally and his colleagues reported that patients with advanced prostate cancer who were treated with LHRH agonists showed a 75% drop in serum testosterone levels, normalization of the acid phosphatase content and a marked reduction in bone pain. As mentioned above, Schally shared the Nobel Prize in 1977 for his work on peptide hormones.

Since then, many different synthetic LHRH agonists have become available. Their main advantage is that, unlike estrogens, they do not lead to an increased risk of thromboembolic complications when used in the treatment of prostate cancer. The various possible methods of androgen ablation, such as orchiectomy and the administration of estrogens or LHRH agonists, have been compared in large-scale randomized trials, which showed that all the different approaches produced comparable results, reducing tumor growth by 70 to 80% in symptomatic patients (Denmeade and Isaacs, 2002).

The androgen receptor was discovered and characterized in the late 1960s by three separate teams, those of Shutsung Liao at the University of Chicago, Nicholas Bruchovsky at the University of Texas Southwestern Medical School in Dallas, and W.I.P. Mainwaring of the endocrinology group at the Imperial Cancer Research Fund in London. This was the first step in the development of antiandrogens. The first drug in this category was cyproterone acetate, which was developed in 1962 by F. Neuman and his team at the central laboratory of the German pharmaceutical company Schering AG in Berlin (taken over by Bayer in 2006, and now called Bayer Schering Pharma). This led to a race among pharmaceutical companies to synthesize other antiandrogens, especially nonsteroidal agents, which are believed to have fewer hormonal side effects (Mainwaring et al., 1987). As a result, flutamide, bicalutamide and nilutamide were developed. Though these drugs are better tolerated by patients than androgen ablation, they have produced results that are worse with regard to total survival rates and progression-free survival.

Ferdinand Labrie, of the Molecular Endocrinology and Oncology Research Center at Laval University, Quebec City, Canada, took the next logical step forward by arguing that combining an antiandrogen such as flutamide with androgen ablation should yield a markedly superior method of treating advanced prostate cancer. His initial clinical results seemed to bear out his assertions, and led to considerable controversy in the medical world about the merits of this combined therapy. Meta-analysis of the numerous randomized trials that have been carried out indicate, unfortunately, that Labrie's combined therapy produces little or no added benefit compared with monotherapy (Denmeade and Isaacs, 2002).

Concluding remarks

A few other matters related to the hormonal treatment of cancer should be mentioned, albeit briefly, before we leave this topic.

In 1929, two teams of physiologists in the United States, F.A. Hartmann and his associates from the University of Buffalo and W.W. Swingle and J.J. Pfiffner from Princeton, prepared extracts from the adrenal cortex that were found to be able to combat the effects of adrenal insufficiency. It was initially hoped that these compounds might be effective in treating burns and certain infections, but when this proved not to be the case interest in this extract waned until 1941. With the shadow of the Second World War coming ever closer to America, the US military authorities approached the National Research Council of the United States with the request that the hormones of the adrenal cortex be made available. Edward C. Kendall (1886-1972), a chemist at the Mayo Clinic in Rochester, Minnesota, was one of the scientists assigned to this work. With his team at the Mayo Clinic, Kendall identified a number of steroids in the adrenal cortex extract, the most interesting of which were provisionally named A, B, E and F. Particular attention was focused on *Compound* E, and by 1944 Kendall and his team had succeeded in isolating and characterizing this compound, which was later named cortisone (Kendall 1950). Kendall shared the Nobel Prize in 1950 with his fellow-American Philip Showalter Hench and with Tadeus Reichstein from Switzerland for "their discoveries relating to the hormones of the adrenal cortex." In 1944, after cortisone was found by F.R. Heilmann and Kendall to be effective in the treatment of lymphosarcoma in mice (Heilmann and Kendall, 1944), it was incorporated into all kinds of therapeutic schedules for the control of lymphoproliferative complaints.

The use of cortisone in the treatment of breast cancer was also investigated for a while. Lawson Wilkins (1894-1963), known as the father of pediatric endocrinology, and his team from The Johns Hopkins Medical School showed in 1952 that the administration of cortisone brought about a reduction in the secretion of estrogen by the adrenal glands, and that prolonged administration ultimately led to atrophy of the adrenal cortex. The administration of cortisone was therefore regarded as a kind of drug-induced adrenalectomy. However, analysis of the results of all past studies of the treatment of breast cancer with corticosteroids must lead to the conclusion that, while cortisone often helps in alleviating subjective complaints, no objective reduction in tumor size can be expected. As a result, corticosteroids are used only as a palliative measure in treatment of the complications of cancer.

It is also known that endometrial carcinomas can react favorably to treatment with progestins. This effect was first described about 1960 (Kistner et al., 1962; 1965).

[8]

The background of targeted therapy and the emergence of a new approach

Introduction

We have known for about thirty years now that the root of cancer lies in the genes. This has led to a massive search for ways of treating cancer that attack it at its roots, which is obviously a much more logical approach than trying to deal with the consequences of faulty functioning of the genes by means such as chemotherapy. The new approach should make it possible to cure the cancer for good while sparing healthy cells.

This "magic bullet," which has remained a dream for centuries, seems at last to be in sight. When Watson and Crick determined the structure of DNA in 1953, many scientists thought that the cure for cancer was just around the corner. But the solution turned out to be more elusive than was initially thought.

When the British Eighth Army under Montgomery defeated Rommel's Afrika Korps at the battle of El Alamein in August 1942, Winston Churchill said, "Now this is not the end. It is not even the beginning of the end. But it is, perhaps, the end of the beginning" (King, 1998). I believe that the new therapeutic strategy internationally known as *targeted therapy* represents the end of the beginning in the centuries-old battle against the massed forces of cancer. Though this new form of treatment was introduced very recently, I am devoting a separate chapter to its description in recognition of its great potential.

Targeted therapy involves the use of a new generation of small molecules and monoclonal antibodies that have been logically designed to block specific transcription and signal-transduction pathways that are essential for the growth and survival of cancer cells. To expand this definition a little: a gene is part of the DNA molecule that causes a cell to produce a specific protein. To this end, the DNA is first transcribed into RNA, which serves as a template for the production of the protein in a part of the cell known as the ribosome. Once created, the protein leaves the ribosome and influences the cell in which it was produced, or another cell, in a way that depends on its own detailed structure. When the protein acts, it first has to bond to a receptor on the cell membrane. This receptor consists of three parts: an extracellular active site, a transmembrane domain and a kinase domain. Once the protein has attached itself to the active site, a cascade of biochemical reactions is initiated, leading to the transmission of a signal to the cell nucleus. This signal acts on the DNA in the nucleus, in the case of cancer, causing the cell to divide. If the signal is interrupted, the cell division is blocked. The passage of the signal from the receptor to the DNA in the nucleus is known as signal transduction (Hobday and Perez, 2005).

Targeted therapy can also be defined as treatment with a drug that specifically attacks a well-defined target or biological pathway, which if inactivated leads to regression or destruction of the malignant process in question – for example, hormone treatment of breast or prostate cancer aimed at the hormone receptor in the tumor cell (see Chapter 6), low-molecular-weight inhibitors of the epidermal growth-factor receptor (EGFR), drugs that block the action of proteins and enzymes that promote processes of invasion and metastasis, and antiangiogenesis agents. Many researchers also regard anticancer antibodies to which cytotoxic radioisotopes, cytostatics or other cytoxic substances have been attached that attack and kill malignant cells with the antigen targeted by the antibody as falling under the heading of targeted therapy (Ross et al., 2004).

Many targeted therapy drugs are currently under investigation. I will restrict myself here to substances that are registered for use in the Netherlands – many of which, of course, will also be in use in other countries throughout the world.

Targeted therapy with monoclonal antibodies

Antibodies are immunoglobulins that recognize antigens and bond to them. Antigens are mostly proteins built up of a sequence of amino acids. When an antibody binds to an antigen, it inactivates it. During the past decade, many monoclonal antibodies that have the ability to stop the growth of specific cells have been produced, and which may thus be included under the heading of targeted therapy. When used as medicaments, such substances always have a name ending in – *mab* (short for monoclonal antibody). The significance and development of these monoclonal antibodies is discussed below, and a definition of this term is included in the Glossary.

Antibody treatment dates back to the end of the nineteenth century, when French physiologists Jules Héricourt and Charles Richet treated patients with advanced melanoma with a serum to combat their tumors that had been prepared in dogs and mules. They commented that in order to be effective, antibody therapy should be combined with radical surgery (Héricourt and Richet, 1895).

The first theoretical description of antibodies was given by Paul Ehrlich, who has been mentioned several times in previous chapters. His *side chain theory*, developed at the end of the nineteenth century, was the first theoretical explanation of the mode of action of what are currently called antibodies. Many attempts were made during the succeeding decades to halt or reverse the progression of cancer with the aid of antisera, but none was effective (for further details, see Chapter 10 on immune therapy).

It was not until Georges J.F. Köhler from the Basel Institute for Immunology and César Milstein from Cambridge developed the hybridoma technique in the 1970s on principles laid down by Niels Jerne (director of the Basel Institute for Immunology from 1969 until his retirement in 1980) that it became feasible to produce antibodies in sufficient quantities to make effective therapy possible. In the hybridoma technique, a mouse myeloma cell line is fused with mouse spleen cells to produce a clone that is "immortal" (that can grow indefinitely in tissue culture) thanks to the properties of the myeloma cell line, while the spleen cells allow it to produce the desired specific type of antibody. These antibodies, which can thus be produced in very large numbers and with precisely identical properties, are called monoclonal antibodies. Jerne, Köhler and Milstein shared the Nobel Prize in Physiology or Medicine in 1984 for this discovery (Grillo-López, 2000). This technique has been used to produce a range of antibodies that influence the growth of tumors, such as trastuzumab, cetuximab, rituximab and bevacizumab. The last member of this list, bevacizumab, stops tumor growth by inhibiting the growth of blood vessels in the tumor; it is therefore classified as an angiogenesis inhibitor. This important subclass of drugs is discussed separately below. To complete the story of angiogenesis inhibitors, we also consider thalidomide, even though it is not an antibody. First of all, however, the discovery and development of the individual monoclonal antibodies will be discussed.

Trastuzumab

A complex sequence of events led up to the development of trastuzumab, a monoclonal antibody that is widely used in the treatment of breast cancer. This story is so instructive, and so important, that we give it in considerable detail here.

Lakshmi Charon Padhy, a postdoctoral student from Bombay who was working in Robert Weinberg's laboratory at MIT, extracted DNA from neurological tumors in the rat in 1979 and injected it into normal mouse cells. This caused them to turn into cancer cells. Padhy discovered that these cancer cells sometimes induced an immune reaction in the mouse due to a particular rat protein on the surface of the mouse cells. This protein was a product of one of the genes of the rat tumor. Weinberg called the gene that made the cancer cells *neu* because it was first discovered in neurological tumors. He then lost interest in this new discovery because at the time he was concentrating on trying to clone the *ras* oncogene. It was not until years later that Ullrich and Slamon discovered the pivotal role played by the *neu* gene in carcinogenesis, as we shall see below.

_____ "I could flagellate myself," Weinberg later commented. "If I'd been more studious and more focused and not as monomaniacal about the ideas that I had at the time, I would have made that connection."

Weinberg could have carried out the key experiment years ahead of his competitors.

_____ "It would have been an overnight experiment. We just didn't do it," he admitted, adding, "That's life. I can't complain or be embittered. It's not as if I didn't have my share of good luck."

In the years to follow, achievements were such that, despite the missed opportunity with *neu*, Weinberg heard from friends that he would share a Nobel Prize with Bishop and Varmus. "Lots of people said to me, 'you're next, Bob'." But when Bishop and Varmus got the award in 1989, there was no third winner. Weinberg, who has won every significant honor in science save the big one, tried to remain philosophical. "How much do you need to make you happy?" he asked. "And in fifty years, who will care who won the Nobel Prize?" (Bazell, 1998).

Another key player in the trastuzumab story was Axel Ullrich, a German biologist. He won a postdoctoral fellowship in the biochemistry department of the University of California, San Francisco (UCSF). When he arrived in 1975, Michael Bishop and Harold Varmus were doing their work on the Rous sarcoma virus, as described in Chapter 2, which would lead to a shared Nobel Prize in 1989 for their discovery of the cellular origin of retroviral oncogenes. Herbert Boyer, the co-founder of Genentech, one of the first biotechnology companies in the world, was also there, discovering that genes from bacteria could be combined with genes from higher organisms. All in all, it was a very stimulating environment for a young researcher. Ullrich's first achievement was the isolation of the gene that codes for insulin. He succeeded in transferring this gene to bacteria, so that the bacteria could produce insulin. This work laid the foundation for recombinant technology, which allows DNA to be transferred to other species – an approach that is of key importance in the biotechnology industry. Indeed, Genentech made wide use of this technology to produce synthetic insulin.

In 1977, Ullrich went to work for Genentech, but dropped his work on insulin. Instead, he moved to the field of cancer and studied epidermal growth factor. This factor had been discovered in 1960 by the American biochemist Stanley Cohen (born 1922) in the department of zoology at Washington University in St. Louis during his investigation of nerve growth factor. The latter had been discovered in the same department by the Italian developmental biologist Rita Levi-Montalcini (born 1909), who had observed that a protein secreted by mouse tumor cells stimulated the growth of nerve fibers in chick embryos. The protein was purified in 1957 by Levi-Montalcini and Cohen from snake venom and mouse saliva extract, and was called nerve growth factor. When Cohen injected an extract of salivary gland into newborn mice, he observed an unexpected speeding up of the animals' development. For example, they opened their eyes early, and their teeth erupted earlier than usual. Cohen explained these observations by suggesting that the extract of salivary gland contained another growth factor alongside the nerve growth factor, which he called epidermal growth factor (EGF) because it showed the ability to stimulate the growth of epithelial cells in the skin and the cornea. Cohen and Levi-Montalcini shared the Nobel Prize in 1986 for their discovery of these growth factors. At the time of writing, Rita Levi-Montalcini is the oldest living Nobel laureate.

EGF resembles hormones in belonging to the class of growth factors that regulate a wide range of bodily functions such as digestion, blood pressure, sleep and respiration in addition to growth. These growth factors do not pass their message on to every cell in the body, but only to those that have a special receptor for them on the surface of the cell. The message is always the same, however: grow and divide. This process is illustrated in Figure 8.1. Unlike hormones, the EGFs are not transported through the body but spread only from one cell to the next.

Many researchers have studied the behavior and properties of EGF. It has been found that EGF is involved in the formation of new blood vessels – a process that is essential for the growth of healthy tissue and also for the growth of malignant tumors – via the production of angiogenetic factors such as vascular endothelial growth factor (VEGF). It was also found that blocking the EGF receptor in tumor cells reduces the expression of VEGF (that is, the amount of VEGF produced) in these cells, so that fewer blood vessels are created and the growth of the tumor is retarded.

In 1983, Ullrich was invited to come and work in London by Michael Waterfield, head of the Protein Chemistry Laboratory at the Imperial Cancer Research Fund (now Cancer Research UK), who believed that he had found evidence of the way oncogenes cause cancer. He told Ullrich that he had managed to purify the protein that functions as the EGF receptor, and thought that it was identical with the protein produced by the oncogene *erb-b*, which causes leukemia in chickens. Ullrich owed the invitation to London to his worldwide reputation as a master cloner, a wizard in the isolation of the DNA fragments that make up a specific gene. Wakefield wanted him to clone the gene for the human EGF receptor by starting from the protein structure and working backwards. Ullrich succeeded in isolating the gene (Bazell, 1998).

The availability of the gene enabled Waterfield, Ullrich and the Israeli protein expert Joseph Schlesinger to be the first to furnish experimental proof of the validity of the theory that growth factors play a key role in the development of cancer, by demonstrating in 1984 that the erb-b oncogene is indeed a mutated form of the gene that codes for the EGF receptor (Ullrich et al., 1984).

Back from London, Ullrich started looking for genes in human DNA that resemble the gene for the EGF receptor. He called the first one he found Her-2, an acronym of *human-epidermal-growth-factor receptor-2*. (The gene he had cloned for Waterfield was Her-1, the first in the series.) There later proved to be a whole family of Her receptors, also known as the ErbB family of tyrosine kinase receptors. Ullrich was able to use existing cloning techniques to determine the protein for which the gene coded. It turned out to be the very same protein that had been found on the surface of mouse cells in Weinberg's laboratory in 1979 and had led to the discovery of the *neu* oncogene. In other words, Ullrich had rediscovered *neu*, starting from a completely different point of departure. Since then, the gene has been known as the *Her-2/neu* gene or *ErbB2*.

Another important player then appeared on the scene: Dennis Slamon, a medical oncologist with a doctorate in cell biology. After graduation, he went to UCLA, where he performed research alongside his clinical work. He built up a collection of fresh tumor tissue from different sorts of cancers. He came to a working agreement with Ullrich: Ullrich would send him DNA samples from his gene collection, and Slamon would check whether they matched the DNA extracts from his tumors. Slamon found that Ullrich's Her-2/neu matched the DNA extracts from certain breast and ovarian cancers. Ullrich and Slamon discovered that this oncogene was not mutated, but that the cells containing the gene produced the corresponding protein in abnormally large quantities – a phenomenon known as overexpression. Further research showed that this protein appeared on the cell surface as a receptor that resembled the EGF receptor (Bazell, 1998). The EGF receptor was also found on other types of cancer cells, such as those from colon cancer, head and neck tumors, cancer of the pancreas, non-small-cell lung cancer, breast, kidney and ovarian cancer, gliomas and bladder cancers. Many of these malignant cells had much larger numbers of EGF receptors than healthy cells. For example, in some cases of breast cancer the number of receptors per cell can be as many as two million while the number in normal cells was found to vary between 50,000 and 100,000 (Herbst and Langer, 2002).

When Slamon discovered this overexpression of Her-2/neu in many breast cancer patients he contacted William McGuire, the renowned researcher from San Antonio who had been studying the influence of hormones on breast cancer for many years (he is mentioned in Chapter 7, in the section on breast cancer and hormones). McGuire had a big collection of frozen tumor tissue, with detailed records of the medical history of the patients from whom the samples were taken. He asked his young assistant Gary Clark to work with Slamon on this problem. In the resulting publication, the authors stated that they had found that cancers with overexpression of Her-2/neu had a poor prognosis, with a higher risk of recurrence, more rapid metastasis and usually a fatal outcome (Slamon et al., 1987).

The next step in Slamon and Ullrich's voyage of discovery involved adding Her-2/neu to normal cells *in vitro*; this was found to turn the normal cells into cancer cells. Ullrich now asked colleagues from the department of immunology at Genentech to make monoclonal antibodies against the Her-2/neu antigen. When Ullrich and Slamon added the monoclonal antibody to breast cancer cells with

FIGURE 8.1 *The growth factors produced and secreted by a tumor cell bond with the receptor on the cell surface to generate a signal passed to the nucleus, telling the cell to proliferate.*

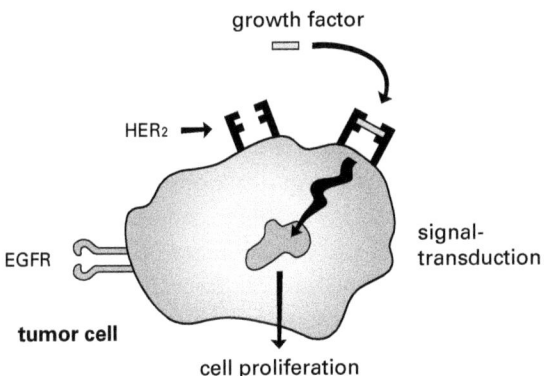

FIGURE 8.2 *When trastuzumab occupies the active site of the HER2 receptor, or cetuximab the active site of the EGF receptor, the relevant growth factor can no longer bond with its receptor, signal transduction to the nucleus is inhibited and the cell stops growing. Other monoclonal antibodies can block the action of other growth factors (not shown here) in a similar way.*

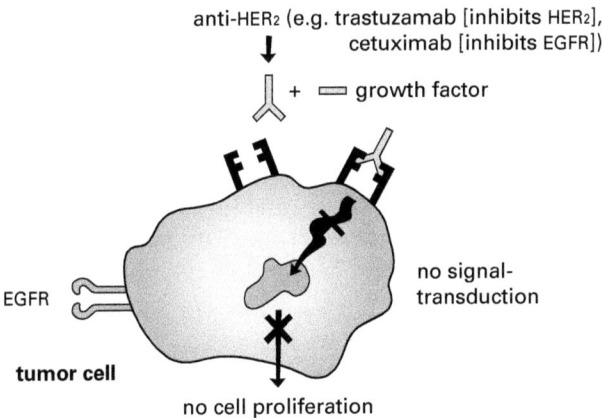

overexpression of Her-2/neu, the cancer cells stopped growing and dividing. This significant finding indicated that a major new anti-cancer drug was in sight.

But a few hurdles still had to be cleared before this discovery could be put to use for therapeutic purposes in humans. In the first place, the monoclonal antibodies that had been developed were derived from mouse genes, which meant that they consisted of mouse proteins. When such antibodies are introduced into the human body, this gives rise to the formation of new antibodies called HAMAs (*human anti-mouse antibodies*) to protect the body against these foreign proteins. When the monoclonal antibodies are administered a second time, the HAMAs neutralize them so that they no longer have the intended effect against the cancer cells; in addition, dangerous allergic reactions can result. Fortunately, another member of the staff at Genentech was able to come to Ullrich and Slamon's assistance. Paul Carter was a 29-year-old Englishman who had learned how to "humanize" monoclonal antibodies at the Medical Research Council's Molecular Biology Laboratory in Cambridge. The objective in this process is to create the biotech equivalent of a wolf in sheep's clothing by making a mouse protein that the body will recognize as human protein. This process can be used to humanize most of the antibody, while still allowing the vital part that bonds with the Her-2 receptor to retain its mouse origin.

Even after the monoclonal antibody had been successfully humanized, another major problem remained: Genentech was hesitant to invest the vast sums required for the development of the monoclonal antibody, fearing that the financial return from the finished drug might not recoup the initial investment. But help came from an unexpected quarter. Slamon, who was fully convinced that he was on the trail of a big new drug, mentioned his problem to Lilly Tartikoff, wife of TV producer Brandon Tartikoff, whom Slamon had treated in the past for Hodgkin's disease. Moved by gratitude for the good care Slamon had given her husband, she started to raise funds to support his research. One of the people she contacted was Ronald Perelman, the chairman and CEO of cosmetics giant Revlon. Perelman was so convinced of the worthiness of this cause that he joined with Lilly Tartikoff to set up the Revlon/UCLA Women's Cancer Research Program. They managed to raise enough money to fund the production of the new monoclonal antibody, which was given the name trastuzumab. The way this drug works is illustrated in Figures 8.1 and 8.2. Clinical trials showed that this monoclonal antibody is a valuable addition to the therapeutic arsenal used in the fight against breast cancer, when administered alone or in combination with cytostatics (Bazell, 1998).

Cetuximab

The mode of action of cetuximab is very similar to that of trastuzumab, but it is active against other types of cancer. Dr. John Mendelsohn from the University of California, San Diego was convinced as long ago as 1980 that the EGF receptor

(EGFR) was an important target for anti-cancer drugs. He and his colleague, the cell biologist and environmental activist Dr. Gordon Sato, a student of the Nobel laureate Max Delbrück, succeeded in producing the monoclonal antibody against the EGFR (Sato et al., 1983). The commercial production of this antibody was entrusted to the biopharmaceutical company ImClone Systems. Like trastuzumab, this was also a mouse antibody and was initially designated IMC C225. It was found to be able to inhibit the growth of tumor cell lines and of tumor xenografts in naked mice that manifested expression of the EGFR (Mendelsohn and Baselga, 2000). In order to avoid the problem of host rejection (HAMAs) discussed above in connection with trastuzumab, a humanized form of the mouse antibody was made. The resultant monoclonal antibody drug was called cetuximab (Goldstein et al., 1995). Further investigation showed that cetuximab could also inhibit the production of a number of angiogenetic factors Preclinical and clinical trials revealed that it can be useful, alone or in combination with the topoisomerase inhibitor irinotecan (discussed in Chapter 6), in the treatment of metastasized colorectal cancer.

Cetuximab also appears to improve the outcome of radiotherapy treatment. Even before this had been shown to be the case, there were indications that it might prove effective to combine cetuximab administration with radiotherapy. Firstly, Ang et al. (2002) demonstrated the prognostic value of the expression of EGF receptors in tumor biopsies from patients with pavement-cell carcinoma of the head and neck. Two large subsequent studies showed the predictive value of the EGF-receptor status for the effect of radiotherapy. A multicenter randomized trial of radiotherapy combined with cetuximab in the treatment of head and neck tumors showed a significant improvement in local control and survival (Bonner et al., 2006).

Angiogenesis inhibitors

Consideration of angiogenesis (the formation of new blood vessels) in tumors is a good starting point for the development of new anti-cancer drugs. As long ago as 1939, A. Gordon Ide, Norman H. Baker and Stafford L. Warren from the University of Rochester postulated that tumors secreted an angiogenetic factor that provided the growing tumor with a network of blood vessels. A few years later, G.H. Algire and H.W. Chalkley from the National Cancer Institute observed that a local increase in blood vessel density preceded rapid tumor growth and concluded that tumors could only grow quickly if they had a plentiful blood supply. There was no new research to report in this field until 1968, when both Melvin Greenblatt and Philippe Shubik from Chicago Medical School and Robert L. Ehrmann and Mogens Knoth from Darmstadt University of Technology in Germany published evidence that tumor angiogenesis is promoted by diffusive factors produced by the tumor cell (Ferrara et al., 2004).

A couple of years later, Judah Folkman (1933-2008), Surgeon-in-Chief at Children's Hospital Boston, published results that showed the potential therapeutic importance of influencing angiogenesis in tumors (Folkman, 1971). This conclusion was based on research he had done on blood vessel growth between 1960 and 1962, while serving as a Lieutenant in the United States Navy. At that time, the United States government was pumping vast amounts of money into scientific research with the aim of achieving significant advances over a wide front. On April 12, 1961, the space race between the US and the Soviet Union was launched when Yuri Gagarin became the first man in space, in a Russian Sputnik. The US was keen to prove that it, too, was capable of major scientific achievements. This objective was largely achieved when the American Neil Armstrong became the first man to set foot on the moon on 21 July 1969.

Folkman's first task in the Navy was to help a heart surgeon by ensuring that a heart-lung machine remained in good working order. He was then asked to try to find blood substitutes that could be used in emergencies. Folkman and a colleague, the pathologist Fred Becker, who had also been drafted into the US Navy, thought that suspensions of hemoglobin might be used for this purpose. In order to test their blood substitutes, they used them to perfuse isolated thyroid glands *in vitro*, since it was known that the thyroid can be kept alive for long periods outside the body if provided with the right nourishment. Folkman was already interested in cancer at this time, so he investigated the effect of adding cancer cells to the perfusion fluid. This proved to lead to the formation of tiny clusters of cancer cells, each about a millimeter in diameter – smaller than the point of a pencil – in the thyroid. The absence of larger tumors was surprising, and suggested the existence of some kind of barrier to tumor growth. When, however, the little clumps of cancer cells were cut out of the thyroid and injected subcutaneously in mice, large tumors were found to develop quite quickly. After a few years, Folkman became convinced that the tumors had remained small in his initial experiment because the perfusion conditions did not allow the blood vessels to function properly. He concluded that a cancer can grow only if the tumor itself makes factors that stimulate the development of a network of blood vessels in the tumor. Such a network is essential for the supply of nutrients and oxygen and the removal of waste products (Cooke, 2001). Prolonged intensive research showed that cancers do secrete a large number of angiogenetic growth factors, and that if angiogenesis is suppressed the cancers can no longer grow.

When this became clear, many substances were tested for their angiogenetic effect. This research finally revealed that vascular endothelial growth factor (VEGF) was probably the most important angiogenesis regulator. The next step was to find substances that could inhibit the action of these angiogenesis regulators.

Bevacizumab

It was the Sicilian-born molecular biologist Napoleone Ferrara who succeeded in isolating VEGF. In 1983, after completing his medical studies at the University of Catania in Italy, he moved to the United States to study endocrinology and was engaged by Genentech in 1988. He was initially set to work on relaxin, a hormone that acts on the human reproductive system. It is Genentech policy to allow employees scope to work on their own personal research interests alongside their official tasks. Ferrara's hobby was the role of antiangiogenesis in cancer treatment. In 1989, he and his team discovered VEGF and succeeded in cloning the VEGF gene, and in 1993 they demonstrated that an antibody against VEGF suppressed angiogenesis and tumor growth in the naked mouse (Kim et al., 1993). This monoclonal antibody was then humanized, and the resultant product was given the name bevacizumab. Experimental trials showed that bevacizumab does indeed inhibit blood-vessel formation in tumors, thus blocking their growth (see Figure 8.3).

After completion of the preclinical trials, bevacizumab was tested on humans. It was found to be active against colorectal cancer, both as a monotherapy and in combination with cytostatics.

Thalidomide

Thalidomide was developed by the German pharmaceutical company Chemie Grünenthal, and put on the market in 1953. Between 1956 and 1961, it was widely prescribed – especially in Europe and Canada – as a sedative and antiemetic in pregnancy. Its teratogenic properties – that is, its tendency to give rise to birth defects – were belatedly recognized in 1961. By that time, about 12,000 "thalidomide babies" had been born worldwide with severe malformations, in particular phocomelia. (This condition, the name of which is derived from the Greek *phoco* meaning seal and *melos* meaning limb, is characterized by extreme shortness or absence of the long bones in the arms or legs, and flipper-like hands and sometimes feet.) Thalidomide was immediately removed from the market. Decades later, in 1994, Robert D'Amato from Judah Folkman's group at the Children's Hospital Boston discovered that thalidomide was a strong angiogenesis inhibitor. This not only explained how it came to cause the malformations notoriously found in thalidomide babies but also suggested that it could be put to good use in fighting diseases. Thalidomide was also found to possess immunomodulating properties (Allard, 2000). Clinical trials have shown that it is effective against multiple myeloma (Singhal et al., 1999) and that it can be used to provide palliative care in patients with Kaposi's sarcoma, one of the illnesses associated with AIDS (Little et al., 2000).

Rituximab

Targeted therapy has also proved effective against non-Hodgkin lymphomas (malignant growth of lymph nodes). There are two types of non-Hodgkin lymphoma, known as B-cell and T-cell lymphoma. The B-cell group is by far the larger, comprising about 85% of all cases. More than 95% of these B-cell lymphomas express the antigen known as the cluster of differentiation 20 (generally abbreviated to CD20). Researchers from IDEC Pharmaceuticals Corporation in San Diego, under the leadership of Nabil Hanna, succeeded in making a monoclonal antibody against CD20 in January 1991, and Darrell Anderson from the same company identified and characterized the protein derived from the serum of mice immunized against CD20, which was provisionally designated IDEC-2B8 (2B8 signifies that this protein was found on plate 2, row B and column 8 of the microplate used to identify it). The mouse produced only three anti-CD20 antibodies, two of which were IgM immunoglobulins while the third was an IgG. The IgG was selected for further study. Roland Newman of IDEC succeeded in creating a humanized version of this antibody.

When sufficient quantities of this monoclonal antibody had been produced, it was given the name rituximab. Clinical trials showed it to be a valuable addition to the drugs available for the treatment of B-cell lymphomas, both as a monotherapy and in combination with chemotherapy (Grillo-López, 2000).

IDEC then tried bonding the radioisotope yttrium-90 to rituximab, with the aim of attacking the lymphoma cells with targeted irradiation as well as with the antibody. This attempt proved successful in 2002, and the new drug was given the generic name 90Y-ibritumomab tiuxetan. Further investigation showed that it was indeed significantly more effective than rituximab alone (Witzig et al., 2002).

Small-molecule targeted therapy

During the past decade, a number of drugs have become available for targeted therapy that are based on much smaller molecules than the monoclonal antibodies discussed above. All these substances act on the kinase domain of the receptor in question. The kinase normally acts as an enzyme, activating its substrates by transferring phosphate groups to them. The new drugs occupy the active site of the kinase, preventing the substrate from bonding with it and thus inhibiting vital processes in the targeted cell. All these small-molecule targeted therapy drugs have names that end in – *nib*. (derived from i**nhib**itor)

Imatinib

The first drug in this class to be discovered was imatinib. As described in Chapter 2, Peter Nowell (a pathologist from Philadelphia) and David Hungerford discovered the Philadelphia chromosome in 1960 in patients with chronic myeloid leukemia (CML). Other researchers subsequently established that this is in fact the fused gene, bcr-abl, which codes for the abnormal bcr-abl protein. Finally, it was shown that this bcr-abl protein causes CML.

Once these facts were known, researchers started looking for substances that could inhibit the action of the bcr-abl protein. It was not until 1992 that the American oncologist Brian Druker succeeded in synthesizing the required inhibitor, in cooperation with research staff from the pharmaceutical company Novartis. After completing his medical studies and a postdoctoral oncology fellowship, Druker was initially engaged as an instructor and researcher at Harvard, where he studied the link between the signaling function of tyrosine kinases and human diseases. Feeling the need for more contact with clinical practice, he moved to Oregon Health & Science University (OHSU) in 1993, where he combined treating leukemia patients with his search for a magic bullet. By this time, Novartis had synthesized a number of kinase inhibitors, making use of the tools Druker had developed in the laboratory. The most promising one was initially designated STI 571 (STI stands for "signal transduction inhibitor"). It was subsequently given the generic name imatinib.

As the initial designation indicates, STI 571 inhibits the signal transduction from the receptor to the nucleus, thus effectively blocking proliferation of the cell in question, as illustrated in Figure 8.3. As a result, it really was the magic bullet Druker – and countless others in the field of oncology – had been looking for, stopping cancerous cells from growing while having little or no effect on healthy cells.

The synthesis of STI 571 was followed by prolonged preclinical and clinical trials, the results of which were so promising that its clinical introduction was eagerly awaited: 95% of the CML patients treated with imatinib were found to have their blood picture normalized, while the cytogenetic defects had disappeared in 60% (Kantarjian et al., 2002). The survival period was increased by four to five years.

Imatinib also proved to give a good outcome in another form of cancer, the rare gastrointestinal stroma cell tumor (GIST), formerly known as leiomyosarcoma of the gastrointestinal tract (Joensuu et al., 2001). Studies by George Demetri and his team at the Dana Farber Cancer Institute in Boston showed that imatinib inhibits the c-KIT receptor, which is expressed by the c-kit proto-oncogene and plays an important role in the development of GIST tumors and is in fact the growth factor for these tumors.

Imatinib was first used to treat a GIST patient in Finland. The results were astonishing. After eight months' treatment, the tumor volume had decreased by 75%. Further trials in a large group of patients showed a decrease in tumor size by more than 50% in more than half of the patients treated, while tumor growth halted in more than one-quarter of the patients. Nearly 90% were symptom-free after 1-2 months' treatment (Demetri et al., 2002). It had been hoped that imatinib might provide a cure for this type of cancer, but unfortunately this proved not to

CHAPTER 8

FIGURE 8.3 *Growth factor receptors in tumor tissue and in tumor vasculature, and the pathway from the receptor to the nucleus, are points where targeted therapy can influence tumor growth in various types of cancer.*

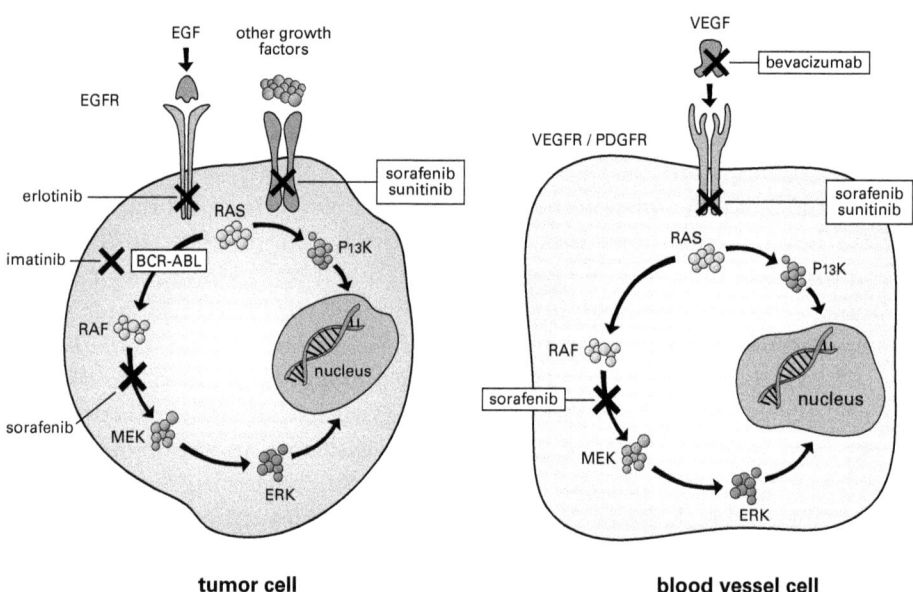

be the case. It does however increase the time to progression by about two and a half to three years.

Sunitinib

Another very interesting small-molecule targeted therapy drug is sunitinib, which was developed through a process of rational drug design by Olga Potapova and her team at the pharmaceutical company Sugen in the United States (later taken over by pharmaceutical giant Pfizer). The particularly interesting feature of sunitinib is that it acts on several different receptors. Apart from being a tyrosine kinase inhibitor, it also targets the vascular endothelial growth factor receptor (VEGFR), the *platelet-derived growth factor receptor* (PDGFR) and the stem cell factor receptor c-Kit (see Figure 8.3). It can be taken orally, and is one of the few drugs that show some activity against the highly therapy-resistant renal cell carcinoma or RCC (Potapova et al., 2006). This fact requires some further explanation. There are five different types of this cancer, depending on the main cell type involved. The most common is the clear-cell type, which occurs in 85% of the cases. The Von Hippel-Lindau (VHL) tumor suppressor gene is inactivated in at least 60% of the cases of clear-cell RCC. This leads to up-regulation of a number of hypoxia-sensitive genes such as those coding for vascular endothelial growth factor (VEGF) and *platelet-derived growth factor* (PDGF), which are assumed to support angiogenesis in the tumor and hence tumor growth.

Bonding of VEGF to the VEGF-2 receptor present on vascular endothelial cells plays a key role in angiogenesis, and PDGF probably plays a role too because its receptors are present on the pericytes that provide structural support for the endothelial cells (Schöffski et al., 2006). The therapeutic effect of sunitinib on RCC can be explained on the assumption that it occupies the active sites on these receptors, thus preventing VEGF and PDGF from promoting angiogenesis and hence tumor growth. About 35% of clear-cell RCC patients showed improvement when treated with sunitinib for a median period of 14 months; this treatment yielded a median survival time of 24 months (Motzer et al., 2007a). In a comparative trial of sunitinib against α-interferon – a widely-used first-line treatment for metastasized cancers – administration of sunitinib to clear-cell RCC patients was found to produce a median progression-free survival time of 11 months, which was significantly longer than the 5 months obtained with interferon. The percentage of patients showing objective improvement was also very significantly higher for sunitinib (31%) than for interferon (6%) (Motzer et al., 2007b).

Since sunitinib also acts on the c-Kit receptor, its effect on patients with imatinib-resistant GIST has been tested. It was found to increase the progression-free survival period to roughly four times longer than that obtained with placebo – 27 weeks as compared with 6 weeks (Demetri et al., 2006, Chow and Eckhardt, 2007). This does not sound like much, and is indeed not very impressive in clinical terms.

It is however highly significant from a scientific perspective, since sunitinib acts on a completely different principle from chemotherapy and because no other systemic therapy has an appreciable effect on this tumor.

Sorafenib

Sorafenib is an oral receptor-kinase and intracellular signal transduction inhibitor. In other words, it blocks tumor cell proliferation and angiogenesis. The main intracellular signal transduction pathway it targets is the MAPK (*mitogen-activated protein kinase*) pathway, which occurs in all cells and includes RAF, MEK and many other proteins; the basic outline of this pathway is illustrated in Figure 8.3. The RAF kinase isoforms occurring near the start of this pathway are enzymes that play an indispensable role in regulating the processes that govern cell proliferation and survival.

In 1989 Usha Kasid, professor of radiation medicine, biochemistry and molecular and cellular biology at the Lombardi Cancer Center at Georgetown University, and her team showed that inactivation of the Raf-1 gene inhibited the growth of human lung, breast and ovarian tumor xenografts in thymusless mice. This was the first indication that the *Raf-1* gene could be an important target for potential anticancer drugs. This was confirmed by joint research carried out by Bayer Pharmaceuticals and Onyx Pharmaceuticals. A project team headed by Barbara Hibner and Bernd Riedl was set up in 1994 with the task of finding a drug that could target Raf-1 kinase activity. In 1995, the team started screening about 200,000 different substances for their ability to inhibit Raf-1 kinase activity. The substance with the greatest activity was sorafenib, which had been synthesized by Roger Smith, a medical chemist working at the Bayer laboratories in West Haven, Connecticut.

After extensive preclinical testing (Wilhelm et al., 2006), sorafenib was tried out in the second-line therapy of renal cell carcinoma. It improved the median progression-free survival time to a period that was twice as long as that found in the placebo group (5.9 months as compared with 2.8 months); 10% of the patients treated with this drug showed a partial remission while the disease remained stable in 74% as compared with 2 and 52% respectively in the placebo group (Oudard et al., 2007).

On the basis of these results, sorafenib is currently used in the second-line treatment of metastasized or advanced renal cell carcinoma. In view of its dual action mechanism, it is also being tested as a possible therapy for other types of tumors.

Erlotinib

Erlotinib was made by James Moyer and colleagues from Pfizer Central Research in Groton, Connecticut; Oncogene Science in Uniondale, New York; and the Storz Cancer Institute in Omaha, Nebraska on the basis of the patent specifications of

Lee Arnold and Rodney Schnur from Pfizer Central Research. The patent rights to erlotinib were subsequently acquired from Pfizer by Roche.

This substance is a specific inhibitor of human epidermal growth factor receptor type 1 (EGFR/HER1) (Moyer et al., 1997). This receptor is a transmembrane glycoprotein belonging to the class of tyrosine kinases. As mentioned above, these tyrosine kinases play a key role in the transmission of signals that are of major importance for cell division and survival of the nucleus. EGFR/HER1 thus plays a crucial role in the growth and progression of cancers (see Figure 8.3).

Since between 40 and 80% of non-small-cell lung cancers show overexpression of EGFR/HER1, it was decided to test the therapeutic powers of erlotinib on patients with this disease.

Preclinical and clinical trials confirmed the drug's activity in the treatment of locally advanced and metastasized non-small-cell lung cancer with overexpression of EGFR/HER1 (Scagliotti, 2007). Erlotinib has been approved by the US Food and Drug Administration for the treatment of this type of cancer and also for the treatment of pancreatic cancer.

Concluding remarks

The explosive increase in our knowledge of the molecular biology of the cancer cell has led to the development of the innovative approach to cancer therapy described in this chapter. The results obtained so far suggest that this targeted therapy may one day replace chemotherapy in the treatment of cancer. We have not yet reached this stage, however. At present, the best results are still obtained by combining these two therapeutic approaches.

In this review, I have so far paid no attention to the side effects of these new drugs. They do have side effects, of course, though in general these are less severe than in traditional chemotherapy. The type of side effect produced by a targeted therapy drug depends on the part of the cell targeted by the drug. For example, substances that target the epidermal growth factor receptor tend to lead to skin complaints and diarrhea. Angiogenesis inhibitors interfere with wound healing and can give rise to hemorrhaging and high blood pressure. The small-molecule drugs that inhibit the c-KIT receptor can lead to bone marrow depression, mainly because they also inhibit the stem-cell factor. And finally, Her-2 inhibitors increase the risk of cardiac arrhythmias.

The field of targeted therapy is still growing rapidly. About 150 monoclonal antibodies are currently undergoing clinical trials (Reichert et al., 2005) and dozens of small-molecule targeted anti-cancer drugs are under investigation. The number of drugs of this type that are approved for clinical use is also growing steadily. I have restricted myself in this review to the substances that have attracted the most attention so far.

The results obtained with angiogenesis inhibitors have thrown a new light on the possibilities for cancer treatment in the future. The aim here is no longer to eradicate the cancer completely but to create a situation where the patient can tolerate the cancer as long as it is held in check – in other words, to turn cancer from a life-threatening disease to a chronic complaint, one with which the patient can live for many years.

[9]

Immunotherapy in the past and the present

Introduction

Attempts to make use of the body's own immune defenses to fight cancer have been going on for more than a century. The initial results tended to be based on anecdotal evidence, and no clear breakthrough was made. Looking back on the past century, we see strong fluctuations in the belief in the efficacy of immunotherapeutic treatment. There were times when it was hoped that immunotherapy would solve the problem of cancer and would become established as one of the four pillars of cancer therapy, alongside surgery, radiotherapy and chemotherapy. At other times, however, any time and effort devoted to research in this field was regarded as wasted.

The striking remissions in cases of inoperable advanced cancer obtained by William Coley and his toxins at the end of the nineteenth century attracted a great deal of attention. His work was previously described in Chapter 4, and will be discussed in somewhat greater detail in the section on aspecific immunotherapy below. This may be regarded as the first serious attempt to use the principles of immunotherapy in the treatment of cancer, though Coley regarded his toxins more as a way of creating hyperthermic conditions (inducing fever) in his patients, which was considered at the time to be a promising means of fighting cancer. However, the results obtained were highly variable, the high fevers induced were not without risk and the cure rate was low. Consequently, the initial enthusiasm for this approach soon evaporated.

Apart from publications describing incidental favorable effects or disappointing results, a number of major hypotheses contributed to the fluctuations in the valuation of immunotherapy.

The renowned scientist Paul Ehrlich, who has been mentioned several times in this book, implied the existence of some form of immunosurveillance when he suggested as early as 1909 that the incidence of cancer would be much higher if the body's immune system did not prevent it. This optimistic view was not shared by other scientists at that time, however (Parish, 2003).

CHAPTER 9

The Australian virologist Sir Frank Macfarlane Burnet (1899-1985), director of the Walter and Eliza Hall Institute of Medical Research in Melbourne, published his theory of acquired immunologic tolerance in 1949. Starting by asking why the body's immune system did not attack its own cells, he hypothesized that the entire immune apparatus is derived from a single pluripotent cell, and that in the course of embryologic maturation the immunologically competent cells that attack the body to which they belong are destroyed. When we are born, all the immunologically competent cells we have left are programmed to attack tissue coming from outside the body. This theory of embryonic maturation and the recognition of self and non-self is known as clonal selection theory.

Clonal selection theory received powerful confirmation from the work of the American geneticist Edward Tatum (1909-1975) on the red bread mold *Neurospora*. Tatum demonstrated that protein production in this unicellular organism is controlled by the DNA of the cell nucleus, and that one single gene or set of genes codes for one specific protein. Antigens are usually proteins, and antibodies always are. This investigation confirmed the one-one relationship between cell and antibody (Richards, 1980). Tatum shared half of the 1958 Nobel Prize in Physiology or Medicine with the American geneticist George W. Beadle (1903-1989) for showing that genes control individual steps in metabolism, while the other half went to Tatum's student, the American molecular biologist Joshua Lederberg (1925-2008), for his discovery that bacteria can mate and exchange genes. Lederberg was a highly versatile scientist, making major contributions in the fields of artificial intelligence and space exploration as well as genetics. Burnet's theoretical model was soon confirmed by experiments performed by Peter Brian Medawar (1915-1987, Mason Professor of Zoology at the University of Birmingham and later Jodrell Professor of Zoology at University College London) and his team. Burnet and Medawar received the 1960 Nobel Prize "for their discovery of acquired immunological tolerance.".

Since this model is based on the assumption that transformed cells cannot be distinguished from the body's own healthy tissue, it gives strong support to the idea that the immune system is unable to protect the body against malignant cells, thus reinforcing the pessimistic mood about the scope for immunotherapy in the treatment of cancer patients that was prevalent at that time.

During the 1960s, the tide turned in favor of immunotherapy again. Ironically enough, Burnet played an important role in changing opinions on this topic. While the immunologic tolerance theory had convinced immunologists that it was unlikely that the body's immune system would be able to recognize tumors, Burnet began to defend the viewpoint that the disposal of malignant cells was one of the main functions of the immune apparatus. He suggested that lymphocytes maintain a continuous check on tissues, probably through recognition of tumor-related antigens, and then eliminate the transformed cells. He coined the term "immunosurveillance" for this process. At about the same time Lewis Thomas (1913-1993), head of pathology at New York University Medical School, postulated that the rejection of a graft reflects the way the body clears up cancers.

The resulting increased readiness to accept the idea of immunotherapy was only short-lived, however. A number of reasons for this change in attitude can be cited. Firstly, it seemed highly unlikely from a theoretical point of view that the immune system would be involved in the recognition and destruction of malignant tumors since acute infections are much more life-threatening – especially for young people – and would thus exert a much stronger selective pressure on the evolution of the immune system. Secondly, an increasing volume of experimental data cast doubt on the validity of the immunosurveillance hypothesis. The strongest argument was that the incidence of primary tumors in athymic naked mice (thought at the time to be T cell-deficient) is comparable with that in syngenic (that is, genetically identical) normal mice. It was discovered later, by the way, that this line of reasoning is invalid because athymic naked mice possess a significant population of functional T cells. Thirdly, scientists began to better understand the process of T cell selection by the thymus: research showed that this organ clears up the T cells targeting the body's own tissue very efficiently. These data reinforced Burnet's immunologic tolerance theory and led to the view held in the 1950s that there were few tumor-specific lymphocytes in the periphery (Parish, 2003).

One of the reasons why people continued to believe in the potential of immunotherapy despite the disappointing results of many studies was the fact that cancers were sometimes found to clear up spontaneously. This was ascribed to an immunologic reaction of the host to the tumor.

The spontaneous regression of cancer is extremely rare, however. A book published in 1966 by Tilden Everson and Warren Cole lists no more than 176 cases recorded in the literature in the period between 1900 and 1965 where the cancer initially observed in patients cleared up spontaneously. Analysis of the data revealed 31 cases of spontaneous remission in renal cell carcinoma (RCC), 29 in neuroblastoma, 19 cases each in melanoma and choriocarcinoma and 13 cases in bladder cancer (Everson and Cole, 1966).

There are however other indications that the patient's own immune system plays an important role in fighting cancer. The fact that a recurrence of cancer may be observed after a lapse of twenty years or more, as sometimes happens in cases of breast cancer or ocular melanoma, suggests that the body's immune system has suppressed the condition for many years. The disappearance of metastases after surgical removal of the primary tumor, which has been described in several cases of RCC, is also ascribed to immunologic effects (Raven, 1990).

Some researchers also believe that the cure of the aggressive metastasized form of choriocarcinoma by simple chemotherapy is due in part to the action of the immune system, as is the observation that administration of a single dose of cytostatic is sometimes enough to cure Burkitt's lymphoma (a tumor of the jaw, mainly found in African boys, mentioned in Chapters 2, 4 and 6).

The pathologic-anatomic changes in the lymph nodes draining a tumor before metastases appear and the presence of leukocytes and in particular macrophages in the tumor are also regarded as signs of an immune reaction by the host (Alexander, 1983).

However, clinical and pathologic-anatomic findings, no matter how interesting they may be, do not provide definitive proof that the action of the immune system can cause cancer to disappear. Data obtained from the study of experimental tumors in animals, where clear evidence has been found that transplantation of a tumor or tumor fragment can lead to the detection of tumor-specific transplantation antigens that can elicit an immune response in the host, are much more important here (Hellström, 1969). The presence of such antigens has sometimes also been demonstrated in in vitro tests (that is, laboratory experiments). Such studies have shown that animals onto which tumors have been grafted have antibodies against the tumor and T-lymphocytes that can have a cytotoxic effect on cultured tumor cells.

A further indication that the immune system plays a role in the suppression of cancer can be derived from the fact that patients with immune deficiencies suffer more often from cancer, mainly from rare types such as non-Hodgkin lymphomas and Kaposi's sarcomas, and the relatively benign skin cancers. These data support the hypothesis that immunosurveillance only applies to cancers in which a virus is involved. In other words, the idea is that it is the virus that is under immunologic surveillance, not the cancer (Alexander, 1983).

The arguments given above are enough to encourage some researchers to persevere in their attempts to look for possible ways of stimulating the immune system to fight cancer. In the rest of this chapter, we will review the historical development of the various treatment methods that have been tried out in the course of time. The presentation is chronological in each section, which means that we regularly jump back in time when we start a new section.

Specific active immunotherapy

Specific active immunotherapy means treatment with tumor cells or extracts of such cells, or with chemically modified tumor antigens specifically targeting the tumor cell. The first group of patients to receive this therapy was described in 1902 by E. von Leyden and F. Blumenthal from the University Hospital in Berlin. These authors used an autologous tumor cell suspension – that is, a suspension of the patient's own tumor cells – as a vaccine. All of the patients treated had advanced metastasized cancer. No objective reduction in the size of the tumor was found in this study, though some subjective improvement was reported in two cases (Von Leyden and Blumenthal, 1902). L. Bertrand, on the other hand, used the same autologous tumor cell vaccine for cancer treatment in 1909 and reported one case of objective tumor regression (Bertrand, 1909). In the same year, Arthur F. Coca (1875-1960) from Cornell University Medical College in New York (who founded the *Journal of Immunology*), working together with P. K. Gilman, treated a number of cancer patients with a vaccine of the same type, and reported tumor regression in several cases. The vaccine they used became known as the Coca-Gilman vaccine. These encouraging results led to a larger trial that was intended to verify the efficacy of the treatment. Five of the forty patients in this trial who received an allogeneic vaccine (one based on tumor cells taken from other patients) showed tumor regression, while none of the 39 patients treated with autologous tumor cell vaccine showed any signs of improvement (Coca et al., 1912).

E.H. Risley, encouraged by the initial optimistic report published by Coca and Gilman, treated twenty patients in the same way in 1911. His patients were divided into two groups, with one group receiving an autologous vaccine and the other an allogeneic vaccine. He did not observe an improvement in any of his patients, however; in fact, he thought that the treatment actually tended to stimulate tumor growth.

J.W. Vaughan of Detroit published data on one hundred patients he had treated with both active and passive immunotherapy in 1914. (Passive immunotherapy is discussed in greater detail in the next section.) The active treatment was based on the use of a tumor extract, which he generally administered intraperitoneally, while he used sheep and rabbit antitumor sera in the passive treatment. There were no controls. Vaughan was clearly an enthusiastic researcher, but the details he gave of the numbers of regressions observed were rather unclear. It must however be concluded from his description that tumor regression was found in some of his patients. He went so far as to claim that 73% of the patients in the group with advanced cancer who were treated by surgery and active immunization showed some degree of regression. A comment he made in this connection is still valid today: "the best results were obtained in those cases where the tumor tissue volume was small and leukocyte differentiation showed a marked response to administration of the cancer protein" (Currie, 1972).

The surgeon Thomas H. Kellock (1863-1922) and the pathologist Helen Chambers (1880-1935) from the Middlesex Hospital in London described twelve patients who had been treated by injecting autologous tumor fragments into the anterior abdominal wall. The tumor fragments had first been irradiated to reduce the risk of tumor growth at the implantation site. This treatment was not found to yield any benefit, however (Kellock and Chambers, 1922).

The pattern sketched above was repeated in subsequent years: a publication describing encouraging results would appear every few years, only to be followed by a series of disappointing reports.

John B. Graham and Ruth M. Graham from Massachusetts General Hospital in Boston described the use of autologous vaccines in the treatment of gynecologic tumors. They treated 232 patients in this way, and concluded that this vaccine therapy could not be recommended as the results it produced were too variable and the benefits obtained were too slight (Graham and Graham, 1959).

In 1960 J.W. Finney, E. H. Byers and R. H. Wilson from the University of Texas Southwestern Medical School in Dallas reported on nine patients with different types of cancer who were treated by intramuscular injection of a tumor homogenate in Freund's adjuvant. The aim of this investigation was not only to test the therapeutic effect but also to determine the nature and extent of the immune reaction to the injection. The vaccine was initially given in three doses on alternate days, with booster injections a few weeks later. All patients showed a rise in "antitumor" antibodies, and the injection of these purified antibodies in subcutaneous metastases gave rise to a spectacular temporary regression in these lesions. However, a rise in these antibodies was also found in another group of five cancer patients who had been treated with radiotherapy only (Finney et al., 1960). The evidence that these antibodies were tumor-specific was thus flimsy.

Norbert Czajkowski and his team at Wayne State University in Detroit tried to boost the immune effect by combining rabbit gamma globulin with human tumor cells. Their initial results were promising: two of the 14 patients with advanced cancer who received this treatment remained tumor-free for about four years and three remained stable or showed very slight progression. Nine patients showed no improvement (Czajkowski et al., 1967). T.J. Cunningham and his team followed the same approach on a group of 42 patients. Unlike Czajkowski, however, they found that only one of the 36 patients for whom the results could be evaluated showed any sign of regression (Cunningham et al., 1969).

Leslie Hughes, professor of surgery at the University of Queensland in Australia, and his team used subcellular tumor extracts for immunization. These "antigen" preparations were combined with whooping cough and typhus vaccine and Freund's adjuvant. Of the twenty patients treated in this way, two reported some subjective response, four showed marginal improvement and only one showed a clear objective response. This study also showed that the vaccine sometimes elicited a cell-mediated immune reaction to the tumor extract, and that its use was safe (Hughes et al., 1970).

L.J. Humphrey from the Harry S. Truman Memorial Veterans' Hospital in Columbus, Ohio, and his colleagues took another approach to the problem. They immunized patients with raw tumor extract, followed by an exchange of plasma and white blood cells between pairs of patients. The vaccine consisted of freeze/thaw-treated tumor homogenate. Thirty-eight patients received this treatment. The two patients in each pair were not required to have the same type of tumor. Eight patients showed some signs of objective improvement, but this was generally transitory. The best results were obtained in patients with small inoperable lesions, a long history of progressive metastasized cancer, or a recurrence of minimal lesions (Humphrey et al., 1971).

The effect of irradiated autologous tumor grafts on melanoma patients has also been investigated, with the aim of studying both the humoral and cell-mediated immune response as well as determining the anti-tumor effect. While it was established that the auto-immunization did give rise to the presence of antibodies and specific cytotoxic lymphocytes in the circulation, not the slightest therapeutic effect could be detected (Currie, 1972).

Reviewing all the different approaches discussed above, it must be concluded that none of them achieved any significant therapeutic benefit.

However, new avenues in specific cellular immunotherapy have opened up in recent decades as our insights into the molecular recognition of antigens and immunoregulation have increased. We have also come to understand why the idea of immunosurveillance as previously formulated is not tenable, and why attempts to vaccinate patients with autologous and allogeneic cancers did not work. The explanation is that when the immune system is presented with a new antigen, it is not necessarily activated. Numerous experiments have shown that when T cells meet antigens, the consequence is determined by the context of the encounter. When the antigen is produced by an inflammation or by tissue destruction caused by a virus or bacterium, the immune system will be activated in accordance with the traditional theory. If however, the antigen arises endogenously, without the danger signals that accompany inflammation and tissue destruction, immunologic tolerance is produced. In other words, the immune response at the T cell level appears to depend on co-stimulatory signals at the moment of antigen recognition (Pardoll, 1998).

New investigations in which the necessary danger signals were added were planned, on the basis of these new insights. David Berd, professor of medical oncology at Thomas Jefferson University in Philadelphia, and his colleagues published the results of a study of this kind, involving 64 patients with metastasized melanoma, in 1990. They gave the patients an autologous melanoma vaccine to which adjuvant BCG vaccine been added three days after a low dose of cyclophosphamide. A significant clinical response was found in about 20% of the patients (Berd et al., 1990).

Malcolm Mitchell and colleagues in Canada set up a phase-III trial, also involving melanoma patients, to compare the effects of Melacine® (a combination of melanoma cell lysates and an adjuvant derived from bacteria) with those of a chemotherapy consisting of dacarbazine, cisplatin, carmustine and tamoxifen. No difference was found between the two treatment groups (Mitchell and Von Eschen, 1997; Mitchell, 1998).

Working at the Vrije Universiteit Hospital, Amsterdam, Jan B. Vermorken, a professor of oncology at the University of Antwerp in Belgium and his team tested a cellular vaccine made of autologous irradiated tumor cells mixed with BCG as adjuvant treatment of patients with stage II and stage III cancer of the colon, and found a significant increase in total survival in stage II patients (Vermorken et al., 1999).

Our greater understanding of the way the immune system works has also led to major changes in vaccine production strategies in recent years. Instead of using tumor cells as a source of antigens it is now possible to use tumor-specific antigens. This approach also makes it possible to follow the impact of vaccination on the immune system.

Now that it has been established that immunologic tolerance is the reason why the immune system does not respond to some new antigens, researchers have been trying to design cancer vaccines that eliminate this tolerance. This requires much deeper insights into the operation of the immune system. Extensive fundamental research has cleared up many issues in this field.

One important finding was that both the CD4 T memory cells and the CD8 T cells (the cytotoxic lymphocytes or CTLs) need to be activated in order to ensure a strong antitumor response. These T cells are activated by special antigen-presenting cells, also known as dendritic cells, which were initially isolated by Ralph Steinman and Zanvil Cohn (1926-1993) from Rockefeller University, New York, in 1973. These dendritic cells are able to present all kinds of antigens in the body to T cells. As mentioned above, antigens are usually proteins. The dendritic cells break these proteins down into their component parts, which are known as peptides. The peptides are presented on HLA (*human leukocyte antigen*) class I molecules on the surface of the dendritic cell. It is this complex of HLA class I molecules and the peptides derived from the tumor antigen that the CTL can recognize with the aid of a special receptor known as the T cell receptor. After making contact with the dendritic cell, these cytotoxic lymphocytes proliferate and look for cells, bearing on their surface the antigen for which they have been programmed by the dendritic cell. When they find these cells, they destroy them.

A variety of vaccine production methods have been designed on the basis of the above insights. The antigens used in such methods are often derived from tumor cells that have been genetically modified to produce co-stimulatory molecules that are essential for T cell activation, or to induce co-stimulatory cytokines that will attract antigen-presenting cells. Tumor-specific antigens may also be used as an alternative (Greten and Jaffee, 1999).

The most promising approach to vaccine production however would seem to be based on the use of a combination of dendritic cells and tumor-specific antigens. The dendritic cells can be obtained by culturing monocytes from peripheral blood. The tumor antigens can be added to these mature dendritic cells. The antigens are then broken down into peptides, which are placed on the surface of the dendritic cells. These charged and activated dendritic cells are administered to patients, where they program the cytotoxic T cells to look for antigens on the surface of tumor cells and then destroy these cells. This approach has been tried with melanoma patients. It is too early to say from the preliminary results obtained so far whether the method is effective.

In general, it may be said that the new generation of immunotherapy methods based on the principles described above still have to be tested, but they seem promising.

There is however one form of cancer immunotherapy that can be characterized as a genuine success story. That is the fairly recent development of vaccines against cancers caused by viruses. A number of human cancers are know to be caused by or are associated with viruses. The best-known example is probably cervical cancer, which is caused by the human papilloma virus (HPV) as discussed in Chapter 2, in the section on viral carcinogenesis. This virus also plays a role in head and neck cancers and in cancer of the penis. Similarly, Burkitt's lymphoma is associated with the Epstein-Barr virus (EBV) and cancer of the liver with the hepatitis B virus. Since an infection with one of these viruses leads to the massive creation of immunogenic proteins in the body, it is to be expected that patients who have a virus-induced tumor would show a clinically important immune response when vaccinated against the virus in question.

Confirmation of this idea was provided by Jeffrey S. Weber, associate professor of medicine at the University of Southern California, and his colleagues. They vaccinated women suffering from intraepithelial cancer of the cervix and the vulva with HPV peptides combined with incomplete Freund's adjuvant, and saw a 50% response rate (Muderspach et al., 2000).

Persistent infection with HPV is recognized to be the greatest risk factor for cervical cancer. Epidemiologic studies have shown that 80% of sexually active young women are infected with this virus. In most cases, the immune system deals with this infection, but if it persists there is a real risk that cervical cancer will develop.

It is now accepted worldwide that HPV vaccination is a highly effective means of reducing the incidence of cervical cancer. Two vaccines, Gardasil and Cervarix, are available on the market and are approved for use in many countries. Despite some reservations expressed about the possible side effects of these vaccines, the health authorities in many countries throughout the world have already decided that mass vaccination of all girls and young women aged 12 to 26 years of age is the goal. Mass vaccination campaigns have already been set up in the US, Canada, Australia, the UK and other European countries. In fact, since 2006 prophylactic HPV vaccination has been available in the Netherlands for all females between 9 and 26 years of age.

The successful use of donor lymphocytes in the treatment of a recurrence of acute lymphoblastic leukemia, mentioned in Chapter 6 on chemotherapy, may also be regarded as an example of specific active immunotherapy. It is certainly active and it may also be regarded as antigen-specific since it is assumed that the lymphocytes react with antigens of the MHC (*major histocompatibility complex*) or the recipient's minor antigens in case of a mismatch.

CHAPTER 9

Specific passive immunotherapy

Specific passive immunotherapy means the therapeutic use of antibodies specifically targeting tumor antigens – in other words, instead of stimulating the body to make its own antibodies against the cancer as in active immunotherapy, the antibodies are presented ready-made. This form of treatment predates specific active immunotherapy by a few years. It involves immunizing animals such as sheep, rabbits, goats or horses with fragments of the patient's tumor and administering the antiserum produced in this way to the patient.

As mentioned in Chapter 8, in 1895 the French physiologists Héricourt and Richet published the results of the treatment of five melanoma patients with antisera produced in dogs and mules. They concluded that their serum therapy did not get rid of the cancer, but was an improvement on any other form of treatment available at the time.

Research into antiserum treatment was stimulated by the finding by the Belgian immunologist and microbiologist Jules Bordet (1870-1961) that immunization with blood of different types led to the production of specific antibodies that were able to destroy red blood cells (Bordet, 1898). Bordet won the Nobel Prize in 1919 (at which time he was Director of the Pasteur Institute in Brussels and a professor at Brussels University. The well-known Institut Jules Bordet in Brussels, a multidisciplinary hospital for cancer treatment and research, is named after him) for his discoveries concerning immunity.

Boeri's 1901 report of tumor regression observed in two melanoma patients he had treated with human antimelanoma serum prepared in goats was also encouraging (Currie, 1972). E. Vidal reported at the second International Congress for Cancer in Paris in 1910 that, using the same technique as Boeri, he had found strong remission of the cancer in three patients and some subjective improvement in a number of other patients (Roberts, 1977).

William N. Berkeley of Cornell University published the results of his three years of experience of the therapeutic use of anti-cancer sera in 1914. He had treated 89 patients, 71 of whom were evaluable. Thirty-two patients had inoperable cancer, and several in this group showed some signs of objective improvement. The other 39 patients had primary tumors that were surgically removed, and received antisera as adjuvant therapy. No survival data were given, but the overall impression left by his description is a pessimistic one (Berkeley, 1914).

Despite the relatively poor results obtained with this approach, researchers kept on trying. In 1958, Gordon Murray (1894-1976) from Toronto, a talented surgeon but a controversial researcher in the field of immunology, published the results he had obtained by treating more than two hundred patients with globulin from horses that had been immunized with a variety of human tumors. He claimed a high frequency of subjective improvement and also sometimes observed objective changes in the tumors (Murray, 1958). His claims were however greeted with skepticism by the medical community. In 1959, Peter Buinauskas from London, Ontario, and colleagues from Austin, Texas, and Chicago used immunoglobulins produced in sheep to treat three breast cancer patients. Once again, the results were disappointing. The only signs of improvement were slight changes in the lymph nodes (Buinauskas et al., 1959).

Researchers now tried a different approach, based on the use of blood from patients in whom spontaneous regression of the cancer had been observed. Wilbur C. Summer and Alvan G. Foraker from the Baptist Memorial Hospital in Jacksonville, Florida, were the first to describe the use of this technique, in 1960. They gave two patients with extensive melanotic metastases transfusions of whole blood from a patient who had experienced regression of a melanoma. One of the patients treated in this way showed spectacular, prolonged regression (Summer and Foraker, 1960). It is doubtful, however, whether the serum alone was responsible for this positive response: since the patients were given a whole blood transfusion they also received lymphocytes from the donor, and these might have brought about the regression of the tumor.

Professor Victor A. Ngu from Cameroon tried the same approach on patients with Burkitt's lymphoma, and reported his results in 1967. He observed temporary regression of the tumors in patients who had been given serum from patients in whom the tumor had disappeared spontaneously. The surgeon Peter Clifford from the Medical Research Laboratory in Nairobi, Kenya, had the opposite experience, however. He treated two patients in the same way in the same year, and found no response in one patient and enhanced tumor growth in the other (Currie, 1972). All in all, this form of treatment did not seem to be very promising.

Isoantibodies, antibodies induced by antigens derived from the same species but not from the same individual, are sometimes used in the treatment of leukemia. John Laszlo and his colleagues from Duke University Medical Center in Durham, North Carolina, described their use of this approach to the treatment of three patients with chronic lymphatic leukemia. The isoantibodies were obtained by immunizing volunteers with lymphocytes. Laszlo's team observed the occurrence of lymphopenia and shrinkage of the lymph nodes in their patients, while normal sera had no effect at all (Laszlo et al., 1968).

Specific passive immunotherapy also includes targeted therapy with monoclonal antibodies against epidermal growth factor, the epidermal growth factor receptor and the vascular endothelial growth factor receptor situated on the tumor cell surface, and treatment with the monoclonal antibody rituximab that targets the cluster of differentiation CD 20 in B-cell lymphomas as discussed in Chapter 8. This form of immunotherapy has already won an established place in the treatment of cancer.

Specific passive immunotherapy has its bizarre variants too. The attempt by E.F. Lewison and colleagues to make use of the protective effect of colostrum in cancer treatment in 1960 is a good example of this. They immunized pregnant cows against human breast cancer by injecting tumor extracts into their udders and collected the colostrum from these cows for the first seven days after the birth of their calves. The colostrum was given orally to the patients whose tumor had been used for the immunization (Lewison et al., 1960). Objective regression of the cancer was not to be expected under these conditions, since antibodies are not absorbed through the wall of the intestines, and it was indeed not observed.

Aspecific immunotherapy

Many different methods have been used to stimulate the reactivity of the immune system in an aspecific way. As described in Chapter 4, William Coley (1862-1936), a bone surgeon at Memorial Hospital in New York, used an extract of *Streptococcus* and *Bacillus prodigiosus* (currently called *Serratia marcescens*) to treat patients with advanced cancer – generally a sarcoma – and achieved objective tumor regression in several patients. This extract, which came to be known as "Coley's toxin", was initially prepared in the Memorial Hospital's own laboratory, but starting in 1899 it was produced and marketed by Parke-Davis - at the time, America's oldest and largest pharmaceutical company. These circumstances are described in a lengthy article by the scientific and medical historian Ilana Löwy (Löwy, 1994).

It may be said in hindsight that Coley's toxin was the first (not very effective) form of aspecific cancer immunotherapy, though as discussed in Chapter 4, Coley's initial objective had been to create conditions of hyperthermia which was thought at the time to play a role in combating cancer. Later researchers intentionally looked for methods of stimulating the patient's own immune system. The first attempts in this direction were made with the aid of antisera targeting the reticuloendothelial system (see "reticuloendothelial system" in the Glossary). Starting from the hypothesis that very low doses of such antibodies would stimulate the target cells instead of killing them, which had been put forward in 1920 by the Russian Nobel laureate Ilya Mechnikov (mentioned in passing in Chapter 6 for his pioneering work on immunity), various researchers prepared antibodies against various components of the human reticuloendothelial system and administered them in very low doses to cancer patients. These preparations were known as antireticular cytotoxic serum (ACS) or reticuloendothelial immune serum (Southam, 1961).

M.P. Fedyushin from the Soviet Union suggested in 1938 that ACS led to regression of metastases and increased survival in some patients. However, Joseph Skapier from the Brooklyn Cancer Institute in New York in 1947 and Davis in 1957 could find no objective tumor regression despite some subjective improvement (Currie, 1972).

Other agents that were thought for a while to be very promising in this connection were BCG vaccine, *Corynebacterium parvum* and levamisole. The results obtained with these agents will be discussed in turn below.

BCG VACCINE

The agent that has been most widely used to stimulate the reticuloendothelial system is BCG vaccine (Bacillus Calmette-Guérin), which is made from avirulent tuberculosis bacilli and is routinely used in most countries of the world – with the notable exception of the United States and the Netherlands – to protect children against tuberculosis. It was developed by the French bacteriologist Albert Calmette and his assistant and later colleague Camille Guérin and was first used on humans in 1921 although mass BCG vaccination did not start until after the Second World War.

The idea that BCG might slow the growth of tumors was first put forward in the context of transplantation studies. Lloyd Old, Donald A. Clarke from the Sloan Kettering Institute and Cornell University Medical School and Baruj Benacerraf at the New York University School of Medicine reported in 1959 that mice infected with BCG showed more resistance to the transplantation of tumors from other mice. They interpreted this as being due to stimulation of graft rejection by the BCG (Old et al., 1959). This finding was confirmed three years later. It is noteworthy that the antitumor activity of BCG was first demonstrated in animal experiments (Löwy, 1994). In fact, this was the first time in the history of cancer immunotherapy that animal trials preceded clinical application.

We have already come across Benacerraf in Chapter 6, in connection with his work on the major histocompatibility complex (MHC) for which he shared the Nobel Prize in 1980. It may also be mentioned that he worked for six years in the 1950s with Bernard Halpern, discussed below in the section on *Corynebacterium parvum*.

The first clinical trial of BCG in the treatment of cancer was carried out by J.E. Sokal and colleagues from Roswell Park Memorial Institute, Buffalo, NY, in the period from 1965 to 1967. The trial involved fifty lymphoma patients. The 25 patients who were given BCG experienced fewer recurrences and a longer mean survival period (25 months) than the control subjects (10.6 months) (Roberts, 1977).

Interest in BCG cancer therapy snowballed when in 1969 Professor Georges Mathé and his team from the Hôpital Paul Brousse in Villejuif near Paris published the spectacular results obtained by treating patients suffering from acute lymphoblastic leukemia with a combination of BCG and irradiated allogeneic leukemic blasts.

As a hematologist, Mathé had long been interested in the experimental study of blood cancers, and he was one of the world leaders in the clinical investigation of cytostatics for the treatment of leukemia. He had also been a member of the team at the Curie Foundation in Paris that had made a widely publicized and largely successful attempt to use bone marrow transplants to save the life of eight workers who had received high doses of radiation after an accident at the nuclear reactor in the Boris Kidrich Institute of Nuclear Physics at Vinča near Belgrade, Yugoslavia in October 1958. He was thus the personification of the link between experimental cancer research, clinical cancer research and the "new immunology" that made the medical miracle of organ and tissue transplantation possible.

Professor Mathé's objective was to use immunotherapy to prolong the remission induced by chemotherapy in leukemia patients. His 1969 article in *The Lancet* described the results obtained with BCG applied to scars in the skin combined with leukemia cells that had been treated with formaldehyde or irradiation. A total of twenty 5-cm scratches arranged in a square grid were made per patient, to which the BCG was applied. Scarification is a fairly painful procedure (as I can testify from first-hand observation). One scar was made every four days for the first month, and then one was added every week until the total of twenty was reached. The irradiated cells were injected subcutaneously every week. It was found that seven of the twelve patients who had received BCG and irradiated allogeneic leukemic blasts were still in remission a year after the treatment, while all of the control subjects had suffered a recurrence within three hundred days (Mathé et al., 1969). In a follow-up trial involving two hundred patients, more than 50% of the patients remained disease-free after four years. Mathé concluded that this was the best form of therapy for leukemia (Mathé et al., 1975). He claimed, moreover, that the results obtained with BCG in leukemia also opened the way to a radically new approach to the treatment of solid tumors. Such a new approach was needed, in his view, because the idea that cancer was a local process was no longer valid. He stated that at the moment when a cancer is discovered, malignant cells have already spread through the body in at least two out of every three cases. Surgery, radiotherapy and even chemotherapy are not enough to eradicate these metastasized cancer cells. "There is," Mathé concluded, "an urgent need to have a new method at our disposal that is capable of eliminating the very last cell or cells" (Löwy, 1994). Since Mathé treated his patients with a combination of irradiated cells and BCG, the results obtained cannot be ascribed solely to BCG.

These excellent results were not repeated in a trial carried out by the Medical Research Council in England following much the same approach. They compared BCG with methotrexate, and with no after-treatment at all following an initial remission produced by chemotherapy, and found BCG to be worse than methotrexate and as good as the controls (Roberts, 1977). Mathé's findings did however receive some support from William Vogler and Yick-Kwong Chan of the United States. They found that BCG treatment produced poor results in children, but prolonged survival in adults with acute leukemia (Vogler and Chan, 1974).

Avrum Bluming and colleagues from the Solid Tumor Center of the Uganda Cancer Institute and Makerere University Medical School in Kampala, Uganda, demonstrated that the way the BCG was applied to melanoma patients had a considerable influence on the final results obtained. They found that the use of large grids of scratches was best, since this allowed a higher dose to be given so that more powerful stimulation of the immune response could be achieved (Bluming et al., 1972).

Another form of BCG treatment for melanoma was also used for a while. This involved direct injection of the BCG into the subcutaneous metastases, giving rise to an inflammation reaction and causing the metastases to be sloughed; it was claimed that even the metastases that were not injected disappeared too. This method was introduced by D.L. Morton and colleagues from the John Wayne Cancer Institute in Santa Monica, California. It seemed however as if the shedding of the metastases was due to the inflammation caused by the BCG rather than an immune reaction, since the melanomas that were not injected did not disappear as I have observed myself.

The only form of BCG cancer treatment that is still in use is the intravesical administration of BCG for the therapeutic, prophylactic or adjuvant treatment of superficial tumors of the bladder.

CORYNEBACTERIUM PARVUM

Corynebacterium parvum (now known as *Propionibacterium acnes*) is also known to cause powerful stimulation of the reticuloendothelial system. Investigation of the clinical application of this effect was sparked by the demonstration in 1963 by Bernard Halpern and his team from the Institut d'Immunobiologie at Hôpital Paul Brousse that *Corynebacterium parvum* inhibited the development of tumors in mice (Roberts, 1977). The use of killed bacteria to treat patients with various forms of metastasized cancer was therefore tested. The results were not particularly encouraging, however. The next idea was to try *Corynebacterium parvum* as an adjuvant. It was given to patients who had been operated on for lung cancer (Woodruff, 1983) and for melanoma; in the latter case, its action was compared with that of BCG (Lipton et al., 1991). The size of the patient group in the lung cancer trial (49) was too small to allow meaningful conclusions to be drawn, while the melanoma study indicated that *Corynebacterium parvum* might be a better adjuvant than BCG. *Corynebacterium parvum* treatment for cancer has never become generally accepted, however.

LEVAMISOLE

Levamisole is a synthetic drug developed by Janssen Pharmaceutica in Belgium that was initially used to treat worm infestations in both humans and animals. It was later found to stimulate the immune system, probably via activation of macrophages. W.K. Amery investigated its effect on lung cancer patients in 1975, and concluded that levamisole inhibited the development of metastases. A.F. Rojas and colleagues also confirmed its effectiveness in patients with advanced breast cancer. They reported that it increased the median disease-free survival period from 9 to 25 months, and raised the 30-month survival rate from 35 to 90% (Roberts, 1977).

The reputation of levamisole was enhanced by a trial in colon carcinoma reported by Laurie et al. in 1989, as described in Chapter 6 in the section on multidisciplinary treatment and adjuvant chemotherapy. An intergroup study under the leadership of Charles Moertel from the Mayo Clinic confirmed these results. This study, in which the North Central Cancer Treatment Group (NCCTG), the Eastern Cooperative Oncology Group (ECOG) and the Southwest Oncology Group (SWOG) participated, showed that levamisol when given in combination with 5-fluorouracil (5-FU) for a year significantly improved the survival of patients with cancer of the colon in Dukes' stage C. The 5-year risk of recurrence fell by 40%, and the mortality rate by 33% after a median follow-up period of 6.5 years (Moertel et al., 1995). This was a very important trial, since it was the first one to demonstrate that adjuvant therapy made sense in colon cancer. The combination of 5-FU with levamisole was however soon replaced by 5-FU with leucovorin, when a large randomized trial showed that the latter produced a 5% rise in the five-year survival rate (Wolmark et al., 1996). Moreover, the treatment period could be reduced to six months with 5-FU with leucovorin, while the efficacy of 5-FU with levamisole was actually found to drop when the treatment period was reduced from twelve months to six (O'Connel et al., 1998).

Cytokines

For a long period it remained unknown how microorganisms such as *Corynebacterium parvum* and those in BCG and Coley's toxin elicited a clinical response in cancer. Research ultimately showed that administration of BCG in the bladder led to inflammation of the bladder that produced substances called cytokines. These cytokines are secreted by cells, and regulate the growth and division of neighboring cells and possibly also of the cells that secrete them. They lead in their turn to an influx of inflammation mediators such as lymphocytes and granulocytes, and it was found that it was a side effect of these inflammation mediators that gives rise to the anticancer activity.

It has been known since 1930 that cells that have been infected with a virus are better able to withstand a subsequent infection. The cytokine responsible for this, interferon (IFN), was finally isolated from experimental cell cultures and later from lymphocytes taken from peripheral blood (Davis et al., 2003). I. Gresser and colleagues from the Viral Oncology Laboratory of the Centre National de la Recherche Scientifique at Villejuif demonstrated in 1969 that IFN can give rise to antitumor effects in mice (Gresser et al., 1969). Once news of this discovery spread, the medical world quickly realized the possibilities for an exciting new therapeutic approach, and many researchers took steps to test this molecule (which in fact turned out to be a family of molecules) in humans.

Some time before, in 1953, Ivan Bennet and Paul Beeson (1908-2006) from the Department of Internal Medicine at Yale had extracted a factor responsible for fever from neutrophil granulocytes in pus. They called it an "endogenous pyrogen" (Bennet and Beeson, 1953). Paul Beeson spent most of his childhood in Anchorage, Alaska, where his father, John Beeson, was a general practitioner and surgeon for the Alaskan Railway. The modern-day world-famous Iditarod dog-sled race from Anchorage to Nome follows the first part of a trail that John Beeson had driven in 1921, four hundred miles on dogsled, to reach an ailing patient in Iditarod. The factor discovered by Bennett and Beeson was subsequently given the name interleukin-1 (Il-1), and was found to be the first of a large family of cytokine molecules. Investigation of interleukin-1 marked the start of modern cytokine biology. Countless studies of these two molecules, IFN and Il-1, quickly followed and laid the basis for much better understanding of the cytokine network. Our increased insights into all these factors – invading pathogens, host cells, cancer cells and a wide variety of signaling molecules – provide a more rational basis for clinical research into cancer and possible ways of combating it (Davis et al., 2003).

In 1984, Jorge R. Quesada and colleagues from the University of Texas described a small group of patients with hairy cell leukemia who had a favorable response to partially purified IFN (Quesada et al., 1984). Since then, IFN has gradually won a place for itself in the therapeutic arsenal used to treat a variety of cancers, such as melanoma, renal cell carcinoma, chronic myeloid leukemia and multiple myeloma. The results obtained have not been outstanding, however.

A team of researchers from the Memorial Sloan-Kettering Cancer Center in New York, including E.A. Carswell and Lloyd Old (mentioned above in connection with his pioneering work on BCG), used a sarcoma model in mice in 1975 to show that administration of BCG to the experimental animals can lead to hemorrhagic necrosis of the tumor. It later proved possible to induce the same effect by administration of lipopolysacharides. The team isolated the responsible factor, which they called tumor necrosis factor (TNF). This factor can also be classified as a cytokine. TNF was subsequently cloned, and its effect on a variety of tumors has been investigated (Davis et al., 2003). It was initially found to be highly toxic and to have little or no therapeutic effect. Later studies showed that it is active, but even more toxic, in high doses. Attempts were then made to get around the toxicity problem through local perfusion. This approach was found to be effective for sarcomas and melanomas confined to the limbs. It allowed high doses to be given without serious systemic side effects, and produced excellent results. Hence, this cytokine finally managed to win an established place in the battery of drugs used in the treatment of these tumors.

The same team first described another important cytokine, known as interleukin-2 (Il-2), in 1976. However, the enthusiasm for immunotherapy research was once again at a low ebb around this time.

CHAPTER 9

In his 1971 State of the Union address, President Nixon had declared "war on cancer" in the following words:

> I will ... ask for an appropriation of an extra $100 million to launch an intensive campaign to find a cure for cancer, and I will ask later for whatever additional funds can effectively be used. The time has come in America when the same kind of concentrated effort that split the atom and took man to the moon should be turned toward conquering this dread disease. Let us make a total national commitment to achieve this goal. America has long been the wealthiest nation in the world. Now it is time we became the healthiest nation in the world.

There was thus plenty of money available for cancer research in the United States. However, the results obtained in the trials of the various forms of immunotherapy were so disappointing that there seemed to be a risk that the funds for further research in this field would soon dry up. In order to revive interest in this topic, some creative researchers coined the concept of "biological response modifiers" – substances or approaches that would modify the relationship between host and tumor in such a way as to create a positive therapeutic benefit. In fact, this is the aim of any immunotherapeutic intervention, simply put. The researchers must have hoped that clothing their projects in such imposing language might increase their chances of continued funding.

But finally, the tide did turn, thanks in large part to the real potential of interleukin-2, the pioneering work of R.T. Prehn and Joan Main from the National Cancer Institute in Bethesda, Maryland, in determining the immunogenicity of primary tumor grafts in syngenic (genetically identical) mice, and the work of the Hungarian biologist George Klein (born 1925) from the Institute of Tumor Biology at the Karolinska Institute in Stockholm on the immune response to autochtonous carcinogen-induced tumors in mice (Mihich, 2000). Klein was mentioned in Chapter 2, in the section on heredity and cancer.

Study of the clinical application of Il-2 started up in 1984. It was found to produce remissions in metastasized melanoma and advanced renal cell carcinoma. Clinical responses were actually rare in these complaints (for example, a response rate of between 4 and 7% was found in melanomas), but if a response did occur it was usually lasting. In the chemotherapy of melanoma patients, on the other hand, a clinical response is often followed by a recurrence. This difference in results suggests that Il-2 changes the body's immune recognition system in such a way that tumor cells that reappear in the affected tissue are quickly recognized and destroyed. Unfortunately, very high doses of Il-2 must be given to achieve such good remissions, and these are associated with such high levels of toxicity that the patients concerned sometimes require intensive care. This toxicity may be caused by the induction of other cytokines, such as TNF, or of molecules like nitric oxide (NO).

In hindsight, the clinical development of Il-2 reflects the style of clinical research common in the 1980s. Since the biology of the cytokines was not yet well understood, the clinical investigation was initially influenced by experience gained in the use of cytostatics, where the doses found to be effective tended to be pharmacologic–that is, much larger than physiologic. A large number of subsequent studies used various doses of Il-2 combined with other agents such as IFN or lymphokine-activated killer cells (LAK cells) and cytostatics. No single combination was found to guarantee effective results, however.

Professor Steven A. Rosenberg of the National Cancer Institute was the great pioneer in the field of LAK cells. He was well aware that many treatments that initially produce promising results turned out to be not so good in the long run. He liked to tell the story of the 58-year-old radiologist who was suffering from extensive melanoma. At that time, Rosenberg was conducting a trial of a form of immunotherapy that had not yet been approved for general clinical use, and he thought it might prove useful for this doctor turned patient. "I sat down with this fellow, to get an informed consent, and I asked him if he wanted to receive the treatment, told him we had had some good results, in patients we had treated before, and was he interested in receiving it – and he looked me straight in the eye and he said something I'll never forget. He said, "Absolutely, doc. I want to receive this new treatment while it's still working." Luckily for the radiologist, the treatment was still working when he got it (Palca, 2007).

Another member of the interleukin family, Il-12, initially looked very promising. It acted on both T cells and NK (natural killer) cells, and also had antiangiogenic properties. Preclinical trials suggested that it might be an excellent anticancer drug. While it seemed perfectly safe in the phase-I trial, unexpected toxic effects, leading to a number of mortalities, were noted during the phase-II trial. Moreover, since the antitumor effect was not as good as expected, this drug has never been approved for clinical use.

The experience with Il-12 did however illustrate one fundamental principle of biological cancer treatment: the maximum tolerable dose need not be the optimum dose. There are in fact indications that lower doses of Il-12 work better than higher ones (Davis et al., 2003).

Many other cytokines have been identified since the discovery and clinical application of Il-2. At the time of writing, thirty-five different interleukin molecules are known and many of these are undergoing clinical investigation at different stages.

Conclusion

More than a century of concentrated work has been devoted to cancer immunotherapy, unfortunately with very limited results. The aim of making immunotherapy one of the four pillars of cancer treatment alongside surgery, radiotherapy and chemotherapy has not been realized. Nevertheless, our vastly increased knowledge of immunology and the availability of powerful new techniques raise the hope that this form of treatment will become a more important therapeutic tool in the future.

There are a few positive exceptions to this rather disappointing conclusion. The use of monoclonal antibodies against growth factors and growth-factor receptors, as described in Chapter 8, a sector that is currently enjoying a great deal of interest, owes its development to immunotherapeutic concepts. The same may be said of monoclonal antibody treatment of B-cell lymphomas involving expression of the cluster of differentiation CD20, and the treatment of recurrences of acute lymphoblastic leukemia with donor lymphocytes. Another success story is the prophylatic use of vaccines to prevent the development of cancers due to viruses, such as cervical cancer, which has achieved worldwide recognition if not yet worldwide implementation.

The great advantage of immunotherapy is that it is based on a physiologic approach and therefore potentially places less of a load on the patient. Moreover, it is systemic, so its effects reach all parts of the body.

The big challenge in this field is the translation of all the potential new benefits of immunotherapy into a clinically applicable protocol. That means formulation of the most promising strategy, careful selection of patients and the planning and execution of effective clinical trials. I look forward to seeing this approach bear fruit in the future.

[10]

The origins of psycho-oncology

Introduction

The diagnosis of cancer, with its threat of a possible fatal outcome and the fears and other emotions that this threat generates, has a whole series of consequences for the patient and those near and dear to him or her. These include the physical symptoms of the disease and the after effects of the treatment given; the need to come to terms with the situation and with the existential dimensions of the disease; worries about the family, on whom the cancer also has a serious impact; and the search for comfort and support in religious, spiritual or philosophical beliefs or in values that give meaning to life and death.

Shakespeare spoke eloquently in *King Lear* of the matters that play a role in a life-threatening illness:

> *We are not ourselves when nature, being oppressed, commands the mind to suffer with the body.* (King Lear, 2.4.115-7)

The new specialism of psycho-oncology, the subject of this chapter, deals with the "suffering of the mind" that arises when the body is attacked by cancer. It addresses the psychological, social, spiritual and existential dimensions of this situation, and tries to help the patient acquire the insight to understand and the strength to bear the presence of this serious disease, an unwelcome intruder that poses a threat to his or her future and to life itself (Holland, 2002). But before psycho-oncology could become common practice, two important hurdles had to be cleared: the stigma associated with cancer itself and the stigma attached to requesting help in coping with one's mental or emotional problems. These two issues will be discussed in turn below.

CHAPTER 10

The stigma of cancer

Psycho-oncology as a discipline within the larger field of oncology is only about thirty years old, since it is only within this period that the stigma attached to the word "cancer" has gradually disappeared so that it finally became possible to speak openly about this dread disease. This is a trend that I have experienced first hand. For example, during my first year of training in internal medicine, in 1967, I diagnosed stomach cancer in one of the patients I had examined. My supervisor, the head of the department where I was working, instructed me to tell the patient that I had good news for her, that she had a gastric ulcer that could be treated by her GP, so she would no longer need to come to our office. She came to see me that afternoon, bringing a couple of baskets of strawberries, and said, "I'm so relieved, doctor. I was afraid that I had cancer." This story reflects a doctor-patient relationship we can look back on only with embarrassment: a paternalistic relationship based on concealment of the true facts in the patient's presumed best interests. At that time it was thought that it would be cruel and inhumane to tell the patient the real diagnosis, because it would cause her to lose all hope, and she would be able to cope with the disease better if she was ignorant of it. Our communication style has changed for the better since then. Patients have become more independent and more assertive. Society rightly rejects an authoritarian stance on the part of the doctor.

This issue has been with us for centuries. A 1996 editorial in the *British Medical Journal*, arguing that even more openness about cancer was needed, mentioned that in 1672 the French physician Samuel de Sorbiere had considered the idea of telling patients with serious diseases the truth about their diagnosis, but thought that it might seriously jeopardize medical practice and concluded that it would not catch on (De Sorbiere, 1672).

Within the past century, a number of prominent authors have expressed their dissatisfaction with the lack of communication between doctor and patient. In his novella *The Death of Ivan Ilych*, published in 1886, Leo Tolstoy wrote (cited here in the translation by Louise and Aylmer Maude):

_____ What tormented Ivan Ilych most was the deception, the lie, which for some reason they all accepted, that he was not dying but was simply ill, and that he only need keep quiet and undergo a treatment and then something very good would result. He however knew that do what they would nothing would come of it, only still more agonizing suffering and death. This deception tortured him ... their not wishing to admit what they all knew and what he knew, but wanting to lie to him concerning his terrible condition, and wishing and forcing him to participate in that lie. Those lies, lies enacted over him on the eve of his death and destined to degrade this awful, solemn act to the level of their visitings ... were a terrible agony for Ivan Ilych.

In her satirically titled book *A Very Easy Death*, published in 1964, Simone de Beauvoir criticized the doctors who had treated her mother for small bowel cancer for keeping the nature of her disease from her. In her book *All Said And Done* – the final part of her five-volume autobiography, which appeared in 1972 – she recounts how her good friend, the Swiss sculptor and painter Alberto Giacometti (1901-1966) was told by doctors that he had a gastric ulcer while in fact he had stomach cancer. Aleksandr Solzhenitsyn paints a similar picture in 1968, in his novel *Cancer Ward*: the hero Pavel Rusanov has a growth on his neck, which his doctor maintains is not cancerous.

This criticism from the world of literature did little or nothing to improve doctor-patient communication, however. Traditionally, the doctor informed the patient's family of a serious diagnosis in confidence. The doctor and the family then maintained a conspiracy of silence, putting up a false façade of hope. The fear of cancer was so great that the family would also keep the bad news from others. Shame and guilt were the prevailing emotions, mixed with fear that the condition was contagious.

After the discovery of anesthesia in the middle of the nineteenth century and of antisepsis and asepsis a little later, the foundation was laid for the gradual development of the surgical treatment of cancer as described in Chapter 4. By the end of the nineteenth century and the beginning of the twentieth, it was possible to operate on many superficial tumors and some deeper tumors too. Moreover, the fear of surgery gradually disappeared thanks to improved methods of pain control, and the introduction of antisepsis and asepsis led to a substantial rise in surgical success rates. If cancer was diagnosed before metastases had time to develop, it was even possible to cure it. At this point, the medical world realized that it was time to tell the public about the importance of consulting a doctor quickly if worrying symptoms were observed. The American Cancer Society (founded in 1913) and the Koningin Wilhelmina Fonds (Dutch Cancer Fund), which had been founded in 1949, began distributing pamphlets with descriptions of the signs people should look for in order to detect cancer early.

Slowly but surely, other therapeutic approaches were developed alongside surgery. Radiotherapy became available in the first quarter of the twentieth century. Initially, however, it was regarded mainly as a palliative measure, to be used only if surgery had failed. And as more information about the health risks associated with radiation became available, people became as apprehensive about radiotherapy as they were about surgery.

During the nineteenth century the willingness to support a good cause and the fear of the dread disease led to growing financial support for research aimed at finding a cure for cancer, and hospitals specializing in the treatment of cancer patients were set up in various countries. In 1851, Dr. William Marsden set up the Free Cancer Hospital in London in memory of his wife Elizabeth Ann, who had died of cancer. It was the first hospital in the world to be devoted to the study and cure of cancer, and was renamed the Royal Marsden Hospital in 1954. The New York Cancer Hospital was found in 1884, renamed the General Memorial Hospital in 1899 and given its current name – the Memorial Sloan-Kettering Cancer Center – in the 1980s, after it had incorporated the Sloan-Kettering Institute. The Roswell Park Memorial Institute in Buffalo was founded in 1898. The Dutch Cancer Institute, the Antoni van Leeuwenhoek Hospital in Amsterdam and the Rotterdam Radiotherapy Institute (later renamed the Daniel den Hoed Clinic) were all founded around 1914. Other countries gradually followed these examples. All of these hospitals were pioneers in combining cancer research with cancer treatment, as was the world-famous Institut Curie in Paris, which was founded in 1909 (Raven, 1990). It might have been thought that the foundation of all these institutions specializing in the treatment of cancer would lead to a lifting of the taboo on the discussion of this disease, but the very low cure rate meant that the time for openness had not yet arrived.

Apart from the facilities offered by the specialized cancer hospitals, most cancer patients were treated in the general wards of general hospitals, by doctors who were not oncology specialists, up until the middle of the twentieth century. The disease received little academic attention because cancer was still not considered to be of any particular scientific interest.

Since the doctors spent little time with cancer patients during their ward rounds, the patients often felt isolated and more or less sentenced to a slow death. The fact that the patients were not told their diagnosis or their prognosis, and that questions that might lead to a discussion on these points, only added to their isolation.

The arrival of cancer chemotherapy after the Second World War changed the situation radically for the better. The prospect of cure, or at least a considerable improvement in the survival period, was now available for diseases such as choriocarcinoma, childhood leukemia, Hodgkin's disease and testicular cancer, the diagnosis of which had previously represented a death sentence. But cytostatic treatment had its drawbacks. It could have major side effects, such as nausea, vomiting and hair loss – or even fatal infections. There was a growing realization that patients should give their consent to such forms of treatment, but first they had to be given enough information about the benefits and risks involved to allow them to come to a well-informed decision. This led to the practice of what is now known as informed consent.

The pressure for more open communication was reinforced by an increased emphasis on human rights, and by the evidence produced by the Nuremberg war crimes trials after the Second World War that during the war people had often been subjected to barbaric medical experiments they were powerless to refuse (Holland, 2004). The risk that patients might be exposed to undesired experimentation – especially in the developing world – made effective communication even more vital.

The introduction of chemotherapy also enhanced the importance of clinical trials, since before a new drug could be approved for clinical use it had to be thoroughly tested, in three phases: to determine the correct dose, to find the side effects produced by its use and to assess its efficacy. During all three phases, the patients taking the drugs are exposed to a variety of risks, the extent of which has not yet been determined. Once again, this makes it essential that the patient give informed consent to the treatment before participating in the trials. This must be based on an open dialogue with the responsible physician about the diagnosis, the treatment options and the pros and cons of each form of treatment.

All the above factors increased pressure on doctors to inform patients with cancer of their diagnosis. In a survey carried out by Donald Oken from the National Institute of Mental Health in 1961, more than 90% of the doctors did not tell patients their diagnosis (Oken, 1961). A similar survey covering the same region carried out in 1977 showed that, at that time, 97% of doctors told patients when they were found to have cancer (Novack et al., 1979). Public knowledge about cancer also increased markedly during the intervening 16 years.

Strangely enough, it had long been the accepted custom for patients who required laryngectomy or mastectomy to be told their diagnosis by the doctor. The consequences of the operation in these cases were so far-reaching that it was no longer possible for the doctor to justify the operation in vague terms, by suggesting for example that the patient was suffering from a troublesome polyp or an inflammation. Psychological investigation had shown in the meantime that patients with breast cancer could on the whole cope well with the diagnosis (Staps, 1983). Moreover, patients' and women's advocacy groups were demanding a less paternalistic approach to the dialogue about diagnosis and treatment. This was in line with a general social trend away from a deferential attitude towards figures of authority, including doctors. The improved cure rates for many forms of cancer also made it easier to talk about the diagnosis and treatment of these conditions.

Politicians finally began to respond to public pressure in these fields. Laws regulating patients' rights, including the right to know one's diagnosis and the various treatment options available, were passed in many countries. The relevant legislation is the Patients Rights Act of 1999 in the US, the Human Rights Act of 1998 in the UK and the *Wet op de Geneeskundige Behandelingsovereenkomst* (Medical Treatment Agreement Act) of 1994 in the Netherlands. There are however many countries that are not yet part of this climate of openness (Surbone and Zwitter, 1997).

As a result of this increased openness of communication, there will be some patients who find it difficult to cope with the news of their diagnosis unaided, especially if it concerns a potentially life-threatening disease such as cancer. They may however find it difficult to call on professional support services for assistance, for the reasons discussed in the next section.

FIGURE 10.1 The Saint John's Dancers in Molenbeek. An etching dated 1642 by the Dutch printmaker Hendrik Hondius the Elder, after a lost original by Pieter Brueghel the Elder (1525-1569). It has been suggested that Brueghel drew this picture from life. This etching is one of a set of three, which Hondius accompanied with a lengthy written description including the following graphic explanation: "Vertooninge Hoe de Pelgerimmen, op s. Jans-dagh, buyten Brussel, tot Meulenbeeck danssen moeten, ende als sy over dese Brugh gedanst hebben, ofte gedwongen werden op desevolgende maniere, dan schijnen sy, voor een jaer, van de vallende Sieckte, genesen te zijn [Images of how the pilgrims, on Saint John's Day, that is Midsummer's Day, outside Brussels, have to dance their way to Meulenbeeck and cross the bridge there, either willingly or by force, and they will be healed from the falling sickness [epilepsy] for a year]. At that time, little difference was seen between epilepsy and what we now recognize as mental illness. (Source: Rijksmuseum, Amsterdam).

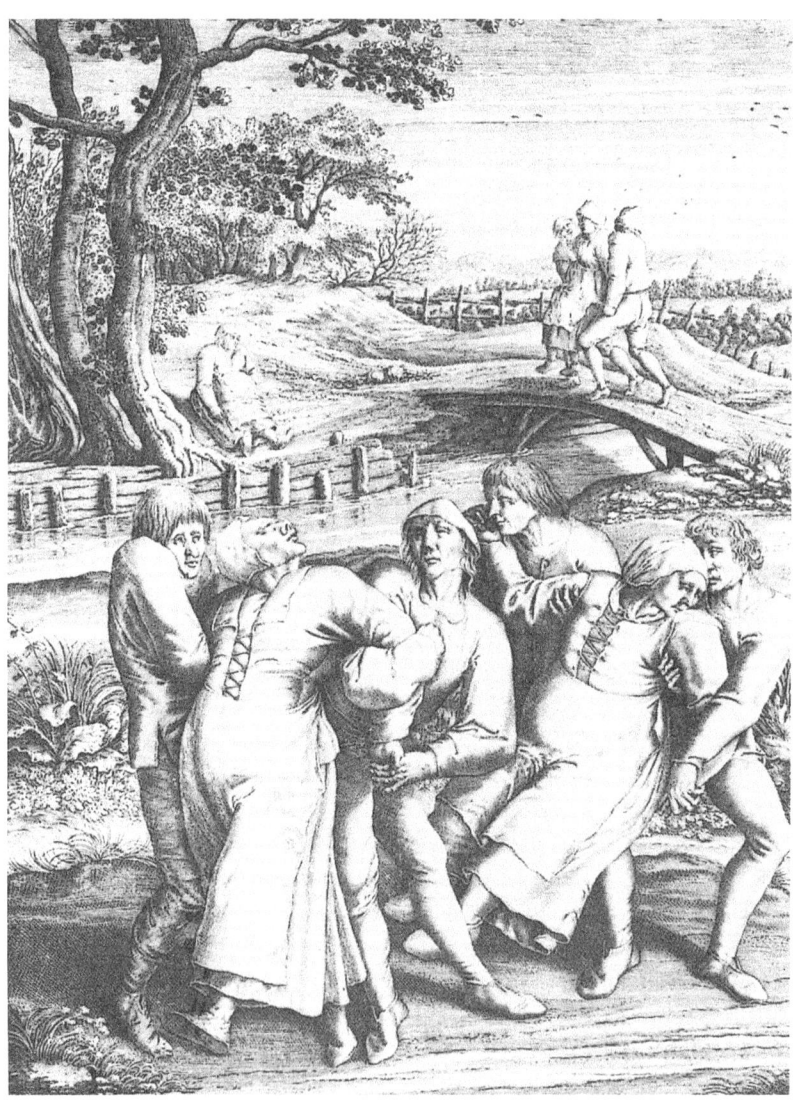

The stigma of mental illness

Even when professional psycho-oncology services are available, patients may be reluctant to make use of them for a number of reasons. They may not wish to allow others such close access to the intimate core of their being; they may wish to avoid being caught up in the mental healthcare "machine" which can involve a loss of independence and the need to submit to intrusive therapies; and above all, a strong feeling still persists that requesting help in coping with the emotional and other consequences of a life-threatening disease such as cancer tarnishes them with the age-old stigma of mental illness.

In an informal sense, psychotherapy can be said to have been practiced through the ages, as individuals received psychological counsel and reassurance from others. Purposeful, theoretically-based psychotherapy was probably first developed in the Middle East during the 9th century by the Persian physician Rhazes or Al-Razi, who was at one time the chief physician of the Baghdad hospital. Among the sayings of Rhazes that have come down to us is the inspiring advice: *Let your first thought be to strengthen your natural vitality.* The knowledge of psychosomatic disorders existed long before this, though physicians had little of no idea how to treat them. For example, the Greek historian Herodotus described how an Athenian soldier, Epizelus, the son of Cuphagoras, who took part in the battle of Marathon in 490 BC, became permanently blind after witnessing the death of a fellow soldier, though he suffered no physical injury himself (Herodotus, Book 6, Passage 117). In the West, however, serious mental disorders were generally treated as demonic or medical conditions requiring punishment and confinement until the advent of moral treatment approaches in the 18th century. This brought about a focus on the possibility of psychosocial intervention – including reasoning, moral encouragement and group activities – to rehabilitate the "insane". [The history of Western psychotherapy has been reviewed by various authors (for example Rudnick, 2002; Bromberg, 1975; Overholser and Bromberg, 2007).]

A telling illustration of the atmosphere that surrounded mental illness in previous centuries is given in Figure 10.1, a reproduction of an engraving by the Dutch printmaker Hendrik Hondius the Elder from the Baroque era. This shows a group of epileptics (at that time, epilepsy was not clearly distinguished from mental illness), each supported by two helpers, who were dancing to the little town of Molenbeek near Brussels on St. John's Day (Midsummer's Day). It was believed that this would cure them of their ailment for a year. This picture shows more clearly than words can tell the typical attitude of the helpers towards their changes: a mixture of amused condescension and affectionate care. It also illustrates the belief that prevailed throughout the Middle Ages in Europe that disease could only be cured through the intervention of God or the saints.

The annual procession of epileptics on the Feast Day of the Nativity of Saint John the Baptist was a real historical event. The type of condition portrayed in the picture seems to have been some form of dyskinesia (which may or may not have been the same as present-day St. Vitus' Dance) that first appeared in the late fourteenth century in a number of mass outbreaks, the first of which was in Aachen on 24 June 1374. The association with Saint John is that he was the patron saint of epileptics, and was therefore invoked for aid by both sufferers and spectators. Dancers would often also be accompanied by musicians as it was believed at that time that music could heal both body and soul. Seizures and fits would often be treated by playing music in an attempt to control the erratic spasms and gyrations of the dancers. (These details are taken from the description of a similar painting by Pieter Brueghel the Younger entitled *The Saint John's Dancers in Molenbeek*, published in the art market information website www.invaluable.com.)

Moving on to more modern times, we find psychoanalysis as perhaps the first specific modern school of psychotherapy, developed by Sigmund Freud (1856-1939) and others in the early 1900s. Trained as a neurologist, Freud began focusing on problems that appeared to have no discernible organic basis, and theorized that they had psychological causes originating in childhood experiences and the unconscious mind. Techniques such as dream interpretation, free association, transference and analysis of the id, ego and superego were developed. The work of Freud has had a revolutionary and lasting influence on the way we think about mental and emotional health, even though many of his basic insights are now largely discredited.

One legacy of Freud's work that has persisted, especially in the US, is the habit of spending large amounts of time and money in consulting psychotherapists (known colloquially as "shrinks"), to provide support and understanding in coping with life's problems. For many decades, many of these therapists were Freudian psychoanalysts. Their popularity is reflected in the TV series *The Sopranos* and in the 1999 film *Analyze This*, both of which are based on the rather incongruous idea of mafia bosses trying to "get in touch with their feelings" through psychotherapy.

There has also been an explosion in the number of mental-health self-help books on the market, of which *I'm OK, You're OK*, by Thomas Harris, MD, is a good example. It offers a practical guide to Transactional Analysis as a tool for solving problems in life. From its first release in 1969, *I'm OK, You're OK* gradually grew in popularity until, in 1972, it made the New York Times Best Seller list and remained there for almost two years. An even earlier worker in this field was the French psychologist Emile Coué (1857-1926), whose books included *Self-mastery through conscious auto-suggestion* (1922). He coined the well-known mantra "Every day, in every way, I am getting better and better."

Another major trend in this field has been the development of an approach to the management of everyday problems now generally referred to as counseling. Carl Rogers was a pioneer in this field. He wrote the book *Counseling and Psychotherapy: Newer Concepts in Practice* in 1942. Three years later he was invited to set up a counseling center at the University of Chicago. It was while working there, in 1951, that he published his major work, *Client-Centered Therapy*, in which he outlined his basic theory. Rogers became the first president of the American Academy of Psychotherapists in 1956. Counseling services are now routinely available to deal with a wide variety of situations – in particular, perhaps, to deal with the psychic trauma generated by emergencies or catastrophes. This is in stark contrast to the attitude expressed during the First World War, for example, when those in command of the soldiers subjected to the horrific bombardments in the trenches in France and Belgium in general expected them to "get a grip on themselves" and punished them if they were unable to do so. During the war, 306 British soldiers were executed for cowardice, many of them victims of what was then known as shell shock. It is a sign of the changing times that on 7 November 2006, the government of the United Kingdom gave them all a posthumous conditional pardon.

To sum up, it may be said that while there has been a growing readiness to engage in some form of mental-health self-help and a growing availability of means to this end over the past century, many people are still hesitant to take a step that will, as they see it, put themselves in the power of the mental healthcare system or expose them to the stigma of mental illness.

To return to our historical review of the development of psycho-oncology, there was a tendency at the end of the nineteenth century to build psychiatric hospitals for the treatment of people with mental illnesses and to set up psychiatric wards in general hospitals, rather than shutting these people up in "lunatic asylums". The importance of teaching doctors and medical students to recognize psychiatric clinical pictures also came to be recognized. This led to a certain degree of interest in psychiatric co-morbidity in patients with internal diseases such as cancer (Holland, 2004).

George Henry, a senior physician at Bloomingdale Hospital at Cornell University Medical School, published the first paper on liaisons between psychiatrists and general medical staff, based on his experience of more than two thousand cases, in 1929. "When psychiatry is first introduced into a general hospital," he wrote, "with very few exceptions there is likely to be indifference or even resistance on the part of the hospital staff....In one hospital, the superintendent rejected the offer of psychiatric support with the comment, 'insanity is hopeless, and there are no insane patients in my hospital.' The director of surgery, on the other hand, said, "I don't know what it's all about, but I guess it won't do any harm." Henry proposed that each general hospital should have a psychopathologic department staffed by at least one psychiatrist (Henry, 1929).

Psychiatry gradually grew in importance. Psychoanalysis was introduced, and a psychosomatic movement grew up within psychiatry that aimed to find a psychological basis for various major chronic diseases such as hypertension, rheumatoid arthritis, peptic ulcers and cancer. From about 1930 to 1960, patients were studied to determine the events or emotions that might be suspected of causing their cancer. It was hypothesized at this time by some followers of the psychosomatic movement that unresolved childhood conflicts could lead to abnormal cell growth and hence to cancer (Bahnson and Bahnson, 1966). Many investigations of this kind were performed in this period, but without the cooperation of the physicians and surgeons in charge of the patients in question. The oncologists were not interested in this approach to the etiology of the disease. This lack of cooperation between the early psychosomatic researchers and the physicians in charge of patients led to a delay of many years – perhaps decades – in the implementation of multidisciplinary prospective studies of the impact of patients' behavior and emotional state on the development of cancer. Such studies have been carried out in the meantime, and have shown that, contrary to the expectations expressed above, features of the patient's personality, depression or stress have no influence on the development of cancer (Dalton et al., 2002).

In the 1950s, psychiatrists at the Memorial Sloan-Kettering Cancer Center in New York under the leadership of Arthur Sutherland and at Massachusetts General Hospital in Boston under the leadership of Jacob Finesinger published a series of papers on the psychological reactions of cancer patients who had been admitted to hospital, though Finesinger had in fact already moved on to set up the Institute of Psychiatry at the University of Maryland, which he would run from 1950 until his premature death in 1959 (Shands et al., 1951; Sutherland et al., 1952; Abrams and Finesinger, 1953). Morton Bard and Sutherland stressed that a one-hour, open-hearted discussion with a patient who was about to undergo mastectomy was of greater benefit than months of postoperative psychotherapy (Bard and Sutherland, 1955).

In 1967, Dame Cicely Saunders founded St. Christopher's Hospice in Sydhenham, southeast London, as a center for the palliative care of terminally ill patients suffering from cancer and other diseases and as a center for education and research. Steven Greer, a lecturer in psychological medicine at King's College Hospital Medical School in London, co-founded the Faith Coultard Unit for Human Studies in Cancer at King's College together with the physician Keith Pettingale and some others in the same year (Holland, 2004), while oncologist and psychoanalyst Loma Feigenberg set up a similar program at the Karolinska University Hospital in Stockholm around the same time (Feigenberg, 1980).

Another key influence in the 1960s was the Swiss-born psychiatrist Elisabeth Kübler-Ross (1926-2004), who published *On Death and Dying* in 1969. In the book she proposed the now famous five stages of grief that apply both to terminally ill patients and to their surviving friends and relatives – denial, anger, bargaining, depression and acceptance – and encouraged the setting up of a hospice care system for the care of the terminally ill. She broke the taboo on talking to cancer patients about their impending death, and challenged doctors and nurses not to avoid these patients but to listen sympathetically to their concerns. Kübler-Ross stimulated both the public and the medical world to recognize the isolation of terminally ill patients, and to respond to their need to talk about their situation (Holland, 2002).

Both Lesley Fallowfield, professor of psycho-oncology at the University of Sussex and Director of the Cancer Research Campaign's Psychosocial Group, and Peter Maguire (1940-2006), professor of psychological medicine at Manchester University, have formulated guidelines on how to break bad news to patients. Many interesting books on this topic have appeared on the market, such as Eric J. Cassell's *Talking with Patients* (1985), and a book of the same name by Philip R. Myerscough from Edinburgh Royal Infirmary (1989) (just two of the countless books and articles that share this evocative title) and *Arzt und Patient. Begegnung im Gespräch* (Doctor and Patient. Encounter in conversation) by the German internist Linus Geisler (1987).

The discipline of psycho-oncology

The conviction gradually grew that psychology had an important contribution to make to the treatment of cancer patients. Despite all the efforts made to improve treatment results, the cure rate continued to hover around 50%. However, the new therapies meant that survival times were increasing, and that patients were living longer with the consequences of the disease and had to learn how to cope with them. They often needed a certain level of psychosocial support in this process – some patients more than others. The social workers, psychologists and psychiatrists working in this field started to campaign for psycho-oncology to be recognized as a separate sub-specialty.

In general, cancer patients are well able to cope with their disease and the treatment they receive with their own resources, backed up by the support of their nearest and dearest and of the medical staff responsible for their treatment. Basically, most of them remain mentally healthy. But they may need some help in the daunting task facing them from professional staff with training and experience in the psychosocial and oncological problems involved.

The discipline of psycho-oncology is concerned with inventorying the effect of the disease on the patient's welfare, the acquisition of insights into the best way to deal with the consequences of the disease and the provision of professional support in coping with the disease, the treatment and its consequences. It also comprises the provision of training and back-up for the professional staff involved, and assistance in teaching patients how to acquire a healthy lifestyle adapted to their circumstances.

Psycho-oncology initially developed formally as a separate sub-specialty in the United States, closely followed by the UK and other Western countries.

The development of psycho-oncology occurred in parallel with a number of important social changes. The public started thinking more positively about cancer, largely because of the growing number of cancer patients who were being cured and who were increasingly ready to tell others about their successful treatment. More and more prominent figures were permitting the media to report on their illness and treatment, such as Betty Ford (born 1918), wife of former US President Gerald Ford, and Margaret (Happy) Rockefeller (born 1926), wife of former Vice President Nelson Rockefeller, who both underwent mastectomies for breast cancer within a few weeks of one another in 1974. They are both still alive at the time of writing–an excellent testimonial to the curative powers of modern oncology. Another important change was the increasing social pressure to respect the human rights of women, consumers and patients. All of these trends helped to bring cancer out into the open and to stimulate research into the psychological dimension of cancer (Holland, 2002).

Social workers and nurses were the first to highlight the psychological and social problems of cancer patients and their families. They had always been in the front line of clinical care and research in the psychosocial domain. They investigated the reactions of children and their parents – both as cancer patients themselves and as the close relatives of cancer patients – the burden placed on caregivers and in particular the requirements of palliative care.

The contribution made by the clergy and pastoral workers to psycho-oncology has only recently been recognized, despite the important role these groups have traditionally played in caring for the sick and dying.

This new discipline has also received input from psychiatry, the behavioral sciences, health psychology, oncology, medical ethics and the reactions of the patients involved, creating a rich and varied mix of information, theoretical models and practical approaches both to research and to clinical applications (Holland, 2004). This diversity has generated psycho-oncology research on a very wide front.

In 1981, the European Organization for Research and Treatment of Cancer set up a Quality of Life study group chaired by the American professor Neil Aaronson from the Division of Psychosocial Research and Epidemiology at the Dutch Cancer Institute in Amsterdam, which drew up guidelines for psycho-oncology research.

Currently, when we evaluate new cancer drugs or forms of cancer treatment, we no longer consider merely the length of the survival period and the disease-free intervals, but also the quality of life as a quantifiable variable. The application of suitable statistical techniques to the combination of quality-of-life and survival data makes it possible to calculate the quality-adjusted survival period; that is, the number of "good" years that a given treatment could be expected to add to a patient's life.

In 1989 David Spiegel, head of the Center on Stress and Health at Stanford Medical School in California, and colleagues published an article in *The Lancet* that attracted a great deal of attention. It gave the results of a randomized prospective study of the influence of psychosocial treatment on the survival of patients with metastasized breast cancer. The treatment, consisting of a 90-minute weekly session of assisted group therapy and self-hypnosis for pain relief, was given to a group of 50 patients. The control group comprised 36 patients. The survival in the group that received the treatment was 36.6 months, as compared with 18.9 months in the control group. This article generated a great number of letters to the editor, and some new studies. A.G.K. Edwards and colleagues from the Division of Nursing at New York University performed a meta-analysis of studies on this topic, and concluded that there is not enough evidence to support the idea that all patients with metastasized breast cancer should be offered psychological group therapy (Edwards et al., 2004)

Researchers and clinicians who are active in the field of psycho-oncology started setting up professional organizations some twenty-five years ago. The International Psycho-Oncology Society (IPOS) was founded in 1984. National associations have been set up in various Western countries, such as the American Psychosocial Oncology Society (APOS), founded in 1986, the British Psychosocial Oncology Society (BPOS), founded by the above-mentioned Steven Greer, and the Dutch Society of Psychosocial Oncology, founded in 1993. Somewhat confusingly, the *Journal of Psychosocial Oncology* is the organ of the Association of Oncology Social Work, based in Philadelphia and founded in 1984.

Every self-respecting discipline needs a handbook of its own. Psycho-oncology has one too – a weighty tome entitled *Psycho-Oncology*, published in 1998 and edited by Jimmie Holland – one of the earliest pioneers of psycho-oncology in the United States, who remains an eloquent advocate for the discipline. She still works at the Department of Psychiatry and Behavioral Sciences at the Memorial Sloan-Kettering Cancer Center in New York, which she helped to set up in 1977.

With a few notable exceptions such as Sloan-Kettering, hospitals were in general slow to recognize the importance of psychosocial support for cancer patients. Much of the early work was left to private initiatives and charities. The past few decades have seen the growth of an appreciable number of day-care and walk-in centers providing such psychosocial support in many Western countries, alongside the expanding network of hospices where a dedicated effort is made to create a positive, live-for-the-day atmosphere for terminally ill patients suffering from cancer and other diseases. In these days of the Internet boom, it is hardly surprising that many flourishing websites offering support and advice for patients with cancer and other diseases have grown up. A good example is Macmillan Cancer Support in the UK, which merged with Cancer Backup in April 2008. The New York-based Association of Cancer Online Resources (ACOR) is an access point for similar services in the US. Such online services have not however replaced telephone helplines, which have burgeoned since Chad Varah (1911-2007), the Anglican vicar of the parish of St. Stephen Walbrook in the City of London, set up the Samaritans in 1953 in the crypt of his church (which had been built by Sir Christopher Wren in 1672-1680 after the previous church on that site had been destroyed by the Great Fire of London in 1666). The Samaritans – the first telephone helpline in the UK, and probably still the best-known – offers non-religious support by phone for people in distress who feel that they have no one to turn to, and who are at risk of suicide (Varah, 1993).

The emotional threshold applying to all mental health issues still slows the development of psychological support for cancer patients. Many patients still fear being branded as mentally ill if they request help in coping with their situation. There can be no doubt, however, that many of these patients do need support. James Zabora, Dean of the National Catholic School of Social Service and Professor of Social Work at the Catholic University of America in Washington, DC, and his team used a brief symptom inventory (BSI) to assess the need for psychosocial support in cancer patients. They estimated that 35% of the 4496 cancer patients seen for the first time at the Sidney Kimmel Cancer Center of the Johns Hopkins Hospital in Baltimore during the period of their study were suffering significant distress, but that fewer than 10% were referred for psychological evaluation and counseling (Zabora et al., 2001). L.E. Carlson from the Department of Oncology of the University of Calgary and the Department of Psychosocial Resources of the Tom Baker Cancer Centre in Alberta, Canada, and colleagues carried out a similar study, and came to comparable conclusions. They estimated that only about half of the patients with serious distress actually requested psychological support, and listed the following main reasons patients gave for not asking for assistance: the feeling that one could cope unaided, ignorance of the resources available and doubt whether the resources provided would really help (Carlson et al., 2004). Dr. Henk K. van Halteren and colleagues from the UMC St. Radboud, Nijmegen, commenting on the results reported by Carlson et al., suggested that the BSI, to be filled in by the patient while waiting to see the specialist, offered a basis for quick assessment of the extent of the distress experienced in any individual case, which the physician could then use as a guideline for recommendation of appropriate support services (Van Halteren et al., 2004).

The NCCN (National Comprehensive Cancer Network), an alliance of all the main cancer centers in the US, set up a multidisciplinary panel in the 1970s to draw up guidelines for the management of psychosocial distress. This panel adopted the following definition:

Distress is an unpleasant emotional experience of a psychological, social, or spiritual nature that may interfere with a patient's ability to cope with cancer and its treatment. Distress extends along a continuum, ranging from common normal feelings of vulnerability, sadness, and fear to problems that can become disabling, such as depression, anxiety, panic, social isolation, and spiritual crisis.

It recommended general use of the term "distress" in this context in preference to such labels as "psychiatric," "psychosocial," or "emotional," which might be experienced as stigmatizing or embarrassing (Holland, 2004).

Conclusion

Psychosocial oncology has made great strides during the past three decades. It is however still far from being generally accepted as an integral part of the treatment of cancer. Both doctors and patients are often reluctant to accept the discipline wholeheartedly. Doctors are frequently unaware of all that this form of support has to offer. This also applies to patients, who are moreover often unwilling to call in the help of professional psychologists or psychiatrists for fear of being labeled mentally ill. Nevertheless, there is a growing understanding of the real contributions this discipline can make in lightening the burden on cancer patients, and it seems likely that it will take its well-deserved place in the treatment of cancer in the foreseeable future.

Glossary

A

Ablation
: Removal of part of a tissue, often by surgical means. However, one may also speak of bone-marrow ablation, where high-intensity chemotherapy and total body irradiation are used to remove bone marrow cells in preparation for a bone-marrow transplant, or of ablation of certain components of the blood such as platelets or white blood cells.

Adnexa
: A medical word for "appendages". In gynecology, the adnexa are the "appendages" of the uterus, i.e. the ovaries and Fallopian tubes.

Apheresis
: (from the Greek for "removal") A medical technique used to remove certain constituents from the blood of a patient before returning the rest of the blood to the circulation.

Allele
: One of a series of two or more variants of a gene occurring in a particular population.

Allogeneic
: Genetically different though belonging to or taken from the same species; often used to describe tissue grafts.

Amino acid
: An acid containing an amino ($-NH_3$) group.

Amorphous
: Shapeless; without a definite crystalline structure.

Anabolic
: Stimulating protein synthesis in the body.

Anaplasia
: When healthy tissue is examined under the microscope, different tissue cells are seen to have clearly different structures. These cells are then said to be structurally differentiated. Loss of structural differentiation is called anaplasia. It is often found in malignant tumors.

Aneurysm
: Local dilatation of an artery.

Angiogenesis
: The formation of new blood vessels.

Anti-emetic
: Substance that suppresses vomiting.

Antigen
: See antibody.

Antibody
: Substance made in the body in response to the introduction of a foreign substance, the antigen. Antibodies adhere to antigens, thus rendering them inactive.

Apoptosis
: Programmed cell death.

Apoptotic bodies
: Small vesicles (membrane-covered compartments) that are visible in cells undergoing apoptosis.

Aspiration
: The sucking up of a fluid.

Atrophy
: The wasting away or decrease in size of an organ. This may be due to reduction in the size of the cells, in their number, or both.

Autochthonous
: Found in the part of the body in which it originated (for example an autochthonous tumor) or in the location in which it originated (for example an autochthonous infection).

Autopsy
: See "Post-mortem examination".

Autosomal dominant inheritance
: In this pattern of inheritance, one of the parents will in principle have the complaint in question. Characteristic features of dominant inheritance are that the disease is found in successive generations and occurs in both males and females; only someone with the disease can transmit it to his or her children; and there is a 50% chance that a child of a person with the disease will also have it.

Autosomal
: Autosomal chromosomes split into two during the reproduction process, unlike the X chromosome.

Avirulent
: Not virulent, pathogenic or giving rise to disease.

B

Basal cell carcinoma
: The most common form of skin cancer.

Base
: A substance that forms a salt when it reacts with an acid. In the context of this book, a base is one of the five building blocks of nucleic acids: adenine, cytosine, guanine and thymine (which occur only in DNA) and uracil (which occurs only in RNA).

Benign tumor
: A mild, unprogressive form of cancer. The tumor cells may displace surrounding tissue but do not invade it. They do not metastasize.

Bias
: Distortion or irregularity; reference or inclination that inhibits impartial judgement, prejudice.

Bone scintigraphy
: Investigation of bones with the aid of radioactive isotopes in order to detect metastases.

C

Cachexia
: Poor general physical condition.

Carcinoma
: A malignant cancer arising from epithelial cells (the cells that line the cavities and surfaces of structures throughout the body).

Case-control study
: A study of two groups of persons who resemble one another as much as possible. One group (the cases) consists of people with a certain disease, while the other group (the control group) consists of people without the disease. The probability that the test subjects in the two groups have been exposed to a certain effect is determined. The ratio of these two probabilities is then calculated, and provides a basis for estimating the likelihood that this effect gave rise to the disease.

Cauterize
: To burn the body to remove or close part of it.

Cell
: A small portion of living tissue enclosed by a membrane, with its own metabolism and DNA. Plants, animals and humans are made up of cells.

Cell cycle
: The cycle in which a single cell produces two cells. It consists of a number of phases, called G(eneration)1, S(ynthesis), G2, and M(itosis).

Cell fusion
: The joining together of two cells into one. See hybridoma.

Chemotherapy
: Use of chemical substances to fight cancer.

Cholecystography
: X-ray investigation of the gall bladder.

Choriocarcinoma
: A form of cancer arising generally from the placenta but sometimes from the ovary.

Chromatin
: The substances in the cell nucleus that can be stained by basic dyes.

Chromosome
: Rod-like body in the cell nucleus that carries the hereditary properties. It is built up of DNA.

Chronic lymphatic leukemia
: Abnormal proliferation of a certain type of white blood cells (lymphocytes), on a long-term basis.

Chronic myeloid leukemia
: Abnormal proliferation of white blood cells, on a long-term basis.

Colectomy
: Surgical removal of all or part of the large intestine (colon).

Colon
: Large intestine.

Colostomy
: A surgical procedure in which the colon is cut and brought to the outside through the wall of the abdomen, thus creating an artificial opening or "stoma". Feces are then collected in a bag called a colostomy bag attached to the opening. Colostomy is usually a temporary measure, but may sometimes need to be permanent.

Colostrum
: The milk produced in late pregnancy and in the first few days after giving birth.

Complete remission
: The complete disappearance of all visible tumors following chemotherapy. This does not necessarily mean that the patient is cured. Microscopic remnants of the tumor may still remain.

Coccynx
: Tail-bone.

Cortisol
: Hormone produced by the adrenal cortex of the adrenal gland.

Cremophor
: ELA solvent widely used to dissolve drugs intended for intravenous administration

Cutaneous stoma
: Opening in the wall of the intestine or the urethra (the tube that takes urine to outside the body).

Cyst
: Body cavity filled with fluid.

Cytology
: The study of living cells.

Cytoplasm
: The viscous fluid contents of a cell.

Cytostatic agent (or Cytostatic drug)
: A substance that inhibits the growth and multiplication of cells.

Cytotoxic T lymphocyte
: Activated T-lymphocyte that attacks antigen-containing cells that are foreign to the body through direct contact.

D

Deletion
In the context of this book, loss of a part of a chromosome.

Deltopectoral flap
A graft used for reconstruction of tissue defects after surgery, including the deltoid muscle (the shoulder muscle) and the pectoral muscle (the muscle of the chest).

Differentiation
See anaplasia.

Distal
Furthest away from the centre of the body. The opposite of proximal.

DNA
(Deoxyribonucleic acid), the carrier of hereditary properties.

Dominant
An allele is said to be dominant if it determines the phenotype in a heterozygotic organism.

E

-ectomy
Surgical removal. This suffix is preceded by the name of the part to be removed; for example, mastectomy is surgical removal of the breast.

Edema
An abnormal accumulation of tissue fluid.

Ego
In the theory of psychoanalysis developed by Sigmund Freud, the part of the psyche that is conscious, most immediately controls thought and behavior, and is most in touch with external reality.

Embryonic cell carcinoma
Malignant tumor arising from poorly differentiated cells produced during various stages of embryogenesis. This type of tumor often occurs in the testicle.

En-bloc resection
Complete removal of the cancer with the surrounding tissue as a whole.

Endotracheal anesthesia
Anesthesia produced by a mixture of gases introduced via a tube inserted into the trachea (windpipe).

Enucleation
Surgical removal of a part of the body without cutting into it, for example because it is affected by a malignant tumor.

Enzyme
A protein that catalyzes a certain biochemical reaction.

Epidemiology
Study of the occurrence (incidence) of a disease in various population groups.

Epithelial cells
The cells that line the cavities and surfaces of structures throughout the body.

Epstein-Barr virus (also known as Human herpesvirus 4)
A virus involved in Burkitt's lymphoma and nose and throat cancers.

Equatorial plane
The plane that separates the two halves of a dividing cell, along which the chromosome pairs arrange themselves. After division, one chromosome of each pair goes to each of the new cells.

Eukaryotes
Eukaryotes are organisms that make up one of the three domains of life. Eukaryotic cells have nuclei and other specialized subunits known as organelles. Fungi, plants and animals are eukaryotes.

Ewing's sarcoma
Malignant tumor of the bone, mainly found in children and adolescents.

Exostosis
Benign bone growth.

F

Femur
: Thigh-bone.

G

Gastrojejunostomy reconstruction
: Surgical connection realized between the stomach and the jejunum, the part of the intestines that follows the duodenum.

Geiger counter
: Instrument for detecting and measuring the intensity of radioactive radiation, named after its inventor Hans Wilhelm Geiger (1882-1945).

Gene
: Part of the DNA polynucleotide chain that codes for a single protein.

Genome
: The entire genetic information contained in a haploid cell. Sex cells (egg cells and sperm cells) are haploid. A diploid cell thus contains two genomes. The term 'human genome' is generally taken to mean the genetic information contained in all human chromosomes (1 - 22 plus X and Y) together with the mitochondrial DNA.

Germline cells
: Sex cells or cells that can develop into sex cells.

Germ-cell mutation
: Mutation in a sex cell or a fertilized egg cell. The mutation is then passed on to all cell in the same germline.

Globulin
: Type of protein present in blood plasma.

Gonad
: Sex gland.

Graft-versus-host disease
: Immune reaction in which the cells of a transplant attack the body of the recipient.

Growth factors
: Proteins that regulate the cell-division process.

Gynecology
: Study of the diseases of women.

H

Half-life
: The half-life of an isotope is the time it takes for half the radioactivity to disappear. The half-life of a cytostatic drug is the time it takes for half of the drug to disappear from the bloodstream.

Hairy cell leukemia
: Malignant proliferation of white blood cells, which have a hairy appearance when viewed under the microscope.

Hematocrit
: The proportion by volume of red blood cells in the blood, expressed as a fraction or a percentage.

Heterozygote
: An organism is said to be heterozygotic for a given gene if it possesses two different alleles of that gene.

Histologic
: Relating to the study of tissues.

HLA (Human leukocyte antigen)
: Another name for the major histocompability complex (MHC); see also Minor antigens.

Hodgkin's disease
: A malignant disease of the lymph nodes. It is distinguished from non-Hodgkin's lymphoma by the presence of a certain cell type.

Hodgkin's lymphoma
: See Hodgkin's disease.

Human papillomavirus (HPV)
: A virus that plays a role in the origin of cervical cancer (cancer of the neck of the uterus).

Hybridoma
: Cell produced by fusion of for example a tumor cell and a B lymphocyte.

Hyperthermia
: Abnormally high body temperature; use of heat to treat cancer

Hypertrophy
: An abnormal increase in the size and weight of an organ due to an increase in the volume of its cells.

Hypopharyngeal carcinoma
: Cancer of the bottom part of the throat.

Hypophysis
: The pituitary gland, a pea-sized gland located at the base of the brain.

Hypothalamus
: A small part of the brain just above the brain stem, with some important functions. It controls the body's status quo, and motivates the basic reactions known as the 'four Fs' (feeding, fighting, fleeing and sexual reproduction (fertility)).

Hypoxic tumor cells
: Cancer cells that contain too little oxygen.

Hysterectomy
: Surgical removal of the womb.

I

Id
: In the theory of psychoanalysis developed by Sigmund Freud, the part of the psyche that is totally unconscious and serves as the source of instinctual impulses and demands for the immediate satisfaction of primitive needs.

Immunoglobulin
: A type of antibody.

Incidence
: The extent to which a given disease occurs in a group of people.

Informed consent
: A basic concept in clinical trials. It means that the patient in question has agreed to take part in the trial, after having been fully informed about the trial procedure and the risks involved.

Intermittent
: Occurring or acting at intervals.

In vitro
: Outside the body (from the Latin for "in glass"). An *in vitro* study is one where the substances under investigation are removed from the body before being subjected to various reactions or other processes.

In vivo
: In a living organism (from the Latin for "in a living body"). An *in vivo* study is carried out inside the body of the patient or experimental animal in question.

Intratracheal insufflation
: Administration of air via the trachea (windpipe) during anesthesia.

Ischemic damage
: Tissue damage due to cutting off of the blood supply.

Isotope
: An element that emits radioactive radiation.

Isotopes
: Isotopes are alternative forms of a chemical element. All isotopes of a given element have the same chemical behavior, because their atomic nucleus contains the same number of protons. They have different numbers of neutrons in the nucleus, however, and hence a different atomic mass. About 80% of the isotopes that occur naturally on Earth are stable. However, if we take the vast number of man-made isotopes into account (about 2760 are known at present), the vast majority of isotopes are radioactive – that is, they emit radiation, turning into other elements in the process. Such isotopes are known as radioisotopes.

K

Kaposi's sarcoma
A malignant disease that occurs in two different forms. The classic type is found mainly in the legs of older people, and the HIV-related type in AIDS patients.

Kinase
Name given to a group of enzymes that can phosphorylate a protein or other molecule (attach a phosphate group to it). A kinase uses (kinetic) energy in this catalytic reaction, hence the name. The phosphorylation often activates the protein in question, thus permitting the control of chemical reactions in the cell and playing a key role in signal transduction. The name of the functional group that is phosphorylated is placed in front of the name of the kinase. For example, tyrosine kinase attaches a phosphate group to a tyrosine molecule in the target protein. Tyrosine is an amino-acid, one of the building blocks of proteins.

L

Lesion
A wound, injury, or localized pathological change in an organ or tissue.

Laparotomy
The opening of the abdominal cavity.

Latency period
Time between first exposure to a carcinogen and the development of clinical signs of cancer.

Laryngectomy
Surgical removal of the larynx (voicebox).

Leucovorin rescue
Administration of a high dose of leucovorin to limit the side-effects during treatment with high doses of methotrexate.

Leukemia
Malignant proliferation of bone-marrow cells, also known as blood cancer.

Leukemic blasts
Young white blood cells which tend to proliferate.

Leukocytes
White blood cells.

Linear accelerator
Type of irradiation equipment that emits artificial high-energy rays.

Lues
Hard chancre (syphilis); a sexually transmitted disease.

Lymphadenectomy
The surgical removal or one or more groups of lymph nodes.

Lymphatic system
A network of vessels that carry lymph around the body, alongside the circulatory system for the blood.

Lymphoblastic leukemia
Proliferation of young lymphocytes.

Lymphocyte
The white blood cells involved in the body's immune response.

Lymphoproliferative disorder
Proliferation of lymphocytes.

Lytic metastases
Metastases in bone that eat away the bone to leave holes in it.

M

Malignant tumor
A cancerous growth from which cells infiltrate into surrounding tissues. This can lead to metastases.

Mammary carcinoma
Cancer originating in the breast.

Mandible
Lower jawbone.

Mastectomy
: Total surgical removal of the breast.

Median
: The half-way value in a series of numbers. If a set of numbers is arranged in order of increasing magnitude, the median is the value with 50% of the values above it and 50% below it.

Melanin
: A dark-colored pigment that occurs in human skin, and also in plants and other organisms.

Melanocytes
: Cells that occur in the epidermis (the upper layer of the skin) and in the iris of the eye. They form the pigment melanin on UV irradiation.

Melanoma
: Cancer formed from melanocytes. This type of cancer usually originates in a birthmark.

Mesenchyme
: Tissue formed by embryonic cells, and originating in the mesoderm (the middle of the three primary germ cell layers).

Mesorectum
: Fatty tissue immediately adjacent to the rectum, which contains blood vessels and lymph nodes. This is a form of mesothelium.

Mesothelioma
: A cancer formed by malignant cells that develop in the mesothelium, the protective lining that covers most of the body's internal organs.

Meta-analysis
: Mathematical analysis of the results of a group of comparable clinical trials. This makes it possible to draw more reliable conclusions about the effectiveness of the intervention or treatment that is the subject of the trials.

Metabolism
: The chemical reactions that occur in living organisms in order to maintain life.

Metastases
: Tumors arising at a distance from the primary cancer, caused by migration and further growth of cells from the primary cancer.

MHC (major histocompatibility complex) proteins
: Proteins on the cell membrane that present foreign antigens to T lymphocytes.

Microbiology
: Biology of micro-organisms such as bacteria.

Microsatellites
: Short pieces of DNA that do not code for proteins, but sometimes have a well-defined function. A microsatellite is often very simple in structure, consisting of two, three or four nucleotides, and is essential for the functioning of a gene.

Microsome
: A small vesicle (enclosed compartment) present within a cell.

Microtubules
: Miniscule tubes that together with other protein filaments form the cytoskeleton (the dynamic structure that gives the cell its rigidity). These tubules undergo a continual process of growth and shrinkage, and have a different form at each stage of a cell's life cycle.

Minor antigens
: Less important antigens, which can still lead to rejection of a transplant even though the HLAs of the donor and the recipient are a perfect match.

Mismatch repair genes
: Errors produced during DNA replication (the copying of strands of DNA) are corrected by the mismatch repair system.

Defects in this system lead to instability of 'microsatellite DNA'. Microsatellites are DNA fragments containing repeating sequences of nucleotides. This microsatellite instability is found in particular in hereditary non-polyposis colorectal cancer (HNPCC), also known as Lynch syndrome.

Mitosis
: Phase during the division of the nucleus where the two chromosomes of each chromosome pair separate.

Monoclonal antibodies
: Monoclonal antibodies are specific antibodies that are identical because they are all produced from one type of immune cell and are all clones of a single parent cell. Cloning is a process widely used in modern biotechnology to produce identical copies of DNA fragments, cells or organisms. The first mammal to be cloned was the world-famous Dolly the sheep.

Morphology
: The theory of the form and structure of organisms.

Mouse myeloma cell
: Malignant plasma cell from a mouse.

MRI
: (magnetic resonance imaging). A widely used modern technique for imaging certain body organs with the aid of strong magnetic fields.

Mucocutaneous zone
: A region on the surface of the body where both skin and mucous membrane are present.

Multicenter randomized study
: A study in which several institutes have participated. ëRandomizedí means that patients are assigned to the group under investigation by chance (or with the aid of a statistical procedure).

Multiple myeloma
: Cancer originating in plasma cells, a particular type of white blood cell that makes antibodies. Also known as Kahler's disease.

Mutagen
: A substance or type of radiation that can give rise to mutations (damage to DNA).

Mutation
: Permanent change in DNA.

Mycosis fungoides
: Malignant skin disease characterized by the presence of inflamed red patches from which mushroom-like solid tumors can grow in extreme cases.

Myeloma cell line
: A cell line is a group of cells formed by division from a single mother cell. The cells keep on dividing endlessly (and are thus ëimmortalí). All cells have the same properties. A myeloma cell line is a cell line derived from a malignant plasma cell.

Myxosarcoma
: A tumor consisting of tissue that resembles mesenchyme (qv.).

N

Naked mouse
: A mutant mouse that has no cellular immunity and hence does not reject transplants.

Nasopharyngeal carcinoma
: Cancer in the region of the nose and throat.

Neurofibroma
: A tumor produced by proliferation of the connective tissue of nerve.

Neurogenic sarcoma
: Tumor originating in nerves.

Nonseminomatous testis tumor
: Cancer originating in the testicle. The most malignant form of testicular cancer as opposed to the seminoma, which is the least malignant form.

Non-Hodgkin lymphoma
: A tumor originating in the lymph nodes. See Hodgkin's disease.

Nucleic acids
: A generic term covering both DNA and RNA.

Nucleoside
: Molecule consisting of a sugar (ribose or deoxyribose), and one of the bases found in DNA and RNA.

Nucleotide
: Molecule consisting of one or more phosphate groups, a sugar (ribose or deoxyribose) and one of the bases found in DNA and RNA.

Nucleus
: The central portion of a eukaryotic cell, containing the chromatin (combination of DNA, proteins and RNA).

O

Omentum
: (from the Latin for "apron"): a fold of peritoneum that hangs down from the stomach.

Oncogene
: A gene that stimulates cells to grow in an uncontrolled manner, leading to the formation of a tumor.

Oncogenic
: Causing cancer; giving rise to tumors.

Orchiectomy
: Surgical removal of the testicles.

Osteosarcoma
: Bone cancer.

Ovariectomy
: Surgical removal of one or both ovaries.

Ovarian cancer
: Cancer originating in the ovaries.

P

Palliative
: Reducing the severity of symptoms, relieving pain or stress.

Papilla of Vater
: Wart-like elevation in the duodenum near the point where it is joined by the bile duct.

Papilloma
: Benign tumor of the skin or mucous membrane, manifesting itself as a wart or cauliflower-shaped growth.

Parametrium
: Fibrous tissue next to the uterine cervix and between the layers of the broad ligament.

Parasitic diseases
: Diseases caused by parasites. A parasite is an organism that maintains its vital functions and multiplies at the expense of another organism, its host.

Pelvic and para-aortal lymph nodes
: Lymph nodes situated in the pelvis and along the aorta.

Perfusion
: The passage of blood through a tissue; in the context of this book, the artificial passage of blood containing a cytostatic drug through a tissue after the normal circulation in the relevant part of the body has been shut down.

Pericyte
: A cell similar in structure to those found in mesenchyme (qv.), associated with the outer wall of the capillaries. Can help to support the capillary, but may also have a range of other important functions.

Peritoneum
: The thin membrane that lines the abdominal cavity and covers most of the organs in this cavity.

PET (positron-emission tomography) scan
> A PET scan provides information about the metabolism in a certain part of the body. Nutrients such as proteins and sugars are consumed in the body cells. A PET camera can show up such substances when they are radioactively labeled. These substances can be administered to a patient, and will then distribute themselves throughout the body in a way that is determined by the metabolism. The distribution can be imaged with the aid of a PET camera and a computer. Tumors can be tracked down by this technique because they have a different metabolism from normal tissues.

Phenotype
> The way in which the alleles present in a given individual are expressed.

Post-mortem examination
> Medical examination of a dead body in an attempt to discover the cause of death.

Platelet-derived growth factor
> A protein produced by the platelets in the blood that stimulates cell growth.

Pavement cell carcinoma
> Cancer of cells in the epidermis (the outer layer of the skin) above the basal layer.

Pneumectomy
> Surgical removal of a lung.

Polyp
> An abnormal growth of tissue from a mucous membrane.

Polycyclic hydrocarbons
> A group of carcinogens, which can be produced during the preparation of food (for example by grilling or frying).

Polycythemia vera
> Malignant increase in the number of red blood cells.

Prehydration
> Administration of fluid before the start of treatment.

Proliferation
> Rapid and often excessive growth of cells.

Proto-oncogene
> A normal gene that can become an oncogene due to mutation or increased expression.

Protozoic disease
> A disease caused by protozoa, unicellular eukaryotes (qv.) that often lead a parasitic existence.

Proximal
> Closest to the centre of the body. he opposite of distal.

Psychosomatic
> Relating to the influence of the mind on the body and the body on the mind, especially with respect to disease.

Psychotherapy
> An interpersonal, relational form of treatment used by trained psychotherapists to help clients to deal with life's problems, often by enabling them to increase their feelings of self-worth and to cope with experiences perceived to be uncomfortable or threatening.

R

Radiotherapy
> Treatment of cancer with radioactive radiation.

Randomization
> The assignment of patients to a group under investigation by chance (or with the aid of a statistical procedure).

Receptor
> Protein in the cell membrane with a specific binding site for substances from outside the cell.

Relapse
> The recurrence of a tumor after it had initially disappeared.

Rectum
: The final part of the large intestine, leading to the anus.

Response
: The response to cancer therapy is the extent to which the therapy causes the signs of the cancer to disappear. A good reaction is generally defined as a 50% or greater reduction in tumor mass. Also known as remission.

Reticuloendothelial system (RES):
: The system comprising all phagocytic cells of the body with the exception of granulocytes. It includes the cells lining the sinusoids of the spleen, lymph nodes, and bone marrow along with the fibroblastic reticular cells of hematopoietic tissues (the tissues responsible for the production of all types of blood cells).

Retinoblastoma
: A cancer of the retina.

Retropubic
: Behind the pubic bone.

Retrospective study
: An investigation based on data collected in the past.

Retrovirus
: A virus with RNA instead of DNA as genetic material.

RNA
: (Ribonucleic acid), plays a key role in the synthesis of proteins in the body.

Rous sarcoma virus (RSV)
: A virus that causes sarcoma in chickens, discovered by Peyton Rous. It is a retrovirus.

S

Sacrum
: Sacred bone; a triangular bone made up of 5 fased vertebrae and forming the posterior section of the pelvis.

Sarcoma
: Cancer originating in subcutaneous tissue such as muscle, blood vessels and connective tissue.

Scrotum
: The bag of skin and muscle containing the testicles.

Segment resection
: Surgical removal of part of a lung lobe.

Sequestration
: Separation of a part from the whole.

Solid tumor
: A cancer the cells of which form a solid mass (swelling), unlike leukemia where the cells remain separate.

Somatic cells
: Cells that do not belong to the germline.

Staging
: Determination of the extent of cancer.

Staging laparotomy
: Abdominal operation performed to determine the extent of cancer.

Stem-cell apheresis
: Removal of stem cells from the blood, for example so that they can be used in bone-marrow transplantation.

Stoma
: Artificial opening to permit excretion of feces or urine, almost always created in the front of the abdomen.

Superego
: In the theory of psychoanalysis developed by Sigmund Freud, the part of the unconscious that is formed through the internalization of the moral standards of parents and society, and that censors and restrains the ego.

Supraglottic laryngeal carcinoma
: Cancer situated above the vocal cords in the larynx (voice box).

Suprapubic
: Above the pubic bone.

T

T cell or T lymphocyte
A kind of white blood cell that plays a key role in the body's immune response. There are three main types of T cells: helper T cells, cytotoxic T cells and suppressor T cells. The stem cells from which all blood cells are formed are situated in the bone marrow. However, the maturation of T lymphocytes takes place in the thymus, an organ situated just behind the breastbone; hence the 'T' in T cell. The process of T-cell maturation is largely completed before the onset of puberty. Immature T cells are as it were 'trained' to distinguish between cells that belong to the body and foreign cells during their stay in the thymus.

Temporal artery
The artery that can be felt in the temple, on the side of the head.

Thalamus
A structure located on the dorsal side of the midbrain (that is, the side closest to the back of the body). It has a number of important functions, including acting as a relay centre for sensory information on its way to the cerebral cortex.

Thymusless mouse
A mouse that has no resistance to human tumor cells.

T lymphocyte
See T cell.

Toxicity
The property of being poisonous.

Tracheobronchial epithelium
The layer of cells covering the trachea (windpipe) and its subdivisions (the bronchi).

Transcranial route
An approach through the skull.

Transference
An effect observed in psychoanalysis in which a person unconsciously redirects feelings from one person to another – for example, a client may experience feelings of love or hate for the therapist that really mirror the feelings he or she has about a parent. Transference was first described by Sigmund Freud. He initially regarded it as a barrier to therapy, but later realized that the proper analysis of transference is in fact a key to successful treatment.

Translocation
In the context of this book, translocation means movement of a fragment of one chromosome to another chromosome.

Transnasal-transsphenoid route
An approach through the nose and the sphenoid bone.

Trial
In the context of this book, a carefully controlled test of the effectiveness of a medical agent or procedure.

Thrombocytes
Blood platelets. They play an important role in the coagulation of blood after an injury.

Tumor
An accumulation of cells due to abnormal cell growth. May be benign or malignant.

Tumor-associated transplantation antigens
Antigens on the surface of tumor cells, which can be detected by transplantation experiments.

Tyrosine kinase
See kinase.

U

Ulcer
A slowly healing sore on the skin, mucous membranes or eye.

Uterus
Womb.

V

Seminal vesicles
Glands at the base of the bladder that provide nutrients for the semen.

Virilization
The development of male characteristics in women, such as deepening of the voice, enlargement of the clitoris and hypertrophy of the muscles.

Virus
Infectious agent consisting of DNA or RNA surrounded by a coat of one or more types of protein, and often by a lipid (fatty) membrane.

X

Xenograft
A surgical graft of tissue from a different species, for example an animal organ transplanted to a human being.

Literature

A

Abrams RD, Finesinger JE. Guilt reactions in patients with cancer. Cancer 1953;6:474-82.

Abul-Hajj YJ, Iverson R, Kiang DT. Aromatization of androgens by human breast cancer. Steroids 1979;33:205-22.

Adair FE, Bagg HJ. Experimental and clinical studies on the treatment of cancer by dichlorethyl-sulphide (mustard gas). Ann of Surg 1931;93:190-9.

Adair FE. The use of the male sex hormone in women with breast cancer. Surg Gynec Obstet 1947;84:719-22.

Aldersey-Williams H. Lucky Jim, Watson and Crick, and the structure of DNA. In: Findings, hidden stories in first-hand accounts of scientific discovery. Norwich: Lulox Books, 2005.

Alexander P. Immunological aspects of malignant disease. Conflicting evidence for immune reactions to human cancer. Cancer Forum 1983;7:60-2.

Allard JW, Thalidomide in the treatment of cancer. Anti-Cancer Drugs 2000;11:787-91.

Ameisen J-C, Chikh A, Bongiorno-Borbone L, Knight RA. Cette mort nécessaire à la vie. J de la Société de Biologie 2005;199:267-76.

Ang KK, Berkey BA, Tu X, Zhang HZ, Katz R, et al. Impact of epidermal growth factor receptor expression on survival and pattern of relapse in patients with advanced head and neck carcinoma. Cancer Res 2002;62:7350-6.

B

Bahnson CB, Bahnson MJ. Role of the ego defenses: denial and repression in the etiology of malignant neoplasm. Ann NY Acad Sci 1966;125:827-45.

Bard M, Sutherland AM. Psychological impact of cancer and its treatment. IV. Adaptation to radical mastectomy. Cancer 1955;8:656-72.

Baum M, Nolvadex Adjuvant Trial Organisation: Controlled trial of tamoxifen as single adjuvant agent in management of early breast cancer; analysis at six years. Lancet 1985;i:836-9.

Bazell R. Her-2, the making of Herceptin, a revolutionary treatment for breast cancer. New York: Random House, 1998.

Beatson GT. On the treatment of inoperable cases of carcinoma of the mamma: suggestions for a new method of treatment with illustrative cases. Lancet 1896;2:104-7, 162-5.

Bennett Jr IL, Beeson PB. Studies on the pathogenesis of fever. J Exp Med 1953;98:493-508.

Beral V, Reeves G. Childbearing, oral contraceptive use, and breast cancer. Lancet 1993;341:1102.

Berd D, Maguire HC Jr, McCue P, Mastrangelo MJ. Treatment of metastatic melanoma with an autologous tumor-cell vaccine: clinical and immunologic results in 64 patients. J Clin Oncol 1990;8:1858-67.

Berenblum I. Experimental inhibition of tumour induction by mustard gas and other compounds. J Pathol Bacteriol 1935;40:549-58.

Berenblum I. The modifying influence of dichlorethyl sulphide on the induction of tumours in mice by tar. J Pathol Bacteriol 1929;32:424-34.

Berkeley WN. Results of three years' observation on a new form on cancer treatment. Amer J Obstetrics and Diseases of Women 1914;69:1060-63.

Bernier J, Hall EJ, Giaccia A. Radiation oncology: a century of achievements. Nature Reviews/Cancer 2004;4:737-47.

Bertrand L. Essais de traitement du cancer par le cancer. Annal. de la Soc. de Med. d'Anvers in 1909: 111-16.

Bett WR. Historical aspects of cancer. In: Cancer. Ed. Raven, London, Butterworth & Co. 1954;1-5.

Biden WM. Stilboestrol for breast tumour. Brith Med J 1943;ii:57.

Bloemers HPJ. Schat uit de keuken van een Duits kasteel. De ontdekking van het DNA 1869-2007. Nijmegen, Valkhofpers: 2007.

Bluming AZ, Vogel CL, Zeigler JL, Mody N, Kamya G. Immunological effects of BCG in malignant melanoma: modes of administration compared. Ann Intern Med 1972; 76: 405.

Boerman OC. Radiochemische oplossingen. Inaugurale rede, 2008.

Bonadonna G. Advances in anthracycline chemotherapy: epirubicin. Milaan: Masson Italia Editori, 1984.

Bonner JA, Harari PM, Giralt J, Azarnia N, Shin DM, et al. Radiotherapy plus cetuximab for squamous-cell carcinoma of the head and neck. N Engl J Med 2006;354:567-78.

Bordet J. Sur l'agglutination et la dissolution des globules rouges par le serum d'animaux injectés de sang défibriné. Annales de l'Institut Pasteur 1898;12:688-95.

Bouchet A. Geschichte der Chirurgie vom Ende des 18. Jahrhunderts bis zur Gegenwart. In: Illustrierte Geschichte der Medizin. Deel 7: 2541-79. Paris, Salzburg, 1983.

Boveri T. Zur Frage der Entstehung maligner Tumoren. Jena: Gustav Fischer, 1914.

Brock N, Hilgard P, Peukert M, Pohl J, Sindermann H. Basis and new developments in the field of oxazaphosphorines. Cancer Investigation 1988;6:513-32.

Budman DR, Meropol NJ, Reigner B, Creaven PJ, Lichtman SM, et al. Preliminary studies of a novel oral fluoropyrimidine carbamate: capecitabine. J Clin Oncol 1998;16:1795-802.

Buinauskas P, McCredie JA, Brown ER, Cole WH. Experimental treatment of tumors with antibodies. A.M.A. Archives Surg 1959;79:432-37.

Burchenal JH. From wild fowl to stalking horses: alchemy in chemotherapy. Cancer 1975;35:1121-35.

Bussemakers MJ, Bokhoven A van, Verhaegh GW, et al. DD3: a new prostate-specific gene, highly overexpressed in prostate cancer. Cancer Res 1999;59:5975-9.

C

Cabanas RM. An approach for the treatment of penile carcinoma. Cancer 1977;39:456-66.

Cabanne F., Gérard-Marchant R., Destaing F. Geschichte des Kebses. In: Illustrierte Geschichte der Medizin. Deel 8: 2849-70. Paris, Salzburg, 1983.

Carlson LE, Angen M, Cullum J, Goodey E, Koopmans J, et al. High level of untreated distress and fatigue in cancer patients. Br J Cancer 2004;90:2297-304.

Carlson RW. The history and mechanism of action of fulvestrant. Clinical Breast Cancer 2005;6:S5-S8.

Cash R, Brough AJ, Cohen MNP, et al. Aminoglutethimide as an inhibitor of adrenal steroidogenesis: Mechanism of action and therapeutic trial. J Clin Endocrinol Metabol 1967;27:1239-48.

Cassell EJ. Talking with patients. Volume 1: The theory of doctor-patient communication. Volume 2: Clinical technique. Cambridge, Massachusetts: MIT Press, 1985.

Cavaliere R, Ciocatto EC, Giovanella B, et al. Selective heat sensitivity of cancer cells. Cancer 1967;20:1351-81.

Char DH, History of ocular oncology. Ophtalmology 1996;103:S96-101.

Chast F. A brief history of drugs: from plant extracts to DNA technology. In: The practice of medical chemistry, Second edition. Ed. CG Wermuth, Amsterdam, Boston, Heidelberg: Academic Press, 2003. p. 3-28.

Chen AY, Liu LF. DNA topoisomerases: essential enzymes and lethal targets. Ann Review Pharmacol Toxicol 1994;34:191.

Chow LQM, Eckhardt SG. Sunitinib: From rational design to clinical efficacy. J Clin Oncol 2007;25:884-96.

Chu E, DeVita jr VT. Principles of cancer management: chemotherapy. In: Cancer, principles & practice of oncology. Ed. DeVita VT jr, Hellman S, Rosenberg SA. 6th Edition, Philadelphia: Lippincott Williams & Wilkins, 2001. p. 289-306.

Cleaves MA. Radium; with preliminary note on radium rays in the treatment of cancer. Med Record 1903;64:501-6.

Coca AF, Dorrance GM, Lebredo MG. 'Vaccination' in cancer. A report on the results of vaccination therapy as applied in 79 cases of human cancer. Zeitschrift für Immunitätsforschung und Experimentelle Therapie. 1912;13:543-85.

Cole MP, Jones CTA, Todd LDH. A new anti-oestrogen agent in late breast cancer, an early appraisal of ICI46474. Brit J Cancer 1971;25:270-75.

Comroe, Jr JH. Retrospectroscope, missed opportunities. Am Review Respir Disease 1976;114:1167-74.

Cooke R. Dr. Folkman's war. Angiogenesis and the struggle to defeat cancer. New York/Toronto: Random House Inc, 2001.

Corman ML. Contributions of eighteenth and nineteenth century French medicine to colon and rectal surgery. Diseases Colon Rectum 2000;43:S1-28.

Cortes JE, Pazdur R. Docetaxel. J Clin Oncol 1995;13:2643-55.

Couch FJ, Weber BL. Breast cancer. In: The genetic basis of human cancer. Eds B. Vogelstein, KW Kinzler. New York/Chicago: McGraw-Hill, 2002. p. 549-81.

Creech O, Krementz ET, Ryan RF, Winblad JN. Chemotherapy of cancer: regional perfusion utilizing an extracorporeal circuit. Ann Surg 1958;148:616-32.

Cunningham TJ, Olson KB, Laffin R, Horton J, Sullivan J. Treatment of advanced cancer with active immunization. Cancer 1969;24:932-37.

Currie GA. Eighty years of immunotherapy: a review of immunological methods used for the treatment of human cancer. Br J Cancer 1972;26:141-53.

Curtin JF, Cotter TG. Historical perspectives. Essays in Biochemistry 2003;39:1-10.

Cvitkovic E. An historical perspective on oxaliplatin: rethinking the role of platinum compounds and learning from near misses. Semin Oncol 1998;25(suppl 5):1-3.

Czajkowski NP, Rosenblatt M, Vazquez J. New method of active immunisation to autologous human tumour tissue. Lancet 1967;ii:905-9.

D

Daley GQ, Etten RA van, Baltimore D. Induction of chronic myelogenous leukemia in mice by the P210bcr/abl gene of the Philadelphia chromosoom. Science 1990;247:824-30.

Dalton SO, Boesen EH, Ross L, Schapiro IR, Johanson C. Mind and cancer: do psychological factors cause cancer? Europ J Cancer 2002;38:1313-23.

Davis IA, Jefford M, Parente P, Cebon J. Rational approaches to human cancer immunotherapy. J Leukoc Biol 2003;73:3-29.

Demetri GD, Mehren M von, Blanke CD, Abbeele AD Van den, Eisenberg B, Roberts PJ, et al. Efficacy and safety of imatinib mesylate in advanced gastrointestinal stromal tumors. N Eng J Med 2002;347:472-80.

Demetri GD, Van Oosterom AT, Garret CR, Blackstein ME, Shah MH et al. Efficacy and safety of sunitinib in patients with advanced gastrointestinal stromal tumour after failure of imatinib: a randomised controlled trial. Lancet 2006; 368: 1329-38??

Denmeade SR, Isaacs JT. A history of prostate cancer treatment. Nature Reviews 2002;2:389-96.

DeVita VT, Lewis BJ, Rozencweig M, Muggia FM. The chemotherapy of Hodgkin's disease. Past experience and future directions. Cancer 1978;42:979-90.

Diamandopoulos GTh: Cancer: an historical perspective. Anticancer Research 1996, 16:1595-602.

Dickson JA. Hyperthermia in the treatment of cancer. Lancet 1979;i:202-5.

Dombernowsky P. Smith I, Falkson G, et al. Letrozole, a new oral aromatase inhibitor for advanced breast cancer: double blind randomised trial showing a dose effect and improved efficacy and tolerability compared with megestrolacetate. J Clin Oncol 1998;16:453-61.

Dufour A. Geschichte der Urologie. In: Illustrierte Geschichte der Medizin. Deel 4. Paris, Salzburg, 1981. p. 1429-81.

Duque-Parra JE. Note on the origin and history of the term 'Apoptosis'. Anat Rec B New Anat 2005;283B:2-4.

E

Ebbell B. The papyrus Ebers: The greatest Egyptian medical document. Copenhagen: Levin and Munksgaard, 1937.

Edwards AGK, Hailey S, Maxwell M. Psychological interventions for women with metastatic breast cancer. Cochrane Database of Systemic Reviews 2004, Issue 2. Art. No.: CD004253. DOI: 10.1002/14651858. CD004253.pub2

Etter LE. Some historical data relating to the discovery of the roentgen rays. Am J Roentgenology 1946;56:220-31.

Evans TRJ, Salle ED, Ornati G, et al. Phase I and endocrine study of exemestane (FCE 24304), a new aromatase inhibitor, in postmenopausal women. Cancer Res 1992;52:5933-9.

Everson TC, Cole WH. Spontaneous regression of cancer. Philadelphia/London: W.B. Saunders, 1966.

Ewing J. Neoplastic diseases. Philadelphia/London: W.B. Saunders Company, 1919.

F

Farber S, Diamond LK, Mercer RD, Sylvester RF, Wolff JA. Temporary remissions in acute leukemia in children produced by folic antagonist, 4-aminopteroylglutamic acid (aminopterin). N Engl J Med 1948;238: 787-93.

Feigenberg L. Terminal care, friendships contracts with dying cancer patients. New York: Brunner/Mazel, 1980.

Ferrara N, Hillan KJ, Gerber HP, Novotny W. Discovery and development of bevacizumab, an anti-VEGF antibody for treating cancer. Nature Reviews/Drug Discovery 2004;3:391-400.

Figdor PP. Philipp Bozzini, der Begin der modernen Endoskopie. Volume 1:2002.

Finney JW, Byers EH, Wilson RH. Studies in tumor auto-immunity. Cancer Research 1960;20:351-56.

Fisher B, Anderson S, Bryant J, et al. Twenty-year follow-up of a randomized trial comparing total mastectomy, lumpectomy, and lumpectomy plus irradiation for the treatment of invasive breast cancer 2002;347:1233-41.

Fisher B, Costantino JP, Wickerham DL, Cecchini RS, Cronin WM, et al. Tamoxifen for prevention of breast cancer: Current status of the National Surgical Adjuvant Breast and Bowel Project. J Nat Cancer Inst 2005;97:1652-62.

Fisher B, Dignam J, Bryant J, et al. Five versus more than five years of tamoxifen therapy for breast cancer patients with negative lymph nodes and estrogen receptor-positive tumors. J Natl Cancer Inst 1996;88:1529-42.

Fisher ER, Hermann CM. Historic milestones in cancer pathology. Semin Oncol 1979;6: 428-32.

Folkman J. Tumor angiogenesis: therapeutic implications. N Engl J Med 1971;285:1182-6.

Ford CE, Hamerton JL, Barnes DWH, et al. Cytological identification of radiation-chimaeras. Nature 1956;177:452-54.

Forgue E, Bouchet A. Die Chirurgie bis zum ende des 18.Jahrhunderts. In: Illustrierte Geschichte der Medizin, deel 3. Paris/Salzburg, 1980. p. 931-1191.

Formigli L, Conti AA, Lippi D. 'Falling leaves': a survey of the history of apoptosis. Minerva Med 2004;95:159-64.

Fuhrman GM. The legacy of Allen Oldfather Whipple. Current Surgery 2005;62:275-6.

G

Gaarenstroom GF. Behandeling van kwaadaardige gezwellen met Röntgenstralen. Ned T v Gen 1915; 59: 1900-21

Geisler L. Arzt und Patient. Begegnung im Gespräch. Frankfurt: Pharma Verlag, 1987.

Giard RWM. Bij de 65e verjaardag van het uitstrijkje: onduidelijke meerwaarde van het bevolkingsonderzoek op baarmoederhalskanker. Ned Tijdschr Geneeskd 2007;151:1268-71.

Gilman A, The initial clinical trial of nitrogen mustard. Am J Surg 1963;105:574-8.

Gocht H. Therapeutische Verwendung der Röntgenstralen. Fortschritte auf dem gebiete der Röntgenstrahlen 1897; 1: 14-22.

Goldstein NI, Prewett M, Zuklys K, Rockwell P, Mendelsohn J. Biological efficacy of a chimeric antibody to the epidermal growth factor receptor in a human tumor xenograft model. Clin Cancer Res 1995;1:1311-18.

Graham FL, Eb AJ van der, Heijneker HL. Size and location of the transforming region in human adenovirus type 5 DNA. Nature 1974;251:687-91.

Graham JB, Graham RM. The effect of vaccine on cancer patients. Surg Gynec Obstet 1959; 114; 131-38

Gray LH, Conger AO, Ebert M, Hornsey S, Scot OCA. The concentration of oxygen dissolved in tissues at the time of irradiation as a factor in radiotherapy. Br J Radiol 1953;26:638-48.

Gresser I, Bourali C, Lévy JP, Fontaine-Brouty-Boyé D, Thomas MT. Increased survival in mice inoculated with tumor cells and treated with interferon preparations. Proc Natl Acad Sci 1969;63:51-7.

Greten TF, Jaffee EM. Cancer vaccines. J Clin Oncol 1999;17:1047-60.

Griffiths CT. Surgical resection of tumor bulk in the primary treatment of ovarian carcinoma. Natl Cancer Inst Monogr 1975;42:101.

Grigg ERN. The trail of the invisible light. Etter LE, ed. Springfield: Charles C. Thomas Publisher, 1965.

Grillo-López AJ. Rituximab: an insider's historical perspective. Semin Oncol 2000;27 (suppl 12)9-16.

Gross R, Lambers K. Erste Erfahrungen in der Behandlung maligner Tumoren mit einem neuen N-Lost-Phosphamidester. Dtsch Med Wschr 1958;83:458-62.

H

Hadju SI. 2000 Years of chemotherapy of tumors. Cancer 2005;103:1097-102.

Hall JF, Lee MK, Newman B, Morrow JE, Anderson LA, Huey B, et al. Linkage of early-onset familial breast cancer to chromosome 17q21. Science 1990;250:1684-89.

Halteren HK van, Bongaerts GPA, Wagener DJT. Cancer and psychosocial distress: frequent companions. Lancet 2004;364:824-5.

Hayes DM, Cvitkovic E, Golbey RB, et al. High dose cis-platinum diammine dichloride. Cancer 1977;39:1372-81.

Heald RJ. Rectal cancer: the surgical options. Eur J Cancer 1998;31A:1189-92.

Heilmann FR, Kendall EC. The influence of 11-dehydro-17-hydroxycorticosterone (Compound E) on the growth of malignant tumor in the Mouse. Endocrinology 1944; 34: 416

Heisterkamp N, Groffen J, Stephenson JR, Spurr NK, Goodfellow PN, et al. Chromosomal localization of human cellular homologues of two viral oncogenes. Nature 1982;299:747-9.

Heisterkamp N, Stephenson JR, Groffen J, Hansen PF, Klein A de, et al. Localization of the c-abl oncogene adjacent to a translocation break point in chronic myelocytic leukaemia. Nature 1983;306:239-42.

Hellström KE, Hellström I. Cellular immunity against tumour antigens. Advances Cancer Res 1969;12:167-223.

Henry GW. Some modern aspects of psychiatry in general hospital practice. Am J Psychiatry 1929;86:481-99.

Henschke UK, Hilaris BS, Mahan GD. Afterloading in interstitial and intracavitary radiation therapy. Am J Roentgenol Radium Ther Nucl Med 1963;90:386-95.

Herbst RS, Langer CJ. Epidermal growth factor receptors as a target for cancer treatment: the emerging role of IMC-C225 in the treatment of lung and head and neck cancers. Semin Oncol 2002;29(suppl 4);27-36.

Héricourt J, Richet Ch. Physiologie pathologique. De la sérothérapie dans le traitement du cancer. C r hebd Séance Acad Sci 1895;121:567-9.

Herodotus, Histories, Book 6, passage 117. Many translations of Herodotus's Histories exist. One of the most recent is: Herodotus, The Histories, Carolyn Dewald (ed.), Robin Waterfield (translator), Oxford World's Classics, OUP, Oxford & New York, reissued 2008. A much older translation, which still reads very well, is that of William Beloe, published in Philadelphia, USA, in 1814.

Hill II GJ. Historic milestones in cancer surgery. Semin Oncol 1979;6:409-27.

Hobday TJ, Perez EA. Molecularly targeted therapies for breast cancer. Cancer Control 2005;12:73-81.

Hodt HJ, Sinclair WT, Smithers DW. A gun for interstitial implantation of radioactive gold grains. Br. J. Radiol. 25:419-420, 1952.

Holland JC. History of psycho-oncology: Overcoming attitudinal and conceptual barriers. Psychosom Med 2002;64:206-21.

Holland JC. IPOS Sutherland memorial lecture: an international perspective on the development of psychosocial oncology: overcoming cultural and attitudinal barriers to improve psychosocial care. Psycho-oncology 2004;13:445-59.

Holsti LR. Development of clinical radiotherapy since 1896. Acta Oncologica 1995;34: 995-1003.

Horwitz KB, McGuire WL. Progesterone and progesterone receptors in experimental breast cancer. Cancer Research 1977;37: 1733-8.

Houtzager HL. Voorwoord: Gezondheidszorg. In: Andel MA van. Chirurgijns, vrije meesters, beunhazen en kwakzalvers. De chirurgijngilden en de praktijk der heelkunde (1400-1800). Tweede druk. 's Gravenhage: Martinus Nijhoff, 1981.

Hsiang Y-H, Hertzberg R, Hecht S, Liu L. Camptothecin induces protein-linked dna breaks via mammalian DNA topoisomerase I. J Biol Chem 1985; 260: 14873-78.

Huggins C. Endocrine-induced regression of cancers. Nobel lecture, 1966.

Hughes LE, Kearney R, Tully M. A study in clinical cancer immunotherapy. Cancer 1970;26:269-78.

Humphrey LJ, Jewell WR, Murray DR, Griffen Jr WO. Immunotherapy for the patient with cancer. Ann Surg 1971;173:47-54.

I

Iveson TJ, Smith IE, Ahern J, et al. Phase I study of the oral non steroidal aromatase inhibitor CGS 20267 in postmenopausal patients with breast cancer. Cancer Res 1993;53:266-70.

J

Jacobson LO, Marks EK, Robson MJ, et al. Effect of spleen protection on mortality following x-irradiation. J Lab Clin Med 1949;34: 1538-43.

Jakobovits I. Jewish medical ethics, a comparative and historical study of the jewish religious attitude to medicine and its practice. New York: Bloch Publishing Company, 1975.

Joensuu H, Roberts PJ, Sarlomo-Rikala M, Andersson LC, Tervahartiala P, et al. Effect of the tyrosine kinase inhibitor STI571 in a patient with metastatic gastrointestinal stromal tumor. N Engl J Med 2001;344: 1052-6.

Jordan VC. The development of tamoxifen for breast cancer therapy: a tribute to the late Arthur L. Pole. Breast Cancer Research and Treatment 1988;11:197-209.

K

Kaae S, Johansen H. Does simple mastectomy followed by irradiation offer survival comparable to radical procedures? Int J Radiat Oncol Biol Phys 1977;2:1163-6.

Kantarjian H, Sawyers C, Hochhaus A, Guilhot F, Schiffer C, et al. Hematologic and cytogenetic responses to imatinib mesylate in chronic myelogenous leukaemia. N Eng J Med 2002;346:645-52.

Kaplan HS. Historic milestones in radiobiology and radiation therapy. Semin Oncol 1979; 6:479-89.

Kardinal CG, Yarbro JW. A conceptual history of cancer. Semin Oncol 1979;6:396-408.

Kardinal CG. Cancer chemotherapy, historical aspects and future considerations. Postgrad Med 1985;77:165-74.

Kardinal CG. Chemotherapy of breast cancer. In: The chemotherapy source book. Perry MC, ed. Baltimore: Williams & Wilkins, 1992. p. 948-88.

Kellock TH, Chambers H. An attempt to procure immunity to malignant disease in man. Lancet 1922;i:217-19.

Kendall EC. The development of cortisone as a therapeutic agent. Nobel prize lecture. December 11, 1950

Kerr JFR, Wyllie AH, Currie AR. Apoptosis: a basic biological phenomenon with wide-range implications in tissue kinetics. Br J Cancer 1972;26:239-57.

Kerr JFR. History of the events leading to the formulation of the apoptosis concept. Toxicology 2002;181-182:471-4.

Kim KJ, Li B, Winer J, Armanini M, Gillett N, Phillips HS, Ferrara N. Inhibition of vascular endothelial growth factor-induced angiogenesis suppresses tumour growth in vivo. Nature 1993;362:841-4.

King MC. Introduction. In: Bazell R. Her-2, the making of Herceptin, a revolutionary treatment for breast cancer. New York: Random House, 1998.

Kinzler KW, Vogelstein B. Lessons from hereditary colorectal cancer. Cell 1996;87:159-70.

Kistner RW, Baginsky S, Craig JM, Bigler P. Effect of progestins on induced endometrial cancer in the rabbit. Surg Forum 1962;13:410-2.

Kistner RW, Griffiths CT, Craig JM. Use of progestational agents in the management of endometrial cancer. Cancer 1965;18:1563-79.

Klein A de, Geurts van Kessel A, Grosveld G, Bartram CR, Hagemeijer A, Bootsma D, et al. A cellular oncogene is translocated to the Philadelphia chromosome in chronic myelocytic leukemia. Nature 1982;300:765-7.

Klijn JGM, Jong FH de. Treatment with a luteinising-hormone analogue (buserelin) in premenopausal patients with metastatic breast cancer. Lancet 1982;1:1213-16.

Kok JB De, Verhaegh GW, Roelofs RW, et al. DD3(PCA3), a very sensitive and specific marker to detect prostate tumors. Cancer Res 2002;62:2695-8.

Kolata G. Frenchman says Nobel panel overlooked his contribution. New York Times. Health ed. 1989, October 11.

Körte W. Erfahrungen über die operative Behandlung der malignen Dickdarm-Geschwülste. In: [B. von Langenbeck's] Archiv für Klinische Chirurgie. Band LXI. Berlin: Verlag von A. Hirschwald, 1900. p. 403-62.

Korteweg R, Thomas F. Tumor induction and tumor growth in hypophysectomized mice. Am J Cancer 1939;37:36.

Krueger G. The formation of the American Society of Clinical Oncology and the development of a medical speciality, 1964-1973. Persp Biol Med 2004;47:537-51.

L

Lacquet L. Persoonlijke mededeling, 2007.

Laszlo J, Buckley CE, Amos DB. Infusion of isologous immune plasma in chronic lymphocytic leukaemia. Blood 1968;31:104-10.

Laurie JA, Moertel CG, Fleming et al. Surgical adjuvant therapy of large-bowel carcinoma: an evaluation of levamisol and the combination of levamisol and fluorouracil. J Clin Oncol 1989; 7: 1447-56

Lena M De, Brambilla C, Valagussa P, Bonadonna G. High-dose medroxyprogesterone acetate in breast cancer resistant to endocrine and cytotoxic therapy. Cancer Chemother Pharmacol 1979;2:175-80.

Lewison EF, Brown RW, Thomas JW, Sykes JF, Ovary Z. 'Protective' colostrum in the treatment of patients with advanced breast cancer. Archs Surg 1960; 8: 176.

Leyden E von, Blumenthal F. Vorläufige Mitteilungen über einige Ergebnisse der Krebsforschung auf der I. medizinische Klinik. Deutsche Mediz Wochenschr 1902;36:637-8.

Li M C. Letter to the Editor, CA Cancer J Clin 1973;23;375-376

Li MC, Hertz R and Spencer DB. Effect of methotrexate therapy upon choriocarcinoma and chorioadenoma. NEJM 1958, 259: 361-66.

Linehan WM, Zbar B, Bates SE, Zelefsky MJ, Yang JC. Cancer of the kidney and ureter. In: DeVita Jr VT, Hellman S, Rosenberg SA. Cancer, principle and practice of oncology. Philadelphia: Lippincott, Williams & Wilkins, 2001. p. 1362.

Lipton A, Harvey HA, Balch CM, Antle CE, Heckard R, Bartolucci AA. Corynebacterium parvum versus bacilli Calmette-Guérin adjuvant immunotherapy of stage II malignant melanoma. J Clin Oncology 1991;9:1151-6.

Litt P. Photon finish. In: The Beaver: Exploring Canada's History, 1 April 2002

Little RF, Wyvill KM, Pluda JM, Welles L, Marshall V, et al. Activity of thalidomide in AIDS-related Kaposi's sarcoma. J Clin Oncol 2000;18:2593-602.

Lorenz E, Uphoff D, Reid TR, et al. Modification of irradiation injury in mice and guinea pigs by bone marrow injections. J Natl Cancer Inst 1951;12:197-201.

Löwy I. Experimental systems and clinical practices: tumor immunology and cancer immunotherapy, 1895-1980. J Hist Biol 1994;27: 403-35.

Lugo TG, Pendergast AM, Muller AJ, Witte ON. Tyrosine kinase activity and transformation potency of bcr-abl oncogene products. Science 1990;247:1079-82.

Lyons AS, Petrucelli RJ. Medicine, an illustrated history. New York: Abradale Press, Harry N Abrams Inc., 1987.

Lyons AS. Medicine in Roman times. In: AS Lyons. RJ Petrucelli. Medicine, an illustrated history. Part 1. New York: Abradale Press, HN Abrams Publ., 1987a. p. 231-64.

Lyons AS. Medicine under Islam. In: AS Lyons. RJ Petrucelli. Medicine, an illustrated history. Part 1. New York: Abradale Press, HN Abrams Publ., 1987b. p. 295-18.

Lyons AS. Women in medicine. In: AS Lyons. RJ Petrucelli. Medicine, an illustrated history. Part 2. New York: Abradale Press, HN Abrams Publ., 1987c. p. 565-76.

M

Maanen H van, Lieverse R, Everdingen J van. De handschoen. In: Uit de oude dokterstas. Amsterdam: Boom Belvédère, 1998. p. 85-7.

Mainwaring WIP, Freeman SN, Harper B. Pharmacology of antiandrogens. In: Furr BJA en Wakeling AE, eds. Pharmacology and clinical uses of inhibitors of hormone secretion and action. London/Philadelphia: Baillière Tindall, 1987. p. 106-31.

Marra G, Boland CR. Hereditary nonpolyposis colorectal cancer: the syndrome, the genes, and historical perspectives. J Natl Cancer Inst 1995;87:1114-25.

Marston Linehan W, Zbar B, Bates SE, Zelefsky MJ, Yang JC. Cancer of the kidney and ureter. In: DeVita VT, Hellman S, Rosenberg SA, eds. Cancer, principles & practice of oncology. 6th ed. Philadelphia: Lippincott, Williams & Wilkins, 2001. p. 1362-96.

Mathé G, Amiel JL, Schwarzenberg L, Hayat M, Pouillart P, et al. Immunothérapie active des leucémies aigues et des lymphosarcomes leucémique. Nouv Presse Méd 1975;4: 1337-42.

Mathé G, Amiel SL, Schwartzenberg L, Schneider M, Cattan A, et al. Active immunotherapy for acute lymphoblastic leukemia. Lancet 1969;1:697-99.

McCarty PJ, Million RR. History of radiation oncology. J Florida M A 1995;82:745-8.

McGuire WP, Rowinsky EK. Paclitaxel in cancer treatment. New York: Marcel Dekker, 1995.

McGurk M, Goodger NM. Head and neck cancer and its treatment: historical review. Br J Oral Maxillofac Surg 2000;38:209-20.

McWhirter R. The value of simple mastectomy and radiotherapy in the treatment of cancer of the breast. Br J Radiol 1948;21:599-10.

Mendelsohn J, Baselga J. The EGF receptor family as targets for cancer therapy. Oncogene 2000;19:6550-65.

Mihich E. Historical overview of biologic response modifiers. Cancer Investigation 2000;18:456-66.

Miller EC, Miller JA. Milestones in chemical carcinogenesis. Semin Oncol 1979;6:445-60.

Mitchell M, Eschen KB von. Phase III trial of Melacine melanoma theraccine versus combination chemotherapy in the treatment of stage IV melanoma. Proc ASCO 1997;16:494a (abstr. 1778).

Mitchell M. Perspective on allogeneic melanoma lysate in active specific immunotherapy. Semin Oncol 1998;25:623-35.

Moertel CG, Fleming TR, Macdonald JS, et al. Levamisole and fluorouracil as effective adjuvant therapy after resection of stage III colon carcinoma: a final report. Ann Int Med 1995;122:321-26.

Montgomery JA. Chemistry and structure-activity studies of the nitrosoureas. Canc Treatm Reports 1976;60:651-64.

Motzer RJ, Michaelson MD, Rosenberg J, Bukowski RM, Curti BD et al. Sunitinib efficacy against advanced renal cell carcinoma. J Urology 2007a; 178: 1883-7.

Motzer RJ, Hutson TE, Tomczak P, Michaelson MD, Bukowski RM et al. Sunitinib versus interferon alfa in metastatic renal-cell carcinoma. NEJM 2007b; 356: 115-24.

Mould RF. Invited review: The early years of radiotherapy with emphasis on X-ray and radium apparatus. Brit J Radiology 1995;68:567-82.

Mould RF. Pierre Curie 1859 – 1906. Current Oncologie 2007; 14:74-82

Moulin D De. A history of surgery, with emphasis on the Netherlands. Boston/The Hague: Martinus Nijhoff, 1988.

Moulin D De. A short history of breast cancer. Boston/The Hague: Martinus Nijhoff, 1983.

Moyer JD, Barbacci EG, Iwata KK, Arnold L, Boman B et al. Induction of apoptosis and cell cycle arrest by CP-358, 774, an inhibitor of epidermal growth factor receptor tyrosine kinase. Cancer Res 1997;57:4838-48.

Muderspach L, Wilczynski S, Roman L, Bade L, Felix J. A phase I trial of a human papillomavirus (HPV) peptide vaccine for women with high-grade cervical and vulvar intraepithelial neoplasia who are HPV 16 positive. Clin Cancer Res 2000;6:3406-16.

Muir, J. The Cancer Curer in South Africa, South African Medical Record, January [year not given, probably 1906 or shortly thereafter], pp. 5-8

Murray G. Experiments in immunity in cancer. Canad M A J 1958;79:249-59.

Muss HB, Case LD, Capizzi RL, Cooper MR, et al. High versus standard dose megestrol acetate in women with advanced breast cancer: a phase III trial of the Piedmont Oncology Association. J Clin Oncol 1990;8:1797-805.

Myerscough PR. Talking with patients, a basic clinical skill. Oxford: Oxford Medical Publications, 1989.

N

Nissen-Meyer R. Castration as part of the primary treatment for operable female breast cancer. A statistical evaluation of clinical results. Acta Radiol, Stockholm, Suppl. 1965;249: 1-133.

Nissen-Meyer R. The role of prophylactic castration in the therapy of human mammary cancer. Eur J Cancer 1967;3:395-403.

Nordenstam JF, Bulander RE, Mellgren AF, Rothenberger DA,. Evolution of surgery for colorectal cancer. In: Gillison W, Buchwald H, eds. Pioneers in surgical gastroenterology, 2007. Ch. 14, p. 237-251.

Novack DH, Plumer R, Smith RL, Ochitill H, Morrow GR, Bennett JM. Changes in physicians' attitudes toward telling the cancer patient. JAMA 1979;241:897-900.

O

O'Connel MJ, Laurie JA, Kahn M, et al. Prospectively randomized trial of postoperative adjuvant chemotherapy in patients with high-risk colon cancer. J Clin Oncol 1998;16:295-300.

O'Shea JS. Specialisation in surgical oncology: Historical perspectives. Ann of Surg Oncol 2004;11:462-64.

Oken D. What to tell cancer patients, a study of medical attitudes. JAMA 1961;175:86-94.

Old LJ, Clarke DA, Benacerraf B. Effects of Bacillus Calmette-Guérin infection on transplanted tumors in the mouse. Nature 1959;184: 291-2.

Oudard S, George D, Medioni J, Motzer R. Treatment options in renal cell carcinoma: past, present and future. Annals of Oncology 2007; 18 (supplement 10):x25-x31.

Overgaard J, Hansen HS, Overgaard M, Basholt L, Berthelsen A, et al. A randomized double blind phase III study of nimorazole as a hypoxic radiosensitizer of primary radiotherapy in supraglottic larynx and pharynxcarcinoma. Results of the Danish Head and Neck Cancer Study (DAHANCA). Protocol 5-85. Radiother Oncol 1998;46:135-45.

Overholser, W. and Bromberg, W. Man above humanity: a history of psychotherapy. Kessinger Publishing, Whitefish, MT, USA, 2007. (New edition of a book originally published by Bromberg in 1954.).

P

Palca J. Gene therapy may bring cancer-killing cells. Research News, August 10, 2007.

Pannuti F, Martini A, Di Marco AR, et al. Prospective, randomized clinical trial of two different high dosages of medroxyprogesterone acetate (MAP) in the treatment of metastatic breast cancer. Eur J Cancer 1979;15:593-601.

Papac RJ. Origins of cancer therapy. Yale J Biol Med 2001;74:391-8.

Pardoll DM. Cancer vaccines. Nature medicine, vaccine supplement 1998;4:S25-S31.

Parish CR. Cancer immunotherapy: The past, the present and the future. Immunol Cell Biol 2003;81:106-13.

Park K. The life of the corpse: Division and dissection in late medieval Europe. J Hist Med Allied Sci 1995;50:111-32.

Patlak M. Targeting leukemia. The FASEB Journal. 2002;16:273.

Patterson JT. The dread disease. Cancer and modern American culture. Cambridge: Harvard University Press, 1987.

Pearson HA. History of pediatric hematology oncology. Pediatric Research 2002;52: 979-92.

Pearson OH, Li C, Maclean JP, Lipsett MB, Wood CD. Management of metastatic mammary cancer. J Am Med Assoc 1955;159:1701-4.

Petrakis NL. Historic milestones in cancer epidemiology. Semin Oncol 1979;6:433-44.

Petrucelli RS. The dark ages. In: AS Lyons, RJ Petrucelli. Medicine, an illustrated history. New York: Abradale Press, HN Abrams Publ., 1987b. p. 279-94.

Petrucelli RS. The middle ages. In: AS Lyons, RJ Petrucelli. Medicine, an illustrated history. New York: Abradale Press, HN Abrams Publ., 1987c. p. 337-68.

Petrucelli RS. The rise of Christianity. In: AS Lyons, RJ Petrucelli. Medicine, an illustrated history. New York: Abradale Press, HN Abrams Publ., 1987a. p. 265-78.

Pierce HL, Miller MA. The evolution of cancer research and drug discovery at Lilly research laboratories. Adv Enzyme Regul 2005;45:229-55.

Platner JZ. Handleiding tot de Chirurgie of Heelkonst. Amsterdam: Uitgever F. Houttuyn, 1764. p. 11.

Potapova O, Laird AD, Nannini MA, Barone A, Li G, et al. Contribution of individual targets to the antitumor efficacy of the multitargeted receptor tyrosine kinase inhibitor SU11248. Mol Cancer Ther 2006;5:1280-9.

Potmesil M. Camptothecins: From bench to hospital wards. Cancer Res 1994;54:1431-9.

Pouw Kraan CTM van der, Dijkstra CD, Verweij CL. Moleculaire ontrafeling van ziekte met DNA-microarrays. Ned Tijdschr Geneeskd 2005;149:626-31.

Proux C. Geschichte der Radiotherapie. In: Illustrierte Geschichte der Medizin. Deel 7. Paris/Salzburg, 1983. p. 2223-41.

Q

Quesada JR, Reuben J, Manning JT, Hersh EM, Gutterman JU. Alpha interferon for induction of remission in hairy-cell leukemia. N Engl J Med 1984;310:15-8.

Qumsiyeh MB, Li P. Molecular biology of cancer: cytogenetics. In: DeVita Jr VT, Hellman S, Rosenberg SA. Cancer, principle and practice of oncology. Philadelphia: Lippincott Williams & Wilkins, 2001. p. 77.

R

Raspail FV. Recherches et physiologique destineés à expliquer, non-seulement la structure et le developpement de la feuille, du tronc, ainsi que de organes qui n'en sont qu'une transformation, mais encore la structure et le développement des tissues animaux. Mem Soc Hist Nat Paris 1827;3:17, 208.

Rather LJ. The genesis of cancer. A study in the history of ideas. Baltimore: Johns Hopkins Univ. Press, 1978.

Raven RW. The theory and practice of oncology, historical evolution and present principles. Camforth, NJ: Parthenon Publising Group, 1990.

Recamier JCA. Recherces sur le traitement du cancer. Parijs: Gabon, 1829.

Reichert JM, Rosensweig CJ, Faden LB, Dewitz MC. Monoclonal antibody successes in the clinic. Nat Biotechnol 2005;23:1073-8.

Remers WA. Mitomycin C and analog development. In: Carter SK, Crooke ST. Mitomycin C, current status and new developments. New York: Academic Press, 1979. p. 27-40.

Ribeiro G, Swindell R. The Christie Hospital tamoxifen (Nolvadex) adjuvant trial for operable breast carcinoma. 7 years results. Eur J Cancer Clin Oncol 1985;21:897-900.

Ribot JG. Geschiedenis van de radiotherapie. Kanker 2005;29:18-23.

Richards V. Current Cancer Immunology. In: Bertino JR. Progress in experimental tumor research. 25 vol. Basel: S. Karger, 1980.

Riskin DJ, Longaker MT, Gertner M, Krummel TM. Innovation in surgery, a historical perspective. Ann of Surgery 2006;244:686-93.

Roberts JA. Immunotherapy in the treatment of cancer. Scot Med J 1977;22:320-30.

Rosenberg B. Fundamental studies with cisplatin. Cancer 1985;55:2303-16.

Rosenberg SA. Principles of cancer management: surgical oncology. In: DeVita VT, Hellman S, Rosenberg SA, eds. Cancer, principles & practice of oncology. 6th ed. Philadelphia: Lippincott, Williams & Wilkins, 2001. p. 253-65.

Ross JS, Schenkein DP, Pietrusko R, Rolfe M, Linette GP, et al. Targeted therapies for cancer 2004. Am J Clin Pathol 2004;122:598-609.

Rowley JD. A new consistent chromosomal abnormality in chronic myelogenous leukaemia identified by quinacrine fluorescence and giemsa staining. Nature 1973;243:290-93.

Rudnick, H. A brief history of Western psychotherapy. Chapter 2 of The links between Western psychotherapy and traditional healing, Doctoral thesis, Rand Afrikaans University 2002. Accessed online via: etd.rau.ac.za/theses/available/etd-05052004-113647/restricted/chap2modern.pdf

Rushman GB, Davies NJH, Atkinson RS. A short history of anaesthesia, the first 150 years. Oxford: Butterworth Heinemann, 1996. p. 9-19.

s

Santen RJ, Worgul TJ, Samojlik E, Interrante A, Boucher AE, et al. Randomized trial comparing surgical adrenalectomy with aminoglutethimide plus hydrocortisone in women with advanced breast carcinoma. N Engl J Med 1981;305:545-51.

Santoro E. The history of gastric cancer: legends and chronicles. Gastric Cancer 2005;8:71-74.

Sato JD, Kawamoto T, Le AD, Mendelsohn J, Polikoff J, Sato GH. Biological effects in vitro of monoclonal antibodies to human EGF receptors. Mol Biol Med 1983;1:511-29.

Savage-Smith E. Attitudes toward dissection in medieval Islam. J Hist Med Allied Sci 1995;50: 67-110.

Scaliotti GV. Potential role of multi-targeted tyrosine kinase inhibitors in non-small-cell lung cancer. Annals of Oncology 2007; 18 (supplement 10):x32-x41.

Schier MJ. University of Texas M.D. Anderson Cancer Center. In: The Handbook of Texas Online 2001.

Schöffski P, Dumez H, Clement P, Hoeben A, Prenen H, et al. Emerging role of tyrosine kinase inhibitors in the treatment of advanced renal cell cancer: a review. Ann Oncol 2006;17:1185-96.

Schubert EL, Hansen MF, Strong LC. The retinoblastoma gene and its significance. Ann Med 1994;26:177-84.

Selikoff IJ, Hammond EC, Churg J: Asbestos exposure, smoking and neoplasia. JAMA 1968;204:106-12.

Shah JP. The making of a speciality. Am J Surg 1998; 176:398-403.

Shands HC, Finesinger JE, Cobb S, Abrams Rd. Psychological mechanisms in patients with cancer. Cancer 1951;4:1159-70.

Sharma R, Beith J, Hamilton A. Systematic review of LHRH agonists for the adjuvant treatment of early breast cancer. The Breast 2005;14: 181-91.

Shimkin MB. Contrary to nature...cancer. US Dept of Health, education and welfare. Public health service NIH. Distributie: Tunbridge Wells: Carlile House Publications LTD, 1979.

Singhal S, Mehta J, Desikan R, Ayers D, Roberson P, et al. Antitumor activity of thalidomide in refractory multiple myeloma. N Engl J Med 1999;341:1565-71.

Skibber JM, Minsky BC, Hoff PO. Cancer of the colon. In: DeVita VT jr, Hellman S, Rosenberg SA, eds. Cancer, principles & practice of oncology. 6th ed. Philadelphia: Lippincott, 2001. p. 1216-71.

Slamon DJ, Clark GM, Wong S, Levin WJ, Ullrich A, McGuire WL. Human breast cancer: correlation of relapse and survival with amplification of the Her-2/neu oncogene. Science 1987;235:177-82.

Sluis RF van der. David van Gesscher. Academisch proefschrift. Nijmegen: Katholieke universiteit Nijmegen, 1990. p. 45-46.

Smith GV, Smith OW. Carcinoma of the breast. Results and evaluation of X radiation and relation of age and surgical castration to length of survival. Surg Gynec Obstet 1953;97:508-16.

Sorbiere S de. Advice to a young physician respecting the way in which he is to conduct himself in the practice of medicine, in view of the indifference of the public to the subject, and considering the complaints that are made about physicians (1672). Quoted in: Katz J. The silent world of doctor and patient. New York: Free Press, 1984:10-2.

Southam CM. Applications of immunology to clinical cancer past: attempts and future possibilities. Cancer Research 1961; 21: 1302-16

Spiegel D, Bloom JR, Kraemer HC, Gottheil E. Effect of psychosocial treatment on survival of patients with metastatic breast cancer. Lancet 1989;ii:888-90.

Squire J, Dryja TP, Dunn J, et al. Cloning of the esterase D gene: a polymorphic gene probe closely linked to the retinoblastoma locus on chromosome 13. Proc Natl Acad Sci 1986;83:6573-77.

Stähelin HF, Wartburg A von. The chemical and biological route from podophyllotoxin glucoside to etoposide: Ninth Cain memorial award lecture. Cancer Res 1991;51:5-15.

Stallworthy J. Progress in gynecology, a personal retrospective view. Gynecol Oncol 1979;8:253-64.

Stam HC. Radiotherapie in Nederland, een historisch perspectief. Utrecht: Bunge, 1993.

Staps T. Psycholoog en kankerpatiënt. Med Cont 1983;38:1457-8.

Stehlin JS jr. Hyperthermic perfusion with chemotherapy for cancers of the extremities. Surg Gynec Obstet 1969;129:305-8

Stoll BA. Hormonal management in breast cancer. London: Pitman Medical Publishing Company, 1969.

Stoll BA. Hormone therapy in relation to radiotherapy in the treatment of advanced carcinoma of the breast. Proc Roy Soc Med 1950;43:875.

Suffness M, Wall ME. Discovery and development of taxol. In: Suffness M, Taxol, science and applications. Boca Raton/New York/London/Tokyo: CRC Press, 1995. p. 3-24.

Summer WC, Foraker AG. Spontaneous regression of human melanoma. Cancer 1960;13:79-81.

Surbone A, Zwitter M. Communication with the cancer patient, Information & Truth. Ann New York Acad Sci 1997;809:1-540.

Sutherland AM, Orbach CE, Dyk RB, Bard M. The psychological impact of cancer and cancer surgery. Cancer 1952;5:857-72.

T

Tanis PJ, Nieweg OE, Valdés Olmos RA, Rutgers EJTh, Kroon BBR. History of sentinel node and validation of the technique. Breast Cancer Res 2001;3:109-12.

Taylor CW, Green S, Dalton WS, et al. Multicenter randomized clinical trial of goserelin versus surgical ovariëctomie in premenopausal patients with receptor-positive metastatic breast cancer: an intergroup study. J Clin Oncol 1998;16:994-9.

Thomas ED. Bone marrow transplantation. Semin Haematol 1999;36(suppl 7):95-103.

Thorwald J. Het magische mes, de fascinerende geschiedenis van 'de eeuw der chirurgen'. Derde druk. (year not given) Utrecht: De Fontein.

Tsuchiya R, Fuhsawa N. Historical survey of carcinoma of the pancreas. Hepatobiliary Pancreat Surg 1999;6:165-70.

U

Ullrich A, Coussens L, Hayflick JS, Dull TJ, Gray A, et al. Human epidermal growth factor receptor cDNA sequence and aberrant expression of the amplified gene in A431 epidermoid carcinoma cells. Nature 1984;309:418-25.

V

Varah, C. Before I die again: the autobiography of the founder of the Samaritans. Constable, London, 1993.

Verdan C. Geschichte der plastischen und wiederherstellenden Chirurgie. In: Illustrierte Geschichte der Medizin. Deel 8. Paris/ Salzburg, 1983. p. 2911-29.

Vermorken JB, Claessen AME, Tinteren H van, et al. Active specific immunotherapy for stage II and III human colon cancer: a randomized trial. Lancet 1999;226:198-206.

Vogel VG, Costantino JP, Wickerham DL, Cronin WM, Cecchini RS, et al. Effects of tamoxifen vs raloxifene on the risk of developing invasive breast cancer and other disease outcomes. The NSABP Study of Tamoxifen and Raloxifene (STAR) P-2 trial. JAMA 2006; 295:2727-41.

Vogler WR, Chan YK. Prolonging remission in myeloblastic leukaemia by Tice strain Bacille Calmette-Guérin. Lancet 1974; 2: 128-31.

Vogt PK, The molecular genetics of cancer, tumour suppressor genes. Helix 1992;3:10-15.

Von Leyden E, Blumenthal F. Vorläufige Mitteilungen über einige Ergebnisse der Krebsforschung auf der I. medizinische Klinik. Deutsche Medicinische Wochenschrift 1902; 36:637-8.

W

Wakeling AE, Bowler J. Steroidal pure antioestrogens. Endocrinology 1987;112:R7-10.

Wall ME, Wani MC. Camptothecin and taxol: Discovery to clinic. Thirteenth Bruce F. Cain Memorial Award Lecture. Cancer Res 1995;55:753-60.

Walsh JJ. The popes and science. New York: Fordham University Press, 1908.

Walshe WH. The anatomy, physiology, pathology and treatment of cancer. Boston: William D Ticknoie, 1844.

Wani MC, Taylor HL, Wall ME, et al. Plant antitumor agents. VI The isolation and structure of taxol: a novel antileukemic and antitumour agent from Taxus brevifolia. J Am Chem Soc 1971;93:2325-7.

Wassink WF. Ontstaansvoorwaarden voor longkanker. Ned Tijdschr Geneesk 1948;97: 3732-47.

Wells C. Bones, bodies and disease. London: Thames and Hudson, 1964.

Wentges RThR. Een keizer zonder stem. In: J.J.E. van Everdingen, et al. Op het lijf geschreven: bekendheden en hun lijfarts. Hoofdstuk 16. Amsterdam/Overveen: Boom, Belvédère, 1995. p. 161-71.

Wertheim Salomonson JKA. Röntgen's-stralen. NTvG 1896;5 Febr. Dl. I: 241-9.

Westermark N. The effect of heat upon rat-tumors. Skandinavische Archiv für Physiologie 1927;52:257-22.

White RJ, Durr FE. Development of mitoxantrone. Investigational New Drugs 1985;3:85-93.

Wilhelm S, Carter C, Lynch M, Lowinger T, Dumas J et al. Discovery and development of sorafenib: a multikinase inhibitor for treating cancer. Nature Reviews 2006;5:835-44.

Witzig Th E, Gordon LI, Cabanillas F, Czuczman MS, Emmanouilides C, et al. Randomized clinical trial of 90Y-labeled ibritumomab immunotherapy for patients with relapsed or refractory low-grade, follicular, or transformed B-cell non-Hodgkin's lymphoma J Clin Oncol 2002;20:2453-63.

Woglom WH. General review of cancer therapy. In: Moulton FR, ed. Approaches to tumor chemotherapy. Washington D.C.: AAAS, 1947. p. 1.

Wold WSM, Green M. Historic milestones in cancer virology. Semin Oncol 1979;6:461-78.

Wolff J. Die Lehre von der Krebskrankheit von den Ältesten Zeiten bis zur Gegenwart. Jena: G. Fischer, 1907.

Wolmark N, Rockette H, Mamoumas EP, et al. The relative efficacy of 5-FU + leucovorin, 5-FU + levamisole, and 5-FU + leucovorin + levamisole in patients with Dukes' B and C carcinoma of the colon: first report of NSABP C-04. Proc Am Soc Clin Oncol 1996;15:205.

Woodruff MFA, Walbaum P. A phase-II trial of Corynebacterium parvum as adjuvant to surgery in the treatment of operable lung cancer. Cancer Immunology Immunotherapy 1983;16:114-6.

Wooster R, Neuhausen SL, Mangion J, et al. Location of a breast cancer susceptibility gene, BRCA2, to chromosome 13q12-13. Science 1994;265:2088.

z

Zabora J, Brintzenhofeszoc K, Curbow B, Hooker C, Plantadosi S. The prevalence of psychological distress by cancer site. Psycho-oncology 2001;10:19-28.

Zaviačić M. Prostate-specific antigen and history of its discovery. Bratisl Lek Listy 1997;98: 659-62.

Zubrod CG. Historic milestones in curative chemotherapy. Semin Oncol 1979;6:490-505.

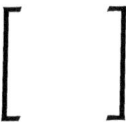

Name Index

A

Aaltonen	54
Aaronson	250
Ablin	197
Adair	155
Adams	109
Aetius	14
Alexander uit Tralles	14
Algire	209
Alibert	31
Allen	155
Altmann	46
Amery	233
Ames	36
Anderson	212
Ang	203
Arcamone	166
Ardenne, John of	63
Areteus of Cappadocia	56
Arnaudet	29
Arnold	157
Aselli	17
Astruc	22
Auer	99
Avenzoar	63
Avery	47
Avicenna	15, 63

B

Baclesse	132
Bagg	155
Bainbridge	148
Baltimore	41, 45
Banting	94
Barclay	172
Bard('s law)	27, 248
Barton	80
Bayon	34
Beard	40
Beatson	184
Beaumont	91
Becquerel	121
Beer	171
Behla	29
Bekkum, Van	177
Bell	88, 101
Belsey	99
Bennet Jr	235
Berd	201
Berenblum	37, 152
Bergenstal	187
Bergmann, Von	87
Berkeley	228
Bernal	47
Bernard, C.	91
Bernard, J.	173
Berthold	196

NAME INDEX

Bertrand	223	**C**	
Best	94		
Bichat	23	Canevazzi	168
Bidloo	148	Carlson	260
Bigelow	84	Carrel	31
bilharzia	29	Carswell	235
Billroth	80 e.v., 149	Carter	207
Birch-Hirschfeld	108	Cash	192
Bishop	43, 204	Cassell	249
Bittner	40	Cavaliere	107
Blair	106	Chadwick	136
Blumenthal	222	Chain	152
Bluming	232	Chambers	223
Boerhaave	22	Chargaff	47
Boeri	228	Chauliac, De	63
Bohr	137	Churchill	99
Bonadonna	166, 174	Clark	206
Bonet	65	Clerico	63
Bordet	2228	Clifford	229
Bourseaux	157	Clowes	150
Boveri	43	Cohen, Solis	103
Bovie	100	Cohen, Stanley	204
Bowler	191	Cohn	226
Boyer	204	Cohnheim	27, 56
Boyle	192	Cole	94
Bozzini	108	Coley	107, 219, 230
Bragg	47	Colton	80
Brenner	59	Cook	36, 40
Bricker	109	Cooper	106
Broca	52	Copher	94
Brock	157	Cordus	81, 147
Brown	55	Cornil	31
Bruchovsky	199	Coutard	132
Brunschwig	65	Creech	113
Buinauskas	229	Crick	48
Burkitt	40, 113	Crile	96
Burnet	220	Curie, Marie	122
Burrows, H.	183	Curie, Pierre	122
Burrows, J.	148	Cushing	100
Burrows, M.T.	31	Czajkowski	224
Bussemakers	198	Czermak	103
Butlin 101		Czerny 109	

D

Daley	45
Dandy	100
Danlos	129
Dausset	177
Davis	230
Davy	80
DeBakey	34
Deming	197
Descartes	19
Desormeaux	108
Despeignes	128
D'Amato	211
D'Argent	112
DiMarco	166
Divis	99
Djerassi	163
Dodds	188
Doering	39
Doll	36
Doisy	197
Domagk	150, 151, 158
Dougherty	155
Dran, Le	20, 79
Druker	45, 213
Duane	139
Dubost	166
Duffy	36
Dukes	192

E

Eb, Van der	42
Ehrlich	149, 202, 219
Ehrmann	209
Einhorn	169
Einstein	137
Eisen	29
Elion	165
Esmarch, Von	91
Esser	106

Etten, Van	45
Ewing	113, 155

F

Führer	25
Fabricius	21
Fallowfield	249
Farber	158, 162, 174
Fauconnet	177
Fedyushin	230
Feigenberg	248
Fermi	137
Ferrara	211
Fibiger	29
Fildes	158
Finesinger	248
Finney	224
Fleming	150
Flemming	58
Fletcher, G.	133
Fletcher, F.	157
Florey	152
Fodor	55
Folkman	210
Franklin	47
Frei	173
Freireich	174
Freund	127
Frieben	38
Fuller	109

G

Gaarenstroom	121
Galenus (Galen)	11, 62, 79, 146
Ganon	41
Geisler	249
Gelmo	151
Gerhardt C.	103
Gerhardt, P.R.	35
Gilman, A.	155

NAME INDEX

Glücksmann	58
Gluckman	178
Gocht	127
Godinot	22, 28
Goldberg	129
Goldin	163, 173
Goldstein, H.	35
Goodman	155
Graham, E.	35, 94, 99
Graham, F.	42
Graham, J.B. & R.M.	224
Grawitz	108
Gray	131
Greenblatt	209
Greer	248
Grein	166
Gresser	234
Griffith	46
Griffiths	111
Grillo	105
Grimmett	138
Groffen	43
Gross	40
Grubbe	126
Gutman	197

H

Haddow	189
Haenszel	39
Hahn	31, 137
Halberstädter	187
Halpern	231
Halsted	87, 90, 96
Halteren, Van	252
Hanaoka	85
Hanau	30
Hanna	212
Hannover	25
Harris	49
Harrison	29
Harvey	17

Haviland	29
Heald	96
Heidelberger	165
Heilmann	200
Heister	182
Heisterkamp	43
Henry	247
Héricourt	202, 228
Herrera	52
Hertz	163
Heyman	139
Hibner	216
Hildanus	65, 77
Hill, A.B.	35
Hill, J.	32
Hippocrates	7, 62
Hitchings	165
Hittorf	115
Hoffmann	182
Holland	251
Holmes	82, 86
Holzknecht	130
Home	24, 101
Hooke	56
Horne, Van	77
Horrax	100
Horsley	100
Horvitz	59
Horwitz, S.	172
Horwitz, K.	183, 184
Houppeville	77
Huggins	187, 197, 198
Hughes	224
Humphrey	224
Hungerford	43, 212
Hunter	19, 196

I

Ibn Sina	15
Ichikawa	34
Ide	209

Ionov	54	Krementz	106
Isaacs	198	Krumbhaar	150

J

L

Jackson	82	Labrie	199
Jacobson	176	Lacassagne	183
Jansen	IX	Laënnec	24
Jensen	183	Lane-Claypon	182
Johannsen	46	Lanfranchi	63, 74
Johnson, I.	171	Langenbeck	108
Johnson, R.	168	Laqueur	189
Joliot	136	Laszlo	229
Joliot-Curie	136	Lathrop	182
Justamond	29	Leeuwenhoek, Van	24
		Leidy	30
		Lembert	91
		Lenard	115, 119

K

		Leonides of Alexandria	62
Kübler-Ross	248	Leriche	94
Kalkar, Van	17	Leuchtenberger	161
Kaplan	139	Levan	43
Karon	171	Levene	46
Kasid	216	Levi-Montalcini	204
Keen	102	Levin	35
Kellock	223	Lewison	229
Kelly	110	Leyden, Von	222
Kendall	200	Li	166
Kerr	58	Liao	199
Kerst	136	Lilienfeld	182
Kidd	168	Lindskog	156
Kienböck	130	Lissauer	149
King	52	Lister	85
Klebs	27	Lloyd Jones	29
Klein	51, 236	Lockshin	56
Knoth	209	Loeb	183
Knudson	51	Lombard	39, 41
Kocher	88	London	129
Köhler	203	Long	81
Kölliker, Von	117	Lorenz	176
Korotneff	29	Louis	101
Korteweg	188	Luft	188
Kraske	93		

NAME INDEX

Lusitanus	28	Moyer	216
Lynch	35, 52	Mulder	42
		Müller('s law)	24, 25
M		Murdock	168
		Murray, G.	228
Müller	24, 34	Myerscough	249
MacKenzie	103		
Macleod	94	**N**	
MacMahon	182		
Maguire	249	Nück	148
Main	236	Nason	29
Mainwaring	199	Nestorius	14
Malpighi	24	Neuman	199
Marchetti	101	Neuss	171
Martin, E.	101	Newman	212
Martin, Hayes	105	Ngu	229
Martin, D.S.	173, 175	Nissen-Meyer	187
Mathé	169, 177, 231	Nitze	108
Maunsell	93	Nowell	43, 212
McDowell	87, 110		
McGuire	184, 206	**O**	
McLellan	197		
McWhirter	96	Oberling	30
Medawar	220	Ochsner	34
Melacine®	225	Oken	243
Meltzer	99	Old	231, 235
Mendel	45	Olivecrona	188
Mendelsohn	207	Oppenheimer	137
Merewether	36	Oribasius	14, 62
Miescher, J.F.	46		
Miescher, P.	177	**P**	
Milstein	203		
Mitchell	225	Padhy	203
Modino de Liuzzi	17	Paget	96
Montgomery	158	Papanicolaou	28
Moore, G.	175	Paracelsus	21, 65, 147
Moore, R.	197	Paré	74
Moreau	30	Pasteur	86
Morgagni	23, 94, 107	Paterson	132
Moniz	100	Paul of Aegina	14, 62
Morton, D.	233	Perutz	48
Morton, W.	81	Petit	79

Petroncello	63
Pettingale	248
Peyrilhe	22, 79
Philips	155
Pillore	92
Pliny the Elder	146
Poincaré	121
Potapova	215
Potier	173
Pott	32
Potter	41
Prehn	236
Priestley	80
Pusey	128

Q

Quesada	235

R

Røjel	41
Ramayana	5, 62
Ramazzini	181
Raspail	24
Récamier	23
Regaud	132
Rehn	34
Remak	26
Reybard	93
Rhoads	156
Richet	202, 228
Riedl	216
Rigoni-Stern	182
Risley	223
Robb, Hunter	87
Roffo	34
Rojas	233
Rood, Van	177
Rosenberg, B.	168
Rosenberg, S.A.	237
Rous	39
Rowley	43
Rudbeck	17
Ruys	25
Roentgen	115

S

Salimbene	16
Sato	209
Sauerbruch	99
Saunders	248
Schabel	173, 175
Schalken	198
Schally	193, 198
Schauta	112
Scheurlen	29
Schiff	172
Schinzinger	184
Schleider	24
Schlesinger	205
Schoental	36
Schultes	77
Schwann	24
Schwartz	131
Scott	198
Scultetus	77
Selikoff	36
Semmelweis	86
Senn	128
Sennert	28
Severinus	21
Shimkin	175
Shope	40
Shubik	209
Sie Kie	16
Simpson	84
Simpson-Herren	175
Sims	110
Sjobring	29
Sjögren	127
Skapier	230
Skipper	173, 175

NAME INDEX

Slamon	203
Slavin	178
Smith, E.	5
Smith, F.R.	41
Smith, G.	187
Smith, R.	216
Smith, W.	35
Sömmering, Von	32
Sokal	231
Spalla	166
Spiegel	250
Squire	51
Staszewski	182
Stehelin	42
Stehlin	107
Steinman	226
Stenbeck	127
Stevenson	38, 182
Stewart	40
Strebel	139
SubbaRow	161
Sulston	59
Summer	229
Sun Simiao	15
Sutherland	248

T

Tatum	220
Temin	41
Terrier	87
Thibodeau	54
Thiersch	26, 86, 91
Thoma	29
Thomas, E. Donnall	177
Thomas, F.	188
Thomas, L.	221
Thomson	115
Tjio	43
Tréfouël	151
Tulp	28

U

Ulhoorn	77
Ullrich	204
Umezawa	167

V

Varmus	43, 204
Vaughan	223
Veer, Van 't	55
Velde, C. van de	96
Vermorken	225
Vesalius	17
Vidal	228
Virchow('s law)	25, 26, 104
Vogel	25
Vogler	232
Vogt, C.	56
Vogt, P.	42
Voigt	126
Volkmann, Von	93
Voorde, Van de	77
Vries, De	177

W

Wakaki	167
Wakeling	191
Waksman	166
Waldeyer, Von	26
Walker	102
Walkhoff	129
Wall	170
Walpole	190
Walshe	28
Walwick	165
Wang	170, 197
Warren, J.C.	88
Warthin	54
Wassink	35

Waterfield	205
Watson, J.D.	47
Weber	227
Weigert	56
Weinberg	203
Wells, H.	80
Wertheim	111
Westermark	107
Whipple	94
White	197
Whiteside	163
Wideröe	135
Wilkins, L.	200
Wilkins, M.	47
Wilkinson	157
William of Saliceto	63
Williams	56
Wintz	132
Witte	45
Woglom	157
Woods	158
Wooster	52
Wyllie	58
Wynder	35

Y

Yamagiwa	34
Yokura	170
Young	109

Z

Zabora	252

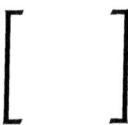

Subject Index

5-fluorouracil (5-FU)	165	anastrozol	192
6-mercaptopurine	165	anatomy	
90Y-ibritumomab tiuxetan	212	pathological	23
		androgen ablation	198
A		androgen receptor	199
		androgens	184, 187, 189
AARC	179	anesthesia	79
ablative hormone therapy	184	angiogenesis inhibitor	209
ABVD therapy	174	anthracyclines	166
acid phosphatase level	197	antiandrogens	199
ACOR	251	antiestrogens	190
actinomycin D	166	antibiotic cytostatics	166
adenomatous polyposis coli (APC) gene	54	antibody	202
adenovirus	40	monoclonal	202
adjuvant chemotherapy	174	antigen	202
adrenalectomy	187, 198	tumor-specific transplantation -s	222
adriamycin	166, 167	antimetabolites	158
aflatoxin B1	36	antisepsis	85
afterloading	139	antraquinones	168
alkylating cytostatics	152	APC gene	54
alpha particle	38	apoptosis	55
American Psychosocial Oncology Society (APOS)	251	APOS	251
		Arab world	14
American Society of cancer Research (AARC)	179	ara-C	165
American Society of Clinical Oncology (ASCO)	179	aromatase inhibotor	192
American Society for Therapeutic Radiology and Oncology (ASTRO)	143	aromatization	192
		artificial radioactivity	136
Ames test	36	asbestos	36
aminoglutethimide	168	Asclepiads	7
aminopterine	161	ASCO	179

SUBJECT INDEX

Association of Cancer Online Resources (ACOR)	251	cancer	12
		bladder	34, 109
ASTRO	143	breast	62, 75, 96, 127, 175, 181, 203
aspecific immunotherapy	230	cervical	41
autografting	31	lung	34, 99
autopsy	15	occupational	32
autologous tumor cell suspension	222	prostate	196
Ayurveda	105	skin-	32
		stigma of	241
B		testicular	169
		Canon of Medicine	15
Bacillus Calmette-Guérin (BCG)	231	capecitabine	165
barber-surgeon	72	carboplatin	169
Bard's law	27	carcinogenesis	37
BCG	231	chemical	32
beta particle	38	gamma	38
bevacizumab	211	multi-step	37
bicalutamide	199	radiation-induced	37
black bile	8, 12, 19	solar	37
bladder cancer	34, 109	UV	37
blastema	25	viral	39
blastema theory	25	X-	38
Blatta bizantina	146	carcinogenic effect	38
bleomycin	167	carcinoma	8
blood transplantation	102	cervical	28, 112
bone marrow transplant	176	endometrial	200
BPOS	251	renal cell	215, 216, 236
brachytherapy	139	carcinos	8
BRCA1 gene	52	castration	197
BRCA2 gene	52	cathode rays	115
breaking bad news to patients	249	cell death, programmed	56
breast cancer	62, 75, 96, 127, 175, 181, 203	cell	55
breast-conserving operation	98	cell, dendritic	226
Bricker procedure	110	Celsus	11, 62, 71, 146
British Association of Radiologists	142	cervical cancer	41
British Psychosocial Oncology Society (BPOS)	251	cervical carcinoma	28, 112
Byzantine Empire	13	cetuximab	207
		chemical carcinogenesis	32
C		chemotherapy	145
		adjuvant	174
Calmette-Guérin, Bacillus	231	combined	173
camptothecin	170	modern	149

SUBJECT INDEX

Chester Beatty group	157
China	15
chirurgeon	71
chloroform	84
chordotomy	101
chromosome	
Philadelphia	43
chronic myeloid leukemia	45
cisplatin	168
clonal selection theory	220
coal	34
cobalt bomb	138
Coley's toxin	107, 230
colon operation	93
colostomy	92
combined chemotherapy	173
commando resection	105
cortisone	170, 173, 187, 200
Corynebacterium parvum	233
crystallography	47
Cushing's clip	100
cyclophosphamide	157
cyproterone acetate	199
cytokines	234
cytology	28
cytosine arabinoside	165
cytostatics	
alkylating	152
antibiotic	166

D

daunorubicin	166
deltopectoral flap	106
dendritic cel	226
deoxyribonucleic acid (DNA)	46
diethylstilboestrol	198
dinosaur	3
Dispensatorium	147
distress	252
DNA	46
chip	55
microarray	55

docetaxel	173
doctor medicinae	71
dosimeter	130
Double Helix	47
double-hit hypothesis	51
doxorubicin	166
duodenum resection	94
Dutch Society of Psychosocial Oncology	251

E

E1 gene	42
Ebers papyrus	5, 61, 79
Edwin Smith papyrus	5, 61
EGF	205
eighteenth century	21
embryologic hypothesis	27
endometrial carcinoma	200
endoscopy	108
endothelial cells	215
epidemiology	38
epidermal growth-factor (EGF)	205
epirubicin	167
epithelium	25
Epstein-Barr virus	40
ErbB2	206
erlotinib	216
ESMO	179
esophagus resection	90
estro	143
estrogen receptor	184
estrogens	187, 188
ether	81
etoposide	170
European Society for Medical Oncology (ESMO)	179
European Society for Therapeutic Radiology and Oncology (estro)	143
exemestane	193
experimental studies	30
extremities	
perfusion of	106
tumor of	106

SUBJECT INDEX

F

Faculty of Radiologists	142
familial adenomatous polyposis (FAP)	52
FAP	52
flutamide	199
Fowler's solution	149
freeze-cut technique	24
fulvestrant	191

G

gamma radiation	38
gamma rays	38
gastric resection	92
gastrointestinal stroma cell tumor (GIST)	213
gastrointestinal tumor	92
gene	32, 183, 201, 204
genome	54
George Ebers papyrus	5, 61, 79
GIST	213
goserelin	193
Greek period	7
growth factor	
epidermal	205
vascular endothelial	205, 215
Gy	131
gynecologic tumor	110

H

Halsted's operation	79
HAMA	207
head-neck tumor	101
Hellenistic period	7
hepatitis-B virus	41
Her-2	206
Her-2/neu gene	206
hereditary nature	52
hereditary non-polyposis colorectal cancer (HNPCC)	52
herpesvirus	40
HNPCC	52
Homo erectus	3
homografting	31
hormone therapy	181
HTLV-1	41
human epidermal growth factor receptor-2	205
humoral theory	8, 12, 26
hyperthermic conditions	106
hypophysectomy	101, 188, 195, 198

I

iatrochemical hypothesis	147
iatrochemistry	147
IFN	234
imatinib	212
immunological tolerance	220
immunosurveillance	219
immunotherapy	219
aspecific	230
specific active	222
specific passive	228
infection	28
initiator	37
interferon (IFN)	234
interleukin-1 (Il-1)	235
interleukin-12 (Il-12)	237
interleukin-2 (Il-2)	235
internal irradiation	139
International Psycho-Oncology Society (IPOS)	251
iphosphamide	158
IPOS	251
irinotecan	170
irradiation	38
internal	139
megavoltage	135
orthovoltage	135
isoantibody	229
isotopes	137

J

Journal of Psychosocial Oncology — 251

K

Kahoun papyrus — 5

L

LAK cells — 237
large intestine — 93
laryngectomy — 90
    partial — 103
L-asparaginase — 168
laughing gas — 80
law
    Bard's — 27
    first law of oncology — 25
    Virchow's — 26
letrozole — 192
leukemia
    chronic myeloid — 45
levamisole — 233
LHRH — 199
LHRH agonist — 193
LHRH analogs — 193
lignite — 34
linear accelerator — 134, 135
lobectomy — 99
lobotomy — 100
lubricating oil — 34
lung cancer — 34, 99
lung resection — 99
lymph theory — 19
lymphokine-activated killer cells (LAK cells) — 237
Lynch syndrome — 54

M

mastectomy — 96
Medical Treatment Agreement Act — 243

Medicine — 15
    Canon of
megavoltage irradiation — 135
Melacine® — 225
melancholy — 12
mental illness
    stigma of — 245
mesorectal excision — 96
mesothelioma — 36
metastasis — 23
methotrexate — 161
microarray — 55
Middle Ages — 16
mitomycin C — 167
mitoxantrone — 168
modern chemotherapy — 149
monoclonal antibody — 202
MOPP regimen — 174
Müller's law — 24
multidisciplinary treatment — 174
multi-step carcinogenesis — 37
mummy — 3
mustard gas — 152

N

National Comprehensive Cancer Network
    (NCCN) — 252
NCCN — 252
neck gland dissection — 102
necrosis — 56
Nederlandse Vereniging
    voor radiologie (NVvR) — 143
    voor Radiotherapy en Oncologie (NVRO) — 143
nephrectomy — 108
neu gene — 206
neu oncogene — 206
neurologic tumor — 100
neurosurgery — 100
neutrons — 38, 136, 137
nilutamide — 199
nineteenth century — 21

SUBJECT INDEX

nitrogen mustard	155
nitrosourea derivates	158
nitrous oxide	80
NVRO	143

O

occupational cancer	32
oncology	
first law of	25
oncogene	43
organ transplantation	113, 232
orthovoltage irradiation	135
ovariectomy	110, 184
overexpression	206
oxaliplatin	169

P

paclitaxel	172
paleopathology	3
pancreas resection	94
pancreaticoduodenectomy	94
papilloma virus	40
papovavirus	40
papyrus	
Ebers	5, 61, 79
Edwin Smith	5, 61
Kahoun	5
paraffin wax embedding	28
parasitic theory	29, 186
parotid tumor virus	40
partial laryngectomy	103
pathological anatomy	23
PCA3 urine test	198
PDGFR	215
perfusion of the extremities	106
Philadelphia chromosome	43
phosphestrol	198
platelet derived growth factor receptor (PDGFR)	215
pneumonectomy	99

polonium	122
polyoma virus	40
post-mortem examination	12, 13, 17, 30
prodrug	157
progesterone receptor	184
progestins	195
programmed cell death	56
promotor	37
prontosil	151
prostate cancer	196
prostatectomy	109
prostate-specific antigen (PSA)	197
protons	38
proto-oncogene	42
PSA	197
psycho-oncology	239

R

rad	131
radiation	126
cathode	115
ultraviolet (UV) solar	37
X-	38, 117, 121
radiation-induced carcinogenesis	37
radioactivity	121
artificial	136
radiobiology	131
radiological Society of North America (RSNA)	142
radiologist	
British Association of -s	142
Faculty of -s	142
Royal College of -s	142
radiotherapists	
Society of -s of Great Britain and Ireland	142
radiotherapy	115
external	130
radium	122
Radium Girls	38, 129
raloxifene	191
reconstructive surgery	105
rectal/rectum resection	93

SUBJECT INDEX

regional flap	106
Renaissance	17
renal cell carcinoma	215, 216, 236
resection	
commando	105
duodenum	94
gastric	92
esophagus	90
lung	99
pancreas	94
rectal / rectum	93
segmental	99
response modifier	236
retinoblastoma	27, 51
retinoblastoma gene	51
retrovirus HTLV-1	41
rhizotomy	101
rituximab	212
Roentgen rays	115
Roman period	11
Rous sarcoma virus	40
Royal College of Radiologists	142
RSNA	142

S

sarcoma	12
scirrhos	8
segmental resection	99
sentinel lymph node	98
SERM	191
signal transduction	201, 202
silver clip	100
skin cancer	32
skin graft	106
smoking	34
Society of Radiotherapists of Great Britain and Ireland	142
Society of Surgical Oncology	113
solar radiation	37
soot	34
sorafenib	216
specific active immunotherapy	222

specific passive immunotherapy	228
spindle poisons	171
src gene	42
stem cell factor receptor c-Kit	215
STI 571	213
stigma of cancer	240
stigma of mental illness	245
sulfanilamide	151
sunitinib	215
surgery	69
breast-conserving	98
neuro-	100
reconstructive	105
thoracic	99
thyroid	90

T

tamoxifen	190, 225
tar	34
targeted therapy	201
taxanes	172
taxol	172
testicular cancer	169
thalidomide	211
thoracic surgery	99
thyroid surgery	90
tinctura vitriolata	148
tioguanine	165
tissue transplantation	232
tiuxetan	212
TME procedure	96
TNF	235
topoisomerase inhibitors	169
topotecan	170
total mesorectal excision (TME)	96
transcription	201
transplantation	30
blood	102
bone marrow	176
organ	113, 232
tissue	232
tumor (fragment)	222

trastuzumab	203
tumor	3, 8
gastrointestinal	92
gastrointestinal stroma cell (GIST)	213
gynecologic	110
head-neck	101
neurologic	100
of extremities	106
transplantation of	222
urologic	107
tumor cell suspension, autologous	222
tumor necrosis factor (TNF)	235
tumor-specific transplantation antigens	222
tumor suppressor gene	51

U

urologic tumor	107
Ultraviolet (UV) radiation	37

V

vaccine	226
VAMP therapy	173
vascular clip	100
vascular endothelial growth factor (VEGF)	205, 215
vascular endothelial growth factor receptor (VEGFR)	215
VEGF	205, 215
VEGFR	215
vinblastine	171
vinca alkaloids	171
vincristine	171
vindesine	171
viral carcinogenesis	39
virus	
adeno-	40
Epstein-Barr	40
hepatitis-B	41
herpes-	40
papilloma	40
papova-	40
parotid tumor	40
polyoma	40
retro- HTLV-1	41
Rous sarcoma	40
Virchow's law	26

W

Wet op de Geneeskundige Behandelingsovereenkomst	243

X

X-radiation	38
X-ray crystallography data	47
X-ray diffraction	47
X-rays	38, 117, 121